AF750740

Cancer Etiology, Diagnosis and Treatments

nova
Medicine & Health
New York

Cancer Etiology, Diagnosis and Treatments

How Plant Flavonoids Affect the Outcome of Hormonal and Biological Cancer Therapies: A Handbook for Doctors and Patients
Katrin Sak, PhD (Editor)
2022. ISBN: 978-1-68507-608-5 (Hardcover)
2022. ISBN: 978-1-68507-698-6 (eBook)

Burkitt Lymphoma: Diagnosis, Risk Factors and Treatment
Douglas V. Berthelot (Editor)
2021. ISBN: 978-1-68507-071-7 (Hardcover)
2021. ISBN: 978-1-68507-083-0 (eBook)

Bridging the Gap: In This Era of Cancer Immunotherapy
Shiu Y. Tsao, FRCR (Editor)
2021. ISBN: 978-1-53619-900-0 (Hardcover)
2021. ISBN: 978-1-53619-983-3 (eBook)

Mesothelioma: Risk Factors, Treatment and Prognosis
Albert K. Martin (Editor)
2021. ISBN: 978-1-68507-075-5 (Softcover)
2021. ISBN: 978-1-68507-134-9 (eBook)

Combination Therapies and their Effectiveness in Breast Cancer Treatment
Manzoor Ahmad Mir, PhD (Editor)
2021. ISBN: 978-1-68507-195-0 (Hardcover)
2021. ISBN: 978-1-68507-247-6978 (eBook)

More information about this series can be found at
https://novapublishers.com/product-category/series/cancer-etiology-diagnosis-and-treatments/

Kulmira Nurgali and
Raquel Abalo
Editors

Platinum-Based Chemotherapy

Clinical Uses, Efficacy and Side Effects

nova
Medicine & Health
New York

Copyright © 2022 by Nova Science Publishers, Inc.
DOI: https://doi.org/10.52305/MPSL2859

All rights reserved. No part of this book may be reproduced, stored in a retrieval system or transmitted in any form or by any means: electronic, electrostatic, magnetic, tape, mechanical photocopying, recording or otherwise without the written permission of the Publisher.

We have partnered with Copyright Clearance Center to make it easy for you to obtain permissions to reuse content from this publication. Simply navigate to this publication's page on Nova's website and locate the "Get Permission" button below the title description. This button is linked directly to the title's permission page on copyright.com. Alternatively, you can visit copyright.com and search by title, ISBN, or ISSN.

For further questions about using the service on copyright.com, please contact:
Copyright Clearance Center
Phone: +1-(978) 750-8400 Fax: +1-(978) 750-4470 E-mail: info@copyright.com.

NOTICE TO THE READER

The Publisher has taken reasonable care in the preparation of this book, but makes no expressed or implied warranty of any kind and assumes no responsibility for any errors or omissions. No liability is assumed for incidental or consequential damages in connection with or arising out of information contained in this book. The Publisher shall not be liable for any special, consequential, or exemplary damages resulting, in whole or in part, from the readers' use of, or reliance upon, this material. Any parts of this book based on government reports are so indicated and copyright is claimed for those parts to the extent applicable to compilations of such works.

Independent verification should be sought for any data, advice or recommendations contained in this book. In addition, no responsibility is assumed by the Publisher for any injury and/or damage to persons or property arising from any methods, products, instructions, ideas or otherwise contained in this publication.

This publication is designed to provide accurate and authoritative information with regard to the subject matter covered herein. It is sold with the clear understanding that the Publisher is not engaged in rendering legal or any other professional services. If legal or any other expert assistance is required, the services of a competent person should be sought. FROM A DECLARATION OF PARTICIPANTS JOINTLY ADOPTED BY A COMMITTEE OF THE AMERICAN BAR ASSOCIATION AND A COMMITTEE OF PUBLISHERS.

Additional color graphics may be available in the e-book version of this book.

Library of Congress Cataloging-in-Publication Data

ISBN: 978-1-68507-972-7

Published by Nova Science Publishers, Inc. † New York

Contents

Preface

According to the Global Cancer Observatory, in 2020 the number of new cases of cancer was 19.3 million people in the whole world, with breast, lung, and colorectal cancer comprising 10-11% each of these figures. In the same year, there were almost 10 million deaths from cancer, with lung cancer being the one leading to more deaths (18%). Unfortunately, these figures are only expected to increase, with an estimated incidence of 30.2 million cases in 2040. (https://gco.iarc.fr, accessed on 31st March 2022). Thus, cancer is a worldwide public health priority, with a high socio-economic impact.

Chemotherapy stands out among the available cancer treatments. Platinum-based chemotherapy is one of the earliest chemotherapeutics introduced to the clinics and it is still the first-line treatment, used alone or in combination with other anti-neoplastic therapy and/or radiation, for many types of cancer in both adults and children. The book "Platinum-Based Chemotherapy: Clinical Uses, Efficacy and Side Effects" offers the reader a general overview of this therapy, as well as an update on some of the most relevant issues specific to this therapy.

The first chapter of the book, "Platinum Analogs from a Chemical and Biological Point of View," summarizes the current knowledge on the chemical and biological characteristics of platinum-based molecules used in chemotherapy. The focus is on their impact on cell function and how this may cause cell resistance to treatment, which is an important drawback of this chemotherapy.

The second chapter, "Role of Cellular Senescence in Resistance to Platinum-Based Chemotherapy," focuses on an important, but often underestimated, aspect of resistance to platinum-based chemotherapy, namely cell senescence. Importantly, therapy-induced senescent cells can re-activate their proliferative potential and lead to cancer recurrence and even metastasis, after the acquisition of a new metabolic stage.

The third chapter, "Main Mechanisms Involved in Major and Minor Side Effects Triggered by Cisplatin-Based Therapy," is a general overview of the many different side effects that cisplatin, the main representative of the platinum-based chemotherapeutics, may cause. The authors distinguish between major side effects, which account for acute morbidity and even mortality, and minor side effects, which do not generally increase mortality but have an important impact on the quality of life of cancer survivors. Both types of side effects require attention and further research efforts because current strategies to palliate or prevent them are mainly symptomatic and of relatively low clinical efficacy.

The remaining chapters focus on some of the side effects of platinum-based chemotherapy. The fourth chapter, "Peripheral Neuropathy and Cognitive Impairment Caused by Platinum-Based Chemotherapy," deals with peripheral and central neurotoxicity, which cause altered peripheral sensations and cognitive impairments, respectively, with an important impact on cancer survivors' quality of life and a significant economic burden. The fifth chapter, "Ototoxicity Induced by Platinum-Based Chemotherapy," focuses on one platinum-induced specific type of neurotoxicity that may cause irreversible sensorineural hearing loss, whose impact is particularly critical in children, who may have long-term difficulties in language and social development. The sixth chapter, "Cardiovascular Side Effects of Platinum-Based Chemotherapy," is focused on one type of major, potentially mortal side effect. In this chapter, the authors point to the fact that most available clinical studies are retrospective and highlight the need for more adequate animal models that may mimic the specific conditions associated with platinum-based chemotherapeutic treatments; these preclinical models are required to identify causes and test treatments and preventative strategies. Finally, the seventh chapter, "Gastrointestinal Side Effects of Platinum-Based and Other Chemotherapeutic Drugs", describes the various side effects of platinum analogs and other chemotherapeutic drugs that may affect the gastrointestinal tract, including painful oral mucositis, distressing nausea, and vomiting, as well as diarrhea and constipation, which do not necessarily cease when chemotherapy cycles cease. In this chapter, the authors also address the issue of the adverse effects that may be caused by the prophylactic and palliative treatments used to counteract those induced by chemotherapy. Importantly, the concept of chemotherapy-induced enteric neuropathy as a leading cause of long-term gastrointestinal sequelae in cancer survivors is deeply discussed.

The editors wish to thank Nova Science Publishers and their team members for the opportunity to publish this book. We are thankful to all authors and reviewers for their contribution and efforts to make the chapters of this book of outstanding quality. We wish to thank also María Montero for her help in formatting the book chapters. Lastly, we thank our family members for their support, encouragement, patience, and unconditional love along this journey.

Editors
Kulmira Nurgali
Raquel Abalo

Chapter 1

Platinum Analogs from a Chemical and Biological Point of View

Mauricio A. Retamal[1,2,3,*], Ignacio A. Cortés-Fuentes[4,5], Juan G. Gormaz[6] and Paola R. Campodónico[7]

[1]Universidad del Desarrollo, Programa de Comunicación Celular en Cáncer, Clínica Alemana Facultad de Medicina, Santiago, Chile
[2]Universidad del Desarrollo, Centro de Fisiología Celular e Integrativa, Clínica Alemana Facultad de Medicina, Santiago, Chile
[3]Department of Cell Physiology and Molecular Biophysics, and Center for Membrane Protein Research, School of Medicine, Texas Tech University Health Sciences Center, Lubbock, TX, USA
[4]Hospital Barros Luco-Trudeau, San Miguel, Santiago, Chile
[5]Departamento de Otorrinolaringología, Facultad de Medicina, Universidad de Chile, Santiago, Chile
[6]Facultad de Medicina, Universidad de Chile, Santiago, Chile
[7]Universidad del Desarrollo, Facultad de Medicina, Instituto de Ciencias e Innovación en Medicina, Centro de Química Médica, Clínica Alemana Universidad del Desarrollo, Santiago, Chile

Abstract

Platinum (Pt) analogues are the most widely used chemotherapeutic agents in oncology, used alone or co-administered with other anti-neoplastic therapy and/or radiation. Pt-based chemotherapies are prescribed to treat a wide spectrum of specific malignancies, including

---

[*]Corresponding Author's Email: mretamal@udd.cl.

In: Platinum-Based Chemotherapy
Editors: Kulmira Nurgali and Raquel Abalo
ISBN: 978-1-68507-972-7
© 2022 Nova Science Publishers, Inc.

digestive, lung, head and neck, prostate, testicular, ovarian, bladder, cervical, breast, sarcomas and melanomas, as well as several hematological cancers. Patients treated with Pt-based chemotherapies suffer significant adverse effects, limiting their use. Management of these toxic effects is a key factor for successful therapy. Considering that relatively few Pt drugs are clinically and broadly used worldwide, understanding the biochemical and biological basis for resistance to Pt drugs is crucial. Thus, our aim is to summarize current knowledge of the chemical and biological features of Pt-based molecules used in chemotherapy, primarily focusing on its effects on cell function and how some of these changes drive cell resistance to Pt-based molecules.

Keywords: cellular resistance, chemotherapy, platinum-based treatments, side effects, toxicity

Introduction

Platinum (Pt) analogues are the most widely used chemotherapeutic agents in modern oncology (administered to nearly half of oncologic patients), considering their use alone or co-administered with another anti-neoplastic therapy and/or radiation. Pt-based chemotherapies are prescribed to treat a wide spectrum of specific malignancies, including digestive, lung, head and neck, prostate, testicular, ovarian, bladder, cervical, and breast sarcomas and melanomas, as well as several hematological cancers.

Patients exposed to Pt-based treatments tend to suffer significant adverse effects, limiting their use. Management of these toxic effects is a key factor for a successful therapy. On the other hand, cancer cells may acquire resistance to this therapy. Therefore, the clinical efficacy of Pt-based treatments is limited both by intrinsic acquired resistance and the therapy's side effects.

The mechanisms through which Pt-based analogues induce their antineoplastic effects and those associated with their toxic effects are not completely understood. To elucidate these differences, it is necessary to understand the chemistry of these compounds and to study the biological effects linked to the interaction of these analogues with cellular macromolecules. This chapter addresses both chemical and biological issues related with Pt mechanisms of action, considering therapeutic approaches as well as side effects from an integrative point of view.

Chemical Aspects of Pt-Derived Compounds Used in Chemotherapy

Cisplatin and Its Derivative Compounds

Compounds with metal ions in their structure have broadly been used in cancer treatment (Borges et al., 2016; Morcelli, Bull, et al., 2016; Morcelli, Kanashiro, et al., 2016). The biological targets of these compounds correspond to: DNA, hormones, enzymes, proteins, etc. (Ali et al., 2013). Platinum complexes react through ligand exchange processes which contribute to their biological effects (Kostova, 2006; Ali et al., 2013). However, these compounds have several side effects which have led to sustained study of drugs based on compounds with metals, specifically new Pt compounds with improved pharmacological properties and a wide spectrum of antitumor effects against cancer.

Cisplatin was synthetized in 1844, and its biological activity was determined in 1965 by Rosenberg et al. (Rosenberg, Van Camp and Krigas, 1965). Cisplatin is more active than transplatin relative to chloride atoms; additionally, transplatin does not have antitumor activity. Both compounds have Pt(II) in a square-planar coordination and do not isomerize under physiological conditions. Also, based on their antitumor difference, cisplatin took the lead over other analogue compounds (Rosenberg et al., 1967; Weiss and Christian, 2012). This drug was approved in 1978, and it is currently used as an antitumor drug for testicular, ovarian, bladder, cervical, head and neck, and small-cell and non-small cell lung cancers (Rosenberg and VanCamp, 1970; Weiss and Christian, 2012; Ali et al., 2013). Figure 1 shows the chemical structure of cisplatin and transplatin compounds, respectively. The chemical structure of cisplatin corresponds to a molecule with centered metal and chlorine, known as leaving groups (LG), and amine, known as non-leaving groups (NLG), as ligands: {*cis*-[$Pt(NH_3)_2Cl_2$]}. Thus, this molecule has two reactive sites associated with Cl- groups under physiological conditions.

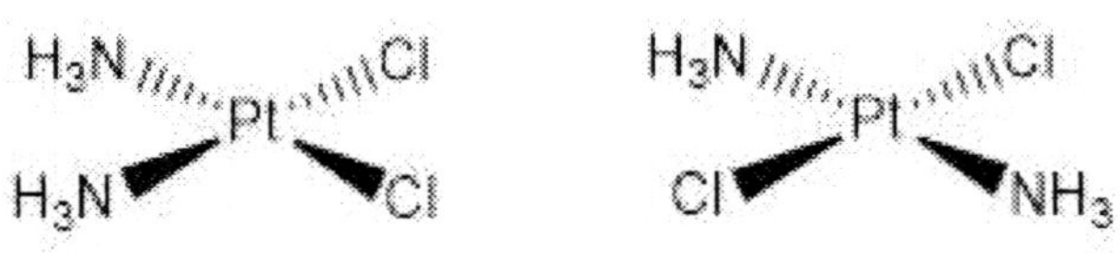

Figure 1. Chemical structure of cisplatin and transplatin compounds.

The Dhara method is used to synthetize cisplatin (see Figure 2 below) (Rebillard, Lagadic-Gossmann and Dimanche-Boitrel, 2008). The first step consists of aqueous $K_2[PtCl_4]$ treated with excess KI to form $K_2[PtI_4]$ (Alderden, Hall and Hambley, 2006; Ghosh, 2019). Then ammonium hydroxide (NH_4OH) is added to precipitate *cis*-$[Pt(NH_2)_2I_2]$. Next, $AgNO_3$ aqueous solution is added to *cis*-$[Pt(NH_2)_2I_2]$ resulting in the formation of soluble $[Pt(NH_3)_2(H_2O)_2]^{+2}$ cation. Finally, $[Pt(NH_3)_2(H_2O)_2]^{+2}$ is treated with excess KCl solution to obtain solid *cis*-$[Pt(NH_3)_2Cl_2]$, which can be purified by recrystallization with hot water containing either 0.1 M HCl or 0.9% NaCl (Hoeschele et al., 1982; Davies et al., 2008). The Reiset method is used to synthetize transplatin by conversion of $K_2[PtCl_4]$ to $[Pt(NH_3)_4]Cl_2$ with ammonia excess. In the second step, the volume is reduced by evaporation and added HCl to obtain transplatin (Natile and Coluccia, 2001; Ghosh, 2019). Finally, the Kurnakov method is used to differentiate cis- and trans- compounds (Kurnakow, 1894; Mellor, 2002). Aqueous cis-/trans- platin compounds react with excess of thiourea (Th), where cisplatin produces a deep yellow water solution while transplatin forms white water insoluble solution (Ghosh, 2019).

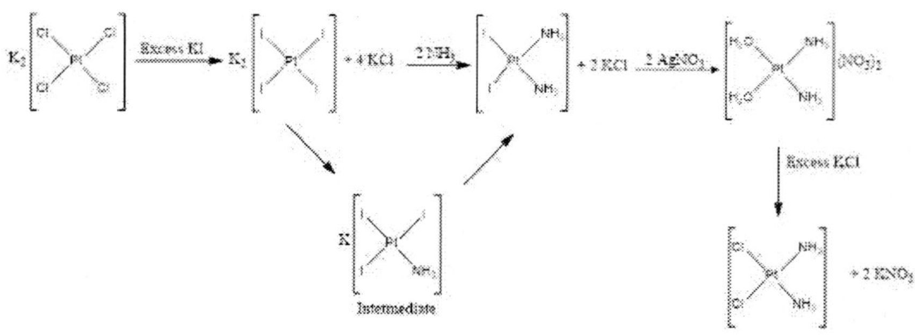

Figure 2. Synthetic route to produce cisplatin by Dhara method (Rebillard, Lagadic-Gossmann and Dimanche-Boitrel, 2008).

The second generation of cisplatin analogues consist of: carboplatin, oxaliplatin and nedaplatin. The compound called diamine-[1,1-cyclobutyldicarboxilato-(2-) O,O′] Pt(II) or carboplatin (approved in 1989) has one bidentate ligand as LG in place of two -Cl groups and biological activity is focused on ovarian, carcinoma, lung, cervical, head and neck cancers (Ali et al., 2013). This drug is more stable than cisplatin, attributable to the chelate effect, and as a consequence interacts less with proteins and thus is excreted more easily through urine. Moreover, carboxylate ligands increase water solubility, improving the drug's ability to cross the blood brain barrier (Pasetto et al., 2006). Oxaliplatin or {[(*1R,2R*)-cyclohexane-1,2-diamine][ethanedioato-O,O′]-Pt(II)} (approved in 1996) has improved antitumor activity in comparison with cisplatin and carboplatin, concerning colon cancer cell lines (Armand et al., 2000). The chemical structure of oxaliplatin shows a single bidentate ligand, when replaced by the amine ligands of cisplatin. Diamine [hydroxy acetate (2-)-O,O′] Pt(II) or nedaplatin shows the highest water solubility, less nephrotoxicity and better anticancer activity than the others (Kawai et al., 2005; Alberto et al., 2009). The third generation of cisplatin comprises lobaplatin and heptaplatin. The IUPAC (International Union of Pure and Applied Chemistry) name of lobaplatin is {[2-hydroxypropanoato (2-)-O1,O2] [1,2-cyclobutanedimethanamine-N,N′]-Pt(II)}. This drug was approved in 2010 for use with myelogenous leukemia, metastatic breast cancer and small cell lung cancers, and it is administered as a diastomeric mixture of S,S- and R,R- configurations ('Lobaplatin: D 19466', 2003). On the other hand, heptaplatin or {[propanedioate (2-)-O,O`] [2-(1-methylethyl)-1,3-dioxolane-4,5-dimethanamine-N,N′]-Pt(II)} (approved in 1999) shows improved anticancer activity in comparison with cisplatin and has high solubility and low toxicity (Gietema et al., 1995; Kim et al., 1995). Figure 3 shows second and third generation cisplatin analogues. In addition, the second and third generation cisplatin analogues are obtained by replacing different chelating agents and LGs, which are more stable (Lippert, 1999; Wheate et al., 2010; Gozelle et al., 2019).

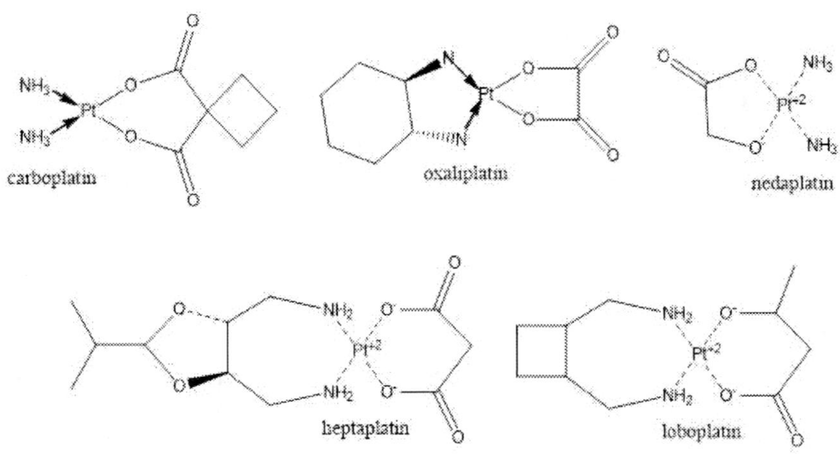

Figure 3. Chemical structure of metal-centered anticancer drugs (Ghosh, 2019).

However, other derivative compounds have been reported and are based on the follow ligands: thiazole, benzoxazole, benzimidazole, imidazole and benzothiazole (Domnina et al., 1983; Mylonas et al., 1988; Muir et al., 1992; Marieke J. Bloemink et al., 1996; Gümüş and Algül, 1997). The key role of these ligands is to attach more specifically to the DNA to achieve more precise activity with lower toxicity (Hydes and Russell, 1988; Murray et al., 1992). Moreover, Pt-based molecules are administered (in general) dissolved in saline solution and thus an important parameter of these drugs is their solubility in water. This parameter is increased by replacing the chlorine groups (cisplatin) with chelating carboxylate, oxalate and glycolate, among others.

Alternatively, drugs such as: iproplatin, tetraplatin and satraplatin are Pt(IV) complexes that have shown anticancer activity (Lebwohl and Canetta, 1998). In general, Pt(IV) complexes act as prodrugs and they need to be reduced to Pt(II) by intracellular or extracellular reducing agents (glutathione (GSH) or ascorbate) to provide biological activity (Ghosh, 2019). These compounds have been discarded in different clinical phase trials with lower toxicities and better physio-chemical properties, but with lower effectiveness than cisplatin (Hall and Hambley, 2002; Ghosh, 2019). Ormaplatin showed neurotoxicity in clinical trials, leading to those trials being suspended (Figg et al., 1997; Kozubík et al., 2005).

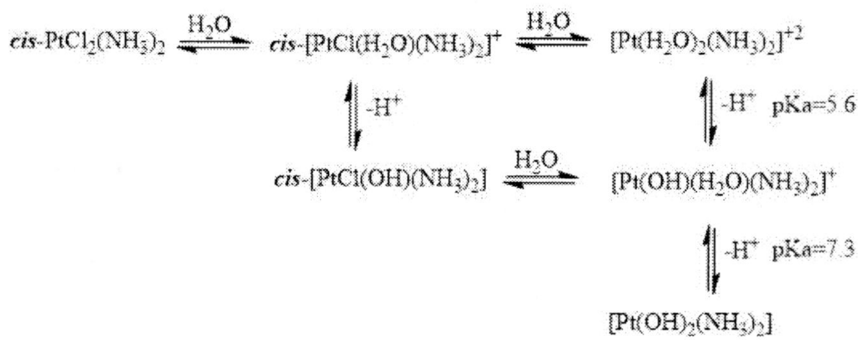

Figure 4. Hydrolysis of cisplatin (Reedijk and Lohman, 1985).

Note that Pt (IV) compounds show an octahedral coordination. The chemical properties of derivative compounds of Pt(II) and Pt(IV) have shown slow ligand-exchange processes -- the reason for the stability of cisplatin -- which shows a low rate of interconversion in solution to transisomer (Davies, Berners-Price and Hambley, 2000). In 1985 Lohman et al. reported the hydrolysis reactions of cisplatin inside the cells (see Figure 4) promoted by the lower concentration of Cl^- anion (4-20 mM compared to ~100 mM in blood) (Ghosh, 2019). The author suggests that the predominant species will be *cis*-$[Pt(NH_3)_2(H_2O)Cl]^+$ which detaches the -Cl group to attack the DNA molecule as *cis*-$[Pt(NH_3)_2(H_2O)]^{+2}$ (water is better LG than -Cl^-) (Davies, Berners-Price and Hambley, 2000) in order to generate an adduct able to establish specific interactions leading to cell killing by overexpression of some proteins and low interstrand-crosslink repairing ability (Reedijk and Lohman, 1985).

Previously, biological molecules such as amino acids, peptides and glucosamines had been used to confer their chemical properties to certain ligands to improve their original properties (Iakovidis and Hadjiliadis, 1994). Thus for example, these biological molecules could be associated with metals as coordination complexes to improve drug toxicities and pharmacological properties (Denny, Rewcastle and Baguley, 1990; Gravatt et al., 1994; Gümüş and Algül, 1997; Gaba and Mohan, 2015). This association occurs because these conjugations induce changes in parameters such as electronic, steric, donor/acceptor properties, hydrogen bond interactions and hydrophobic action. Additionally, Gao et al. reported that Pt(IV)-based compounds used as pro-drugs increased the response of human tumor cells to Pt(II) drugs in pre-clinical studies (Matesanz, Leitao and Souza, 2013; H et al., 2018; Moreira et al., 2019). In summary, the negative side effects of cisplatin have been reduced with the second and third generation of analogues. However, a few compounds have been approved and others have been discontinued during clinical trials due to therapeutic dose, side effects, effectivity and other reasons, opening a new area for developing drugs with highlighted biological activity and a broader activity spectrum. For instance, satraplatin, a Pt drug, completed Phase III clinical trial in patients with prostate cancer and Phase I clinical trial of the combination with gemcitabine in patients with advanced solid tumors (Sternberg et al., 2009; Paola et al., 2012).

In order to develop new Pt-based drugs, it is important to consider chemical stability, bond interactions with the biological target, biological reaction mechanisms, physical chemistry properties and drug delivery systems, among other parameters. In this area, synthesis and characterization of new compounds incorporating biological tests and DFT (Density Functional Theory) plus SMD (Simulation Molecular Dynamic) studies must be considered in a rational search. Thus, if the mechanism of the biological reaction is known, the interaction could be simulated and optimized by recognizing the molecular interactions of the ligands. Usually the synthetized compounds must follow an efficient synthetic route, and they must be highly pure, stable in the air and soluble in polar solvents (Gaba and Mohan, 2015). Furthermore, these compounds should be structurally characterized by using melting points, elemental analysis, and ^{1}HNMR, IR and HRMS spectra. Bond lengths and angles of the molecules could be obtained if any compound is crystallized and analyzed by X-ray. Afterward, a distorted square-planar geometry for Pt(II) compounds can be described. Other compounds without X-ray structure could be analyzed by DFT calculations using an available molecule of known X-ray structural parameters. To mimic this, the medium is incorporated in an implicit solvent (water) model able to reproduce the structural parameters given low energy conformations. Otherwise, if the biological mechanism and target are known, it is possible to do a docking study to obtain orientations and interactions with the biological target. Moreover, computational and empirical experiments can be used in order to develop Pt-based drugs attached to the chemical carrier to increase their biological activity (Tchounwou et al., 2021). Thus for example, using these techniques has made possible the creation of an asplatin attached to p-sulfocalix[4]arene (PSC4) which, *in vitro*, present a higher cytotoxicity in MCF-7 cells, HeLa and A549 cell lines (Fahmy et al., 2022). These studies could lead to designs for new drugs with superior efficiency and that provide new therapeutic strategies in cancer treatment (Moreira et al., 2019).

Biological Aspects of Pt-Derived Compounds Used in Chemotherapy

Biological Effects of Pt-Derived Compounds

DNA Damage

One of the main Pt-based drug mechanism of action on cancer cells is through the chemical modification of purine bases in the DNA, but the drug can also react with the amino acids of certain proteins, such as cysteines (Ishida et al., 2002). Regarding interactions between Pt-based compounds and DNA, it is well known that DNA adducts can be formed, specifically with the imidazole ring of two adjacent guanines or adenine and guanine, both at position 1,2 and 1,3 intrastrand. Finally, these DNA modifications can form intra- and interstrand crosslinks (Fichtinger-Schepman et al., 1985; Saris et al., 1996; Wang and Lippard, 2005). Interestingly, formation of DNA adducts by carboplatin is 230-fold less effective, as compared to the same cisplatin concentration (Blommaert et al., 1995). A similar phenomenon was observed using lobaplatin and oxaliplatin in vitro; however, in vivo the formation of DNA adducts induced by different Pt-based drugs was similar, suggesting that there are cytoplasmic conditions in vivo that favor lobaplatin and oxaliplatin-induced DNA adducts (Saris et al., 1996). Interestingly, although cisplatin tends to form DNA adducts more easily than oxaliplatin, these are more efficiently repaired than those induced by oxaliplatin (Hector et al., 2001). Both intra- and interstrand crosslinks are toxic for cells because they are highly effective blocking the mRNA transcription and DNA replication. Therefore, cells that do not have an efficient DNA-repairing mechanism enter in apoptosis (Brown, Kumar and Tchounwou, 2019). However, nuclear DNA damage alone cannot be the cause of cell death, and it has been proposed that Pt-based modification in the mitochondrial DNA (mtDNA) is needed to observe cell death consistently (Yang et al., 2006). The production of mtDNA adducts is strongly associated with mitochondrial malfunctioning (Marullo et al., 2013) and lack of mtDNA adducts was associated with cisplatin resistance of head and neck cancer cells, which was a GSH-concentration dependent mechanism (Yang et al., 2000).

Mitochondria Dysfunction

In addition to mitochondrial DNA adduct formation, cisplatin affects several other mitochondrial functions, most of which are linked to reactive oxygen species (ROS) production (Marullo et al., 2013). Thus, in mice lymphoid leukemia L1210 cells, application of cisplatin at 1 μg/ml decreased mitochondrial membrane potential, which was correlated with ROS production measured as changes in dichloro-dihydro-fluorescein diacetate (DCFH-DA) and tetramethylrhodamine methyl ester perchlorate (TMRE) fluorescence fluorescence (Franskevych et al., 2016). Similarly, cisplatin-induced renal tubular-cell apoptosis, via ROS production in the mitochondria, was associated with decreased mitochondrial cell volume (Shen et al., 2021). The effect of cisplatin on the mitochondria has been prevented by using Penicillium B, which activates the adenosine monophosphate-activated protein (AMP) kinase (Shen et al., 2021) and by DIDS (4,4'-Diisothiocyanatostilbene-2,2'-disulfonate), which is an inhibitor of the mitochondrial outer membrane protein voltage-dependent anion-selective channel 1 (VDAC1) (Luo et al., 2021), suggesting that the effect of Pt-based drugs can be pharmacologically modulated. Consistent with the importance of mitochondria in the final effect of cisplatin, the drug was recently shown to be more efficient in eliminating cells with higher mitochondrial content, because they produce larger amounts of ROS (Kleih et al., 2019). Based on these results, molecules have been developed to join Pt-based drugs to molecules with affinity for mitochondria, thus enhancing its toxic effect on this organelle. (Bera et al., 2021; Muhammad et al., 2021).

In summary, there is a correlation between the number of mitochondria and higher ROS production, which in turn correlates with Pt-based chemotherapy efficiency. However, the problem is not so simple, and results in vitro should be taken carefully. Thus, for example, it is well known that solid tumors tend to be hypoxic because they lack blood irrigation and, it was recently suggested that a hypoxic condition significantly reduces ROS production by mitochondria, which in turn mediates the acquisition of cisplatin resistance by a human carcinoma cell line (Kim et al., 2021). Nevertheless, in head and neck squamous tumor cells, hypoxia promotes cell death induced by cisplatin (Wu et al., 2021). Thus, the role of mitochondria in cancer cell death induced by Pt-based drugs can be complex and, therefore, in vitro and in vivo results must be contrasted.

ROS Production

As mentioned earlier, it is well known that cisplatin enhances ROS production via mitochondrial dysfunction through a decrease in GSH concentration and disruption of antioxidant enzyme activity (Bompart, 1989). However, cisplatin can increase ROS and H_2O_2 production through an increase of oxidative enzymes activity such as that of nicotinamide adenine dinucleotide phosphate (NADPH) oxidase (Itoh et al., 2011). In this case it is not known whether cisplatin can directly or indirectly modify the NADPH oxidase activity, but at least it was not due to an increase of NADPH oxidase expression (Itoh et al., 2011). On the other hand, aldehyde dehydrogenase (ALDHs) is a family of proteins that help to eliminate aldehydes produced by oxidative stress (Yadav, Choudhary and Bodakhe, 2018). Interestingly, in mice knockout for ALDH2, cisplatin induced more ROS production compared to cells from wild type mice, suggesting that ALDH2 may contribute to cisplatin sensitivity (Kim et al., 2017). Despite the potential link of ROS production with the cisplatin net effect, it is not known whether ROS production can also be part of cisplatin cell resistance. Thus, for example, exposure of cisplatin to H460 (a lung carcinoma cell line), increases H_2O_2 levels, which in turn activates autophagy, an apoptotic resistance associated mechanism (Sumkhemthong et al., 2021). To the contrary, in oral squamous cell carcinoma cell lines, cisplatin-induced autophagy is linked to increased cell apoptosis (Magnano et al., 2021).

Therefore, the effect of cisplatin or other Pt-based drugs in terms of autophagy could be cell dependent. Not only can Pt-based drugs be connected to autophagy, but they can also be associated with other cellular mechanisms. Thus, for example, ROS induce the epithelial-to-mesenchymal transition of mesothelioma cells (Kim, Cui and Kim, 2013), which can be linked to a more malignant cell phenotype.

As a result of this relationship between ROS production and cisplatin-induced resistance, some strategies have been developed to modulate ROS production or its bioavailability to enhance cisplatin-mediated effects. For example, Aldo-keto reductases (AKRs) are enzymes involved in cell detoxification because they eliminate some ROS such as lipid peroxides and other carbonyl groups. In several human tumors, an increase of these proteins has been reported, and the use of AKRs inhibitors have been associated with decreased drug resistance and cisplatin anticancer effect enhancement (Penning et al., 2021). Another strategy used to decrease cisplatin-induced ROS production is to load the cells with l-2-oxothiazolidine-4-carboxylic acid (OTC), which increases the GSH content in the cells and therefore increases antioxidant defenses. The use of OTC resulted in a significant reduction of ROS, nuclear factor κ-light-chain-enhancer of activated B cells (NF-κB) translocation into the nucleus, intercellular adhesion molecule 1 (ICAM-1), caspase 3 activity, and the infiltration of macrophages into kidneys (Lee, Moon, et al., 2006). Thus, ROS levels can both help or worsen the final effect of Pt-based compounds on cell viability, which may depend on the ROS production source (i.e., mitochondria or cytoplasm) or the cell type, or both.

Inflammation

Inflammation is a cellular process mounted by a tissue to protect itself from an insult (e.g., pathogens, tissue damage, etc.). There are two classes of inflammatory responses: acute and chronic. While the acute response lasts from hours to a few days, a chronic response can last even several years, as in cancer. Generally speaking, inflammation is mediated by pro-inflammatory molecules, such as cytokines (e.g., TNF-α (Tumor necrosis factor), INF-γ (Interferon-gamma), interleukin-1 (IL-1), etc.), metabolites (arachidonic acid, prostaglandins, lipoxins, etc.) and nitric oxide, among others. In mice, cisplatin induces renal failure, which is associated with a significant increase in serum, kidney, and urine levels of TNF-α; moreover, mice deficient in TNF-α production do not present renal failure induced by cisplatin (Ramesh and Reeves, 2002). A more detailed study demonstrates that the TNF receptor 2 (TNFR2) but not TNFR1, mediates this phenomenon (Ramesh and Reeves,

2003). Accordingly, the use of rosiglitazone, which can regulate production of inflammatory mediators, decreased renal damage in mice after cisplatin injection (Lee, Kim, et al., 2006). This phenomenon was correlated with a decrease of activated NF-κβ in HK-2 cells (Lee, Kim, et al., 2006). These results suggest that cisplatin can induce substantial systemic inflammation, which is the principal mediator of organ damage.

Activation/Inhibition of Intracellular Pathways

Cisplatin has been reported to activate cell pathways related to several processes described above; for example, it activates protein kinase C (PKC) and extracellular signal-related kinase (ERK)-dependent pathways, which are linked to an increase of TNF-α production, mitochondrial dysfunction, and the activation of caspases in mice renal cells (Nowak, 2002; Jo et al., 2005). Similarly, cisplatin-induced renal failure is associated to p38 mitogen-activated protein kinase (MAPK) activation mediated by ROS production (Ramesh and Reeves, 2005), activation of mitogen-activated protein kinase kinase 3/6 (MKK3/6) (Hernández Losa et al., 2003) and phosphorylation of c-Jun N-terminal kinase (p-JNK) (Francescato et al., 2007). In Pam 212 mouse keratinocytes, cisplatin activates JNK, due to increased enzymatic activity more than an increase in protein levels, which correlates to a higher phosphorylation of p-JNK (Sánchez-Perez, Murguía and Perona, 1998). Additionally, the over expression of ERK phosphatase (CL100/MKP-1) in 293T cells drastically reduced JNK activation induced by cisplatin, which was associated with an increase of cell survival after cisplatin treatment (Sánchez-Pérez et al., 2000). Regarding Jun, cisplatin also increases its expression by activating its promoter through a Src-dependent pathway (Rabo et al., 1996). An increase of c-Jun impacts the signaling mediated by NF-κβ, resulting in decreased 293T survival induced by cisplatin (Sánchez-Pérez et al., 2002), but cisplatin not only activates certain proteins related to cell death. Thus, in an oral squamous cell carcinoma cell line (KOSC-2), cisplatin inhibited the expression of X-chromosome-linked inhibitor of apoptosis protein (XIAP), which is an endogenous inhibitor of several caspases (Matsumiya et al., 2001). Therefore, cisplatin can induce cell death or even cell survival related pathways. This difference in cell response may depend on cell type, cell metabolism or other unknown mechanisms.

On the other hand, it is well known that Pt-derived drugs can directly modulate the activity of certain proteins. Thus for example, in bacteria, both cis- and trans-Pt(NH3)2Cl2 interact with thymidylate synthetase sulfhydryl groups. As a result, it was not a surprise that this interaction would be βmercaptoethanol sensitive (Aull, Rice and Tebbetts, 1977). Similarly, cis-diamminedichloroPt reacts with cysteine groups of rat kidney proteins present in mitochondria and cytoplasm as well (Levi et al., 1980). In addition to cysteine groups, cisplatin can form adducts with methionine of alpha 2-Macroglobulin (Pizzo et al., 1986). Additionally, cisplatin inhibits mitochondrial malate and lactate dehydrogenases, and this inhibition was decreased by the presence of ATP, RNA and DNA in the media, suggesting that ATP concentration (Friedman et al., 1978), and therefore the cell metabolism and ROS-defenses, can impact the final cisplatin effect. In this regard, GSH content of renal cells has been shown to modulate cisplatin-induced kidney damage (Zunino et al., 1989). Other proteins that have been shown to bind Pt-based drugs include: Na^+/K^+ ATPase and Mg^{2+} ATPase (Daley-Yates and McBrien, 1982), mitochondrial phosphate transport (Tkacova and Kuzela, 1985), transferrin (Sykes, TR, Stephens-Newsham and Noujaim, 1985), human albumin (Momburg et al., 1987), proteins involved in ubiquitination (Isoe et al., 1992), and glutaredoxin (Wells et al., 1991). However, it appears that cisplatin does not interact with dopamine-D2, histamine-H1 and acetylcholine-muscarinic receptors (Peroutka, 1987). In summary, much more information is needed on the mechanism by which Pt-derived drugs modulate the activity of certain intracellular signaling pathways, not discarding direct or indirect modifications mediated by ROS or inflammatory mediators.

Resistance Mechanisms

Transporters

One main feature of cancer cells is that they can become resistant to chemotherapy drugs, which correlates with low drug levels in their cytoplasm. Cancer cells have developed several ways to become resistant (Lohan-Codeço et al., 2022), some of which will be presented in this section. One explanation for Pt-based drug resistance is that cancer cells present low levels of transporters that could allow the entry of drugs into the plasma membrane (Amable, 2016). Thus, for example, in cervical and ovarian human carcinoma cell lines, there is a correlation between those cells that are sensitive to cisplatin and high levels of copper transporter 1 (CTR1) mRNA (Zisowsky et al., 2007), which has been postulated as a cisplatin transporter in yeast and mammalian cells (Ishida et al., 2002; Johnstone et al., 2016). Accordingly, the use of copper chelator in a mouse model of human cervical cancer enhanced cisplatin uptake and therefore DNA adducts and cell death (Ishida et al., 2010). Promising results have been obtained using the Cu^{2+} chelator (trientine) in patients as well (Kuo et al., 2021). Moreover, clinical studies have demonstrated that CTR1 expression correlated with Pt concentration and patients' clinical outcomes (Kilari, Guancial and Kim, 2016). Cisplatin has also been shown to induce the internalization and proteolysis of CTR1, which in time will produce resistance (Holzer, Manorek and Howell, 2006). This interaction is mediated by direct interaction between cisplatin and kiteplatin with two methionine-rich domains at the extracellular amino terminal of the CTR1 (Guo, Smith and Petris, 2004; Barbanente et al., 2022). It is important to note that despite that all these results support a correlation between CTR1 expression/activity and Pt-based drugs transport. There are other studies that have questioned that CTR1 is directly involved in the Pt transport into the cells (Larson et al., 2009; Makovec, 2019). Therefore, more experiments are needed in order to solve these discrepancies.

Of course, CTR1 is not the only transporter that could mediate cisplatin transport into the cytoplasm; thus other transporters have been mentioned, such as glucose transporter 1 and transmembrane protein 205 (TMEM205) (Shen et al., 2012) as well as organic cation transporters implicated in oxaliplatin transport (Johnstone et al., 2016). In conclusion, several transporters seem to participate in Pt internalization and externalization and in consequence they are involved in the process of Pt-based drug resistance acquisition in cancer cells.

Another explanation for low drug levels in resistant cells is the presence of ATP-binding cassette (ABC)-transporters in their plasma membrane, which have the ability to actively remove drugs from the cytoplasm (Prieto-Vila et al., 2017), in turn decreasing the effective concentration of chemotherapy drugs (Shanker et al., 2010). In particular, ABCA1, ABCC2 and ABCC6 are directly involved in Pt-based drug efflux from cancer cells (Ween et al., 2015). The clinical implication is that, for example, in colon cancer, the expression levels of the ABCC transporters are well correlated with the cancer grade, response to chemotherapy, and disease-free interval (Hlavata et al., 2012). Therefore, ABC transporter expressions (or at least some of them) can be useful for predicting the treatment response in cancer patients. Other ABC-transporters involved in drug resistance are the P-glycoprotein and multidrug resistance-associated protein 1 (MRP1) (Altenberg, 2004). Interestingly, despite cisplatin not being mobilized through P-glycoprotein transporters, it can enhance its expression (Demeule, Brossard and Béliveau, 1999) via the interaction with sulfiredoxin (SRX) (Takami, Sakamoto and Yamamoto,

2003). Therefore, Pt-based drugs can enhance drug-resistance mechanisms used in chemotherapy (Hamaguchi et al., 1993).

DNA Repair

Another way that cancer cells overcome the damage induced by Pt-based compounds is through DNA repair (Kiss, Xia and Acklin, 2021). As previously mentioned, one main Pt mode of action is via formation of DNA adducts, which alter its replication and mRNA production, and both changes ultimately induce cell death. Cancer cells can express proteins that can repair these DNA modifications. Furthermore, these proteins can be involved directly in DNA repair or as part of intracellular pathways that can activate DNA damage response (DDR) proteins. Thus, for example, drugs used in chemotherapy have been shown to activate phosphatidylinositol 3-kinase/protein kinase B (PI3k/AKT) dependent pathways (including breast cancer susceptibility gene 1 (BRCA1), high mobility group box 1 (HMGB1) and p53, among others), which in turn activate discoidin domain receptor (DDR), thus increasing damaged DNA restoration (Alemi et al., 2021). In this context, several proteins are needed for DNA reparation, which can be grouped in nucleotide excision repair (NER), homologous recombination repair, nonhomologous end joining, and translation synthesis or post-replication repair (Kryczka et al., 2021). The use of cisplatin conjugated to a poly (ADP-ribose) polymerase 1 (PARP-1) inhibitor (a protein associated with DNA repair) has shown high effectiveness, thus inducing death of malignant pleural mesothelioma cells (Gabano et al., 2021). Similar effects were observed by Rev-1 inhibition, a scaffold of the Y Pol family (Yoon et al., 2021). As mentioned earlier, DNA modification occurs by intra- and interstrands and the repair mechanism points to excise the segment presenting the adduction, subsequently filling the gap with a new DNA strand. When feasible, the undamaged sister chromatin is used as a template. Interestingly, the molecular circadian clock has a profound effect on the effect of cisplatin-induced cell death. Thus, for example, when the circadian clock molecular machinery is pharmacologically enhanced, cells present decreased cisplatin-induced DNA damage restoration (Anabtawi, Cvammen and Kemp, 2021). Therefore, it appears that a correct sleep-wake cycle could be helpful in chemotherapy treatment; however, more studies are needed in order to provide well-studied and appropriate chrono-chemotherapy regimens (Yanyan Yang et al., 2021).

Pt-Related Compounds Inactivation

A well-known cell detoxification mechanism is mediated by GSH and the enzymes that use it to deactivate oxidative molecules. Thus, in the early 1990s, cells presenting a high resistance to H_2O_2 were observed also to be highly resistant to cisplatin-induced cell death (Spitz et al., 1993). In particular, cisplatin-resistant cells show higher concentration of GSH, which was associated with less DNA damage (Spitz et al., 1993). As expected, the inactivation of cisplatin was associated with the formation of GSH-cisplatin conjugated, which is why decreased GSH intracellular content increases cisplatin effectiveness (Komiya et al., 1998). With this in mind, it is no surprise that there is a good correlation between GSH peroxidase - especially GPX1 -- and a poor prognosis of patients with oral squamous cell carcinoma (Lee et al., 2017). In the same type of cancer an overexpression of cysteine transporter (SLC7A11) was also correlated with poor patient prognosis (Lee et al., 2018). Moreover, simultaneous inhibition of GSH and thioredoxin reductase (TRX)-mediated metabolism synergically enhance cell death induced by cisplatin in head and neck squamous cell carcinoma cells (Sobhakumari et al., 2012). This cell death indicates that cysteine either is a GSH building block and/or is a structural component of several antioxidant proteins and thus a key factor in Pt cell resistance.

Epigenetics Factors

microRNAs (miR) have been shown to be key players in the development of chemoresistance and miR can influence some aspects of the mechanism of resistance described above. Thus, for example, the downregulation of miR-130a-3p, miR-148a-3p, miR-125a-5p, and miR-1226-3p in esophageal squamous carcinoma results in more cisplatin-sensitive cells (Lindner et al., 2018). One molecular explanation (among many possible ones) is that, for example, in esophageal-derived cancer stem cells which are highly cisplatin resistant, they present high levels of miR-130a, which negatively regulates CTR1 levels (Lindner et al., 2018; Lohan-Codeço et al., 2022) and as mentioned before, could modify cisplatin intracellular levels. Alternatively, high levels of miR-630 and miR-224 in non-small cell lung cancer cells, correlate with low levels of p53, which is a key cisplatin resistance regulator in this type of cell (Kryczka et al., 2021). Thus, these examples clearly show that miRs are important factors promoting cancer relapse and chemoresistance, and future studies could produce deeper understanding in this regard.

Another epigenetic factor involved in cancer chemoresistance is DNA methylation, which is commonly associated to gene silencing. Chemotherapy-resistant cancer cells have also been well documented to present a high degree of DNA methylation (Shen et al., 2012). It is believed that genes involved in controlling cisplatin cytotoxicity are often hypermethylated (Chang et al., 2010). Accordingly, gene analyses of different non-small lung cancer cell lines, revealed that the insulin-like growth factor-binding protein-3 promoter is hypermethylated, which perfectly correlated with their cisplatin sensitivity (De Caceres et al., 2010). On the other hand, genes associated with Src-kinase-dependent pathways are hypermethylated in xenograft preclinical models of high-grade serous ovarian cancer (Tomar et al., 2016). Therefore, DNA methylation represents a good patient prognosis biomarker. In this regard, there are DNA methylation panels to detect gene hypermethylation for esophageal cancer, which can be used as prognosis predictors and could help to determine the best treatment, in a sort of precision medicine (Wang et al., 2021). Additionally, the use of DNA methylation inhibitors has been recommended to re-sensitize cancer cells to (for instance) Pt-derived drugs (Wang et al., 2021). Thus there are preclinical studies using demethylating agents, azacitidine and decitabine, which have shown promising results for high-grade serous ovarian cancer treatment (Matthews, Bowden and Wong-Brown, 2021). These results open a promising window to develop new therapies against cancer.

Finally, histone acetylation has been associated with changes in the expression of proteins involved in cisplatin resistance (Shen et al., 2012). Thus, for example, in lung cancer cell lines, the histone acetylase (TIP60) is overexpressed, and this was correlated with cell sensitivity to cisplatin (Miyamoto et al., 2008). One possible mechanistic explanation, given by Wang et al. (2020), is that cancer cell lines that are chemotherapy resistant present high levels of JNK/c-Jun, which in turn increase histone acetylation by decreasing the expression of histone deacetylase 3 (HDAC3) (Wang et al., 2020). However, in gastric cancer cells, HDAC3 overexpression was correlated with increased PI3k/Akt-mTOR activity and increased chemotherapy resistance (Ren and Tang, 2021). According to the last study, treatment of ovarian carcinoma cell line (A2780) with HDAC3 inhibitors and DNA methylation, sensitized these cells to cisplatin (Steele et al., 2009). Moreover, HDAC3 inhibitors tend to increase p21 expression which in turn induce cell cycle arrest, primarily at the G1 phase, and increase the expression of proapoptotic genes and decrease the expression of anti-apoptotic ones (Lu and Chao, 2012).

All these results strongly suggest that drugs directed against epigenetic factors associated to the gain in chemoresistance, could be used to enhance the cytotoxic effects of Pt-based drugs on cancer cells.

Pt-Based Compound Side Effects and Reflections on Several Mechanisms of Action

Ototoxicity

Pt-based treatments generate irreversible damage along the auditory system from the cochlea to the auditory nerve. It has been reported that apoptosis is triggered on different cells, including hair cells, supporting cells, stria vascularis, and spiral ganglion cells (Devarajan et al., 2002; Laurell et al., 2007). Accordingly, children exposed to cisplatin and carboplatin drugs in utero (for their mother's cancer treatments) tend to develop hearing loss, though interestingly, none of them present this problem when their mothers were treated with oxaliplatin (Finch and Cardonick, 2021). However, in adults, this Pt-derived drug can (rarely) induce irreversible unilateral hearing loss (Oh et al., 2013; Güvenç et al., 2016). Consistent with these results, in a mice model of hearing loss, treatment with cisplatin induced ototoxicity, whereas carboplatin and oxaliplatin did not (Gersten et al., 2020). These results, correlated with the concentration reached into the cochlea, and thus the levels of carboplatin and oxaliplatin were much lower than that of cisplatin (Gersten et al., 2020). Experimental data have shown that copper transporter-1 and organic cation transporters play a key role in Pt-based drug uptake in auditory cells (cisplatin is more efficiently transported, compared with oxaliplatin and carboplatin) (Perde-Schrepler et al., 2020) and this may explain why oxaliplatin exerts less ototoxicity as opposed to cisplatin. Outflow of the drug by the ATP7A/7B has also been reported to influence their toxic effects (Ding et al., 2018; Petruzzelli and Polishchuk, 2019).

DNA injury caused by Pt-based drugs has an important role in ototoxicity. However, toxic ROS production accounts for the key event in auditory cell death. Different ROS sources have been described as contributing to cell damage such as mitochondrial damage and subsequent electron chain leakage, lipid-peroxidation, increased NOX3 activity with superoxide production, and decreased antioxidant potential (Tang et al., 2021). Superoxide production leads to oxidation of lipid membranes causing aldehyde 4-hydroxynonenal, which is highly toxic. NOX3, an isoform of NADPH oxidase, is especially produced in the inner ear (Bánfi et al., 2004). Its activity seems to be mediated by the transient receptor potential vanilloid 1 channel pathway associated with Ca^{+2} overload and subsequent activation of STAT1 (Kaur et al., 2011), a key transcriptional factor involved in caspase-mediated outer hair cell death (Mukherjea et al., 2011; Lu et al., 2019). ROS production is also related to reactive nitrogen species production triggering S-nitrosylation of several proteins. Cisplatin may generate protein nitration leading to downregulation of LIM domain only 4 (LMO4) and promoting p53-mediated apoptosis in cochlear cells (Jamesdaniel, Rathinam and Neumann, 2016).

Ototoxicity has triggered intensive research about the mechanisms involved and potential targets for its prevention. As a result, other reported mechanisms involved in ototoxicity include: inhibition of the thioredoxin enzyme system, endoplasmic reticulum stress-generation (Zong et al., 2017), and iron- and autophagy-related pathways (Dammeyer et al., 2014; Jian et al., 2021). For a more comprehensive review of this matter see other chapters in this book.

Cardiac Toxicity

During the last three decades, many clinical studies have reported that several cancer survivors treated with Pt-analogues are associated with significantly increased risk of major cardiovascular events, with cisplatin-induced cardiotoxicity being an increasing concern (Herradón et al., 2017). Other cardiovascular complications, especially hypertension, dyslipidemias and atherosclerosis have been also associated with Pt-based chemotherapy, but with minor frequency. In the past, it was noted that these side effects do not appear to be dose dependent as they were able to occur during treatment, days or weeks after treatment, or in some cases months or years following completion of Pt-exposition (Pai and Nahata, 2000). The mechanism associated with cardiac toxicity associated to Pt-analogue chemotherapy is complex and not fully understood. However, oxidative stress is recognized as a major mechanism underlying these side effects (Demkow and Stelmaszczyk-Emmel, 2013; Dugbartey, Peppone and de Graaf, 2016). Basic studies revealed that in isolated hearts exposed to cisplatin, clinical manifestations were associated with increased ROS concentrations and lipid peroxidation that can be attenuated by co-administration of n-acetyl cysteine, a precursor of glutathione with antioxidant capacity (Rosic et al., 2016). It had previously been reported that both glutathione and antioxidant enzymes levels were diminished in cardiac tissue of rats exposed to cisplatin (El-Awady et al., 2011). In that study cardiac damage was associated with mitochondrial membrane depolarization and mitochondrial ultrastructural abnormalities.

These manifestations were reduced when antioxidants were co-administrated with cisplatin. Consistent reports revealed that cisplatin accumulation in the mitochondrial matrix affected the mitochondrial electron transport chain, triggering excessive endogenous ROS production (Kruidering et al., 1997; Davis, Nick and Agarwal, 2001; Nishikawa et al., 2001; Townsend et al., 2009). The important amount of mitochondria in cardiac tissue and the fact that heart physiology is highly dependent on mitochondrial capacity may account for the predisposition of this organ to Pt-analogue toxicity (Dugbartey, Peppone and de Graaf, 2016). According to other studies, cisplatin is a potent inhibitor of fatty acid oxidation (Chang et al., 2002; Portilla et al., 2002; Dzagnidze et al., 2007), resulting in mitochondrial dysfunction with additional ROS overload. The latter produced ATP depletion and consequently energy depletion, hindering the ability to sustain the endogenous antioxidant system (Dugbartey, Peppone and de Graaf, 2016).

As in other organs, inflammatory response seems to occur after cell or tissue damage due to oxidative stress associated with Pt-analogue exposure in the cardiac tissue (Xing et al., 2019), leading to the synthesis and release of myriads of inflammatory cytokines and chemokines, highlighting translocation of NF-κB from the cytosol to the nucleus, with subsequent TNF-α production (Topal et al., 2018).

Renal Toxicity

As mentioned, Pt-based drugs are broadly used against cancer cells, but their side effects have hindered their use. Early studies demonstrate that cisplatin causes human renal failure, distal convoluted tubules and collecting-duct necrosis, dilatation of convoluted tubules, and formation of casts (Gonzales-Vitale et al., 1977). These changes persisted as long as 29 days after cisplatin therapy (Gonzales-Vitale et al., 1977), but, interestingly, some of these changes can be prevented by the diuretic furosemide (Ward et al., 1977). To decrease kidney side-effect severity, some Pt-derived compounds with reduced side effects have been tested. In one of these studies, the effect of Pt(IV)-nitroxyl complex (PN149) was tested in a renal cell line ciPTEC (immortalized human proximal tubule epithelial cells). PN149 was observed to increase ROS production in these cells without an inflammatory response, which has been suggested as the main source for Pt toxicity in human kidneys (Schoch et al., 2021). Additionally, natural compounds have been tested as kidney protectors against cisplatin. As in humans, cisplatin induces renal failure in mice, which was determined by an increase of real ROS and protein content in the urine. All these modifications were decreased by administration of an *Acacia hydaspica* extract (Afsar et al., 2021). Interestingly, despite the fact that cisplatin-induced ROS production was decreased by this extract, the size of the tumors was diminished (Afsar et al., 2021), suggesting that at least in this model, ROS does not mediate cisplatin-induced cell death. Similarly, an extract of *Salvia miltiorrhiza* reduced blood content of urea nitrogen, creatinine, ROS, and proinflammatory cytokines enhanced by cisplatin in mice. This phenomenon was mediated by nuclear factor E2-related factor 2/heme oxygenase 1 (Nrf2/HO-1) activation and inhibition of the NF-κB pathway (Yu et al., 2021). On the other hand, in the last decade, speculation that gut microbiome is very important to human health is growing in acceptance. Thus, deregulation of gut microbiome is now known to impact proper organ functions (Murphy et al., 2021; Salinas et al., 2021; Schächtle and Rosshart, 2021) and is even related to cancer development (Grover et al., 2021; Li et al., 2021; Murphy et al., 2021). Accordingly, regarding the role of gut microbiome in health modulation, in a recent set of experiments, the administration of probiotics (*Lactobacillus reuteri* and *Clostridium butyricum*) to cisplatin-treated rats reduced inflammation, suppressed uremic toxin production and enhanced butyrate production, all of which correlates with renal function restoration (Hsiao et al., 2021). Thus, it can be concluded that renal damage is mostly related to a higher level of ROS and proinflammatory cytokines produced by Pt-based drugs.

Nervous System Toxicity

As is well known, neurons do not divide; therefore, Pt-based compounds are not expected to alter these cells through such division. However, like cells in the human body, neurons need to maintain their functions through the activity of many different types of proteins, which under normal conditions are constantly created and degraded in special organelles such as lysosomes and proteosomes. To maintain proper protein levels, they are constantly translated from mRNAs, which in turn are transcribed from genes. Referring to Pt-induced neuronal damage, it is well known that during chemotherapy a peripheral neurotoxicity can be induced (Kanat, Ertas and Caner, 2017), mostly due to damage of sensory neurons such as those located in the dorsal root, trigeminal and nodose ganglia. This damage can be produced in several ways, reflecting the broad spectra of actions that Pt-analogues have. Thus, in dorsal root sensory neurons, cisplatin can form adducts with their DNA (Meijer et al., 1999; McDonald et al., 2005; Dzagnidze et al., 2007) and therefore can inhibit mRNA formation. This phenomenon can be caused by blocking the RNA polymerase binding to the DNA (Ang, Myint and Lippard,

2010), interfering with the binding of some transcription factors to gene promoter regions (Treiber et al., 1994; Zhai et al., 1998) and activation of mRNA transcription repressors (Gilder et al., 2011; Calkins, Iglehart and Lazaro, 2013). Protein production inhibition can be the cause for the reduction of both neuronal size and axonal communication (Yan et al., 2015). Additionally, cisplatin can induce mtDNA damage in sensory neurons (Podratz et al., 2011), which in turn can be associated with higher ROS production and decreased ATP cellular content (Podratz et al., 2011) that undoubtedly can be associated with neuronal malfunction. On the other hand, cisplatin induces substantial changes in shape, size and number of mitochondria of the dorsal root ganglion (DRG) neurons, which may result in their swelling and vacuolization (Bobylev et al., 2018).

Contrary to what has been observed in inner ear cells, oxaliplatin shows significant impact on neurons. As this molecule is commonly known to induce peripheral neuropathy, it can have an important impact on patients' quality of life (Yang Yang et al., 2021; Peng et al., 2022). Interestingly, neuropathic pain has been correlated with a downregulation of potassium channels (K2P and Kv), as a consequence of increased histone deacetylase (Pereira et al., 2021). Reduction of these ion channels should result in a loss of the negative resting membrane potential values. On the other hand, oxaliplatin applied intracellularly decreases the amplitude of action potentials (Grolleau et al., 2001), which could be explained by the fact that oxaliplatin modifies Na^+ currents (Yang Yang et al., 2021).

Decreasing oxaliplatin-induced neuropathic pain has been achieved after HDAC-inhibitor treatment, in a mice cancer model (Lamoine et al., 2021). However, we would like to point out that the neurotoxic effect of oxaliplatin is much more complex and seems to involve several molecular mechanisms. Thus, for example, in an *in vitro* model of neurotoxicity-suppressed neurite growth, it was restored by renin-angiotensin-aldosterone system inhibitors in a ERK1/2-dependent manner (Uchida et al., 2022). Additionally, oxaliplatin induces p38 phosphorylation and downregulation of JNK/Sapk, which are stress signals in DRG neurons (Ta et al., 2006; Yang Yang et al., 2021). Consequently, the nerve growth factor (NGF) increase of JNK/Sapk pathways is a factor protecting against oxaliplatin-induced toxicity in DRG neurons (Meijer et al., 1999). Thus, at least oxaliplatin-induced neuronal damage depends on several intracellular-pathway activation or repression, and modulation of these pathways could be used as inhibitors of the deleterious effects induced by this drug.

In summary, Pt-based molecules can alter sensory neuron activity as a result of significant changes in protein expression caused by DNA adduct production on the cell nucleus and in the mitochondria. For a more comprehensive review of this matter see other chapters in this book.

Conclusion

This chapter provides a general view of the basis for chemical and biological effects of Pt-based drugs on various cells. Pt-based drugs, especially cisplatin, are long-standing, clinically used drugs with interesting chemical behaviors and several well-known biological effects in standard models. Although there are common mechanisms suitable for multiple cell models, the biological effects of Pt drugs and interactions with each cell type and their genetic profile need to be further determined. This aspect of Pt-analogues is especially relevant in those non-tumoral cells, which account for Pt-drug side effect profiles. However, some data obtained from non-cancer models limit the potential to extend these conclusions.

Undeniable progress in survival of cancer patients has been made as a result of the extensive use of Pt drugs worldwide, but this same use has been also associated with increased sequelae in those patients. As a result, intensive research about how to decrease side effects is occurring with clinical testing of various drugs. However, in some cases, chemical and biological effects of cisplatin have been overlooked, leading to decreased antitumoral effects.

Considering that relatively few Pt drugs are clinically and broadly used worldwide, understanding the biochemical and biological basis for resistance to Pt drugs is crucial. Research seeking to understand these issues aims to develop strategies to overcome drug-resistance and their unfavorable clinical effects. Therefore, translational approaches are needed for designing interventions related to increasing oncologic effectiveness of Pt drugs and/or to ameliorate side effects.

References

Afsar, T. et al. (2021) 'Acacia hydaspica R. Parker ethyl-acetate extract abrogates cisplatin-induced nephrotoxicity by targeting ROS and inflammatory cytokines', *Scientific Reports*, 11(1), 17248.

Alberto, M. et al. (2009) 'The second-generation anticancer drug Nedaplatin: a theoretical investigation on the hydrolysis mechanism', *The journal of physical chemistry. B*, 113(43), 14473–14479.

Alderden, R. A., Hall, M. D. and Hambley, T. W. (2006) 'The Discovery and Development of Cisplatin', *Journal of Chemical Education*, 83(5), 728–734. doi: 10.1021/ED083P728.

Alemi, F. et al. (2021) 'Molecular mechanisms involved in DNA repair in human cancers: An overview of PI3k/Akt signaling and PIKKs crosstalk', *Journal of Cellular Physiology*.

Ali, I. et al. (2013) 'Platinum Compounds: A Hope for Future Cancer Chemotherapy', *Anti-Cancer Agents in Medicinal Chemistry*, 13(2), 296–306.

Altenberg, G. (2004) 'Structure of multidrug-resistance proteins of the ATP-binding cassette (ABC) superfamily', *Current medicinal chemistry. Anti-cancer agents*, 4(1), 53–62.

Amable, L. (2016) 'Cisplatin resistance and opportunities for precision medicine', *Pharmacological Research*, 106, 27–36.

Anabtawi, N., Cvammen, W. and Kemp, M. G. (2021) 'Pharmacological inhibition of cryptochrome and REV-ERB promotes DNA repair and cell cycle arrest in cisplatin-treated human cells', *Scientific Reports*, 11(1), 17997.

Ang, W., Myint, M. and Lippard, S. (2010) 'Transcription inhibition by platinum-DNA cross-links in live mammalian cells', *Journal of the American Chemical Society*, 132(21), 7429–7435.

Armand, J. et al. (2000) 'Oxaliplatin in colorectal cancer: An overview', *Seminars in Oncology*, 27(5 SUPPL. 10), 96–104.

Aull, J. L., Rice, A. C. and Tebbetts, L. A. (1977) 'Interactions of Platinum Complexes with the Essential and Nonessential Sulfhydryl Groups of Thymidylate Synthetase', *Biochemistry*, 16(4), 672–677.

Bánfi, B. et al. (2004) 'NOX3, a superoxide-generating NADPH oxidase of the inner ear.', *The Journal of biological chemistry*, 279(44), 46065–72.

Barbanente, A. et al. (2022) 'Interaction of Copper Trafficking Proteins with the Platinum Anticancer Drug Kiteplatin', *ChemMedChem*, 17(1).

Bera, A. et al. (2021) 'Oxoplatin-B, a cisplatin-based platinum(IV) complex with photoactive BODIPY for mitochondria specific "chemo-PDT" activity', *Journal of Inorganic Biochemistry*, 223, 111526.

Blommaert, F. A. et al. (1995) 'Formation of DNA Adducts by the Anticancer Drug Carboplatin: Different Nucleotide Sequence Preferences in Vitro and in Cells', *Biochemistry*, 34(26), 8474–8480.

Bobylev, I. et al. (2018) 'Depletion of Mitofusin-2 Causes Mitochondrial Damage in Cisplatin-Induced Neuropathy', *Molecular Neurobiology*, 55(2), 1227–1235.

Bompart, G. (1989) 'Cisplatin-induced changes in cytochrome P-450, lipid peroxidation and drug-metabolizing enzyme activities in rat kidney cortex', *Toxicology Letters*, 48(2), 193–199.

Borges, L. J. H. et al. (2016) 'In vitro and in vivo studies of the antineoplastic activity of copper (II) compounds against human leukemia THP-1 and murine melanoma B16-F10 cell lines', *European Journal of Medicinal Chemistry*, 123, 128–140.

Brown, A., Kumar, S. and Tchounwou, B. (2019) 'Cisplatin-Based Chemotherapy of Human Cancers.', *Journal of cancer science & therapy*, 11(4).

Calkins, A. S., Iglehart, J. D. and Lazaro, J. B. (2013) 'DNA damage-induced inhibition of rRNA synthesis by DNA-PK and PARP-1', *Nucleic Acids Research*, 41(15), 7378–7386.

Chang, B. et al. (2002) 'L-Carnitine inhibits cisplatin-induced injury of the kidney and small intestine', *Archives of Biochemistry and Biophysics*, 405(1), 55–64.

Chang, X. et al. (2010) 'Identification of hypermethylated genes associated with cisplatin resistance in human cancers', *Cancer research*, 70(7), 2870–2879.

Daley-Yates, and McBrien, D. (1982) 'The inhibition of renal ATPase by cisplatin and some biotransformation products', *Chemico-biological interactions*, 40(3), 325–334.

Dammeyer, et al. (2014) 'Cisplatin and oxaliplatin are toxic to cochlear outer hair cells and both target thioredoxin reductase in organ of Corti cultures', *Acta Oto-Laryngologica*, 134(5), 448–454.

Davies, M. S. et al. (2008) '[1H, 15N] Heteronuclear Single Quantum Coherence NMR Study of the Mechanism of Aquation of Platinum(IV) Ammine Complexes', *Inorganic Chemistry*, 47(17), 7673–7680.

Davies, M. S., Berners-Price, S. J. and Hambley, T. W. (2000) 'Slowing of cisplatin aquation in the presence of DNA but not in the presence of phosphate: Improved understanding of sequence selectivity and the roles of monoaquated and diaquated species in the binding of cisplatin to DNA', *Inorganic Chemistry*, 39(25), 5603–5613.

Davis, C. A., Nick, H. S. and Agarwal, A. (2001) 'Manganese superoxide dismutase attenuates cisplatin-induced renal injury: Importance of superoxide', *Journal of the American Society of Nephrology*, 12(12), 2683–2690.

De Caceres, I. I. et al. (2010) 'IGFBP-3 hypermethylation-derived deficiency mediates cisplatin resistance in non-small-cell lung cancer', *Oncogene*, 29(11), 1681–1690.

Demeule, M., Brossard, M. and Béliveau, R. (1999) 'Cisplatin induces renal expression of P-glycoprorein and canalicular multispecific organic anion transporter', *American Journal of Physiology - Renal Physiology*, 277(6 46-6).

Demkow, U. and Stelmaszczyk-Emmel, A. (2013) 'Cardiotoxicity of cisplatin-based chemotherapy in advanced non-small cell lung cancer patients', *Respiratory Physiology and Neurobiology*, 187(1), 64–67.

Denny, W. A., Rewcastle, G. W. and Baguley, B. C. (1990) 'Potential Antitumor Agents. 59. Structure-Activity Relationships for 2-Phenylbenzimidazole-4-carboxamides, a New Class of "Minimal" DNA-Intercalating Agents Which May Not Act via Topoisomerase II', *Journal of Medicinal Chemistry*, 33(2), 814–819.

Devarajan, et al. (2002) 'Cisplatin-induced apoptosis in auditory cells: role of death receptor and mitochondrial pathways.', *Hearing research*, 174(1–2), 45–54.

Ding, D. et al. (2018) 'Cisplatin-induced vestibular hair cell lesion-less damage at high doses', *Journal of otology*, 13(4), 115–121.

Domnina, E. S. et al. (1983) 'Synthesis and antitumor activity of complex compounds of Pt(II), Pt(IV), and Pd(II) with 1-vinylazoles', *Pharmaceutical Chemistry Journal 1984 17:6*, 17(6), 426–429.

Dugbartey, G. J., Peppone, L. J. and de Graaf, I. A. M. (2016) 'An integrative view of cisplatin-induced renal and cardiac toxicities: Molecular mechanisms, current treatment challenges and potential protective measures', *Toxicology*, 371, 58–66.

Dzagnidze, A. et al. (2007) 'Repair capacity for platinum-DNA adducts determines the severity of cisplatin-induced peripheral neuropathy', *Journal of Neuroscience*, 27(35), 9451–9457.

El-Awady, E. S. E. et al. (2011) 'Cisplatin-induced cardiotoxicity: Mechanisms and cardioprotective strategies', *European Journal of Pharmacology*, 650(1), 335–341.

Fahmy, S. A. et al. (2022) 'Synthesis, Characterization and Host-Guest Complexation of Asplatin: Improved In Vitro Cytotoxicity and Biocompatibility as Compared to Cisplatin', *Pharmaceuticals 2022, Vol. 15, Page 259*, 15(2), 259.

Fichtinger-Schepman, A. M. J. et al. (1985) 'Adducts of the Antitumor Drug cis-Diamminedichloroplatinum(II) with DNA: Formation, Identification, and Quantitation', *Biochemistry*, 24(3), 707–713.

Figg, W. D. et al. (1997) 'Pharmacokinetics of elemental platinum (ultrafiltrate and total) after a thirty minute intravenous infusion of ormaplatin', *Biopharmaceutics and Drug Disposition*, 18(4), 347–359.

Finch, L. E. and Cardonick, E. H. (2021) 'Incidence of childhood hearing loss after in utero exposure to platinum agents', *Prenatal diagnosis*, 41(11), 1467–1474.

Francescato, H. D. C. et al. (2007) 'Effect of JNK inhibition on cisplatin-induced renal damage', *Nephrology Dialysis Transplantation*, 22(8), 2138–2148.

Franskevych, D. V. et al. (2016) 'Modulation of cisplatin-induced reactive oxygen species production by fullerene C60 in normal and transformed lymphoid cells', *Ukrainian Biochemical Journal*, 88(1), 44–50.

Friedman, M. E. et al. (1978) 'Interactions of Cis- and Trans-platinum(II) complexes with dehydrogenase enzymes in the presence of different mono- and polynucleotides: Evidence for a ternary complex', *Bioinorganic Chemistry*, 8(4), 341–353.

Gaba, M. and Mohan, C. (2015) 'Development of drugs based on imidazole and benzimidazole bioactive heterocycles: recent advances and future directions', *Medicinal Chemistry Research 2015 25:2*, 25(2), 173–210.

Gabano, E. et al. (2021) 'Unsymmetric cisplatin-based pt(Iv) conjugates containing a parp-1 inhibitor pharmacophore tested on malignant pleural mesothelioma cell lines', *Molecules*, 26(16).

Gersten, B. K. et al. (2020) 'Ototoxicity and Platinum Uptake Following Cyclic Administration of Platinum-Based Chemotherapeutic Agents', *Journal of the Association for Research in Otolaryngology : JARO*, 21(4), 303–321.

Ghosh, S. (2019) 'Cisplatin: The first metal based anticancer drug', *Bioorganic Chemistry*, 88, 102925.

Gietema, J. A. et al. (1995) 'Phase II and pharmacokinetic study of lobaplatin in patients with relapsed ovarian cancer', *British Journal of Cancer*, 71(6), 1302–1307.

Gilder, A. et al. (2011) 'Coilin participates in the suppression of RNA polymerase I in response to cisplatin-induced DNA damage', *Molecular biology of the cell*, 22(7), 1070–1079.

Gonzales-Vitale, J. et al. (1977) 'The renal pathology in clinical trials of cis-platinum (II) diamminedichloride', *Cancer*, 39(4), 1362–1371.

Gozelle, M. et al. (2019) 'Studies on the synthesis, characterization, cytotoxic activities and plasmid DNA binding of platinum(II) complexes having 2-subsituted benzimidazole ligands', *Polyhedron*, 161, 298–308.

Gravatt, G. L. et al. (1994) 'DNA-Directed Alkylating Agents. 6. Synthesis and Antitumor Activity of DNA Minor Groove-Targeted Aniline Mustard Analogues of Pibenzimol (Hoechst 33258)', *Journal of Medicinal Chemistry*, 37(25), 4338–4345.

Grolleau, F. et al. (2001) 'A possible explanation for a neurotoxic effect of the anticancer agent oxaliplatin on neuronal voltage-gated sodium channels', *Journal of Neurophysiology*, 85(5), 2293–2297.

Grover, K. et al. (2021) 'A discussion of the gut microbiome's development, determinants, and dysbiosis in cancers of the esophagus and stomach', *Journal of Gastrointestinal Oncology*, 12, S290–S300.

Gümüş, F. and Algül, Ö. (1997) 'DNA binding studies with cis-Dichlorobis (5(6)-non/chlorosubstituted-2-hydroxymethyl-benzimidazole) platinum(II) complexes', *Journal of Inorganic Biochemistry*, 68(1), 71–74.

Guo, Y., Smith, K. and Petris, M. J. (2004) 'Cisplatin stabilizes a multimeric complex of the human Ctr1 copper transporter: requirement for the extracellular methionine-rich clusters', *The Journal of biological chemistry*, 279(45), 46393–46399.

Güvenç, M. G. et al. (2016) 'Sudden hearing loss due to oxaliplatin use in a patient with colon cancer', *Journal of chemotherapy (Florence, Italy)*, 28(4), 341–342.

H, C. et al. (2018) 'Effective platinum(IV) prodrugs conjugated with lonidamine as a functional group working on the mitochondria', *Journal of inorganic biochemistry*, 180, 119–128.

Hall, M. D. and Hambley, T. W. (2002) 'Platinum(IV) antitumour compounds: their bioinorganic chemistry', *Coordination Chemistry Reviews*, 232(1–2), 49–67.

Hamaguchi, K. et al. (1993) 'Cross-Resistance to Diverse Drugs Is Associated with Primary Cisplatin Resistance in Ovarian Cancer Cell Lines', *Cancer Research*, 53(21), 5225–5232.

Hector, S. et al. (2001) 'In vitro studies on the mechanisms of oxaliplatin resistance', *Cancer Chemotherapy and Pharmacology*, 48(5), 398–406.

Hernández Losa, J. et al. (2003) 'Role of the p38 MAPK pathway in cisplatin-based therapy', *Oncogene*, 22(26), 3998–4006.

Herradón, E. et al. (2017) 'Characterization of Cardiovascular Alterations Induced by Different Chronic Cisplatin Treatments', *Frontiers in Pharmacology*, 0(MAY), 196.

Hlavata, I. et al. (2012) 'The role of ABC transporters in progression and clinical outcome of colorectal cancer', *Mutagenesis*, 27(2), 187–196.

Hoeschele, J. D. et al. (1982) 'Analysis and Refinement of the Microscale Synthesis of the 195m Pt-labeled Antitumor Drug, czs-Dichlorodiammineplatinum(1l), cis-DDP', *Radiochimica Acta*, 31(1–2), 27–36.

Holzer, A. K., Manorek, G. H. and Howell, S. B. (2006) 'Contribution of the major copper influx transporter CTR1 to the cellular accumulation of cisplatin, carboplatin, and oxaliplatin', *Molecular pharmacology*, 70(4), 1390–1394.

Hsiao, Y. et al. (2021) 'Administration of lactobacillus reuteri combined with clostridium butyricum attenuates cisplatin-induced renal damage by gut microbiota reconstitution, increasing butyric acid production, and suppressing renal inflammation', *Nutrients*, 13(8).

Hydes, C. and Russell, M. J. H. (1988) 'Advances in platinum cancer chemotherapy', *Cancer and Metastasis Reviews 1988 7:1*, 7(1), 67–89.

Iakovidis, A. and Hadjiliadis, N. (1994) 'Complex compounds of platinum (II) and (IV) with amino acids, peptides and their derivatives', *Coordination Chemistry Reviews*, 135–136(C), 17–63.

Ishida, S. et al. (2002) 'Uptake of the anticancer drug cisplatin mediated by the copper transporter Ctr1 in yeast and mammals', *Proceedings of the National Academy of Sciences of the United States of America*, 99(22), 14298–14302.

Ishida, S. et al. (2010) 'Enhancing Tumor-Specific Uptake of the Anticancer Drug Cisplatin with a Copper Chelator', *Cancer Cell*, 17(6), 574–583.

Isoe, T. et al. (1992) 'Inhibition of different steps of the ubiquitin system by cisplatin and aclarubicin', *BBA - General Subjects*, 1117(2), 131–135.

Itoh, T. et al. (2011) 'Cisplatin induces production of reactive oxygen species via NADPH oxidase activation in human prostate cancer cells', *Free Radical Research*, 45(9), 1033–1039.

Jamesdaniel, S., Rathinam, R. and Neumann, W. L. (2016) 'Targeting nitrative stress for attenuating cisplatin-induced downregulation of cochlear LIM domain only 4 and ototoxicity', *Redox Biology*, 10, 257–265.

Jian, B. et al. (2021) 'Autophagy-dependent ferroptosis contributes to cisplatin-induced hearing loss', *Toxicology Letters*, 350, 249–260.

Jo, S. et al. (2005) 'MEK inhibitor, U0126, attenuates cisplatin-induced renal injury by decreasing inflammation and apoptosis', *Kidney international*, 67(2), 458–466.

Johnstone, T. C., Suntharalingam, K., & Lippard, S. J. (2016). The Next Generation of Platinum Drugs: Targeted Pt(II) Agents, Nanoparticle Delivery, and Pt(IV) Prodrugs. *Chemical reviews*, 116(5), 3436–3486.

Kanat, O., Ertas, H. and Caner, B. (2017) 'Platinum-induced neurotoxicity: A review of possible mechanisms', *World Journal of Clinical Oncology*, 8(4), 329.

Kaur, T. et al. (2011) 'Short interfering RNA against STAT1 attenuates cisplatin-induced ototoxicity in the rat by suppressing inflammation', *Cell Death and Disease*, 2(7), e180.

Kawai, Y. et al. (2005) 'Relationship between cisplatin or nedaplatin-induced nephrotoxicity and renal accumulation', *Biological and Pharmaceutical Bulletin*, 28(8), 1385–1388.

Kilari, D., Guancial, E. and Kim, E. S. (2016) 'Role of copper transporters in platinum resistance', *World Journal of Clinical Oncology*, 7(1), 106–113.

Kim, D. K. et al. (1995) 'Pharmacokinetics and antitumor activity of a new platinum compound, cis-malonato[(4 R,5 R)-4,5-bis(aminomethyl)-2-isopropyl- 1, 3-dioxolane]platinum(II), as determined by ex vivo pharmacodynamics', *Cancer Chemotherapy and Pharmacology*, 37(1–2), 1–6.

Kim, J. et al. (2017) 'Aldehyde dehydrogenase 2∗2 knock-in mice show increased reactive oxygen species production in response to cisplatin treatment Tse-Hua Tan', *Journal of Biomedical Science*, 24(1).

Kim, M. C. et al. (2021) 'Reduction in mitochondrial oxidative stress mediates hypoxia-induced resistance to cisplatin in human transitional cell carcinoma cells', *Neoplasia (United States)*, 23(7), 653–662.

Kim, M. C., Cui, F. J. and Kim, Y. (2013) 'Hydrogen peroxide promotes epithelial to mesenchymal transition and stemness in human malignant mesothelioma cells', *Asian Pacific Journal of Cancer Prevention*, 14(6), 3625–3630.

Kiss, R. C., Xia, F. and Acklin, S. (2021) 'Targeting DNA damage response and repair to enhance therapeutic index in cisplatin-based cancer treatment', *International Journal of Molecular Sciences*, 22(15).

Kleih, M. et al. (2019) 'Direct impact of cisplatin on mitochondria induces ROS production that dictates cell fate of ovarian cancer cells', *Cell Death and Disease*, 10(11).

Komiya, S. et al. (1998) 'Role of glutathione in cisplatin resistance in osteosarcoma cell lines', *Journal of Orthopaedic Research*, 16(1), 15–22.

Kostova, I. (2006) *Platinum Complexes as Anticancer Agents | Bentham Science*, *Recent Patents on Anti-Cancer Drug Discovery*.

Kozubík, A. et al. (2005) 'High effectiveness of platinum(IV) complex with adamantylamine in overcoming resistance to cisplatin and suppressing proliferation of ovarian cancer cells in vitro', *Biochemical Pharmacology*, 69(3), 373–383.

Kruidering, M. et al. (1997) 'Cisplatin-induced nephrotoxicity in porcine proximal tubular cells: Mitochondrial dysfunction by inhibition of complexes I to iv of the respiratory chain', *Journal of Pharmacology and Experimental Therapeutics*, 280(2), 638–649.

Kryczka, Jolanta et al. (2021) 'Molecular mechanisms of chemoresistance induced by cisplatin in NSCLC cancer therapy', *International Journal of Molecular Sciences*, 22(16).

Kuo, M. T. et al. (2021) 'Targeting the Copper Transport System to Improve Treatment Efficacies of Platinum-Containing Drugs in Cancer Chemotherapy', *Pharmaceuticals (Basel, Switzerland)*, 14(6).

Kurnakow, N. (1894) 'Ueber complexe Metallbasen; Erste Abhandlung', *Journal for Praktische Chemie*, 50(1), 481–507.

Lamoine, S. et al. (2021) 'The Class I HDAC Inhibitor, MS-275, Prevents Oxaliplatin-Induced Chronic Neuropathy and Potentiates Its Antiproliferative Activity in Mice', *International journal of molecular sciences*, 23(1).

Larson CA, Blair BG, Safaei R, Howell SB. (2009). The role of the mammalian copper transporter 1 in the cellular accumulation of platinum-based drugs. *Mol Pharmacol*, 75(2) : 324-30.

Laurell, G. et al. (2007) 'Effects of a Single High Dose of Cisplatin on the Melanocytes of the Stria Vascularis in the Guinea Pig', *Audiology and Neurotology*, 12(3), 170–178.

Lebwohl, D. and Canetta, R. (1998) 'Clinical development of platinum complexes in cancer therapy: an historical perspective and an update', *European Journal of Cancer*, 34(10), 1522–1534.

Lee, J. R. et al. (2017) 'Overexpression of glutathione peroxidase 1 predicts poor prognosis in oral squamous cell carcinoma', *Journal of Cancer Research and Clinical Oncology*, 143(11), 2257–2265.

Lee, J. R. et al. (2018) 'Overexpression of cysteine-glutamate transporter and CD44 for prediction of recurrence and survival in patients with oral cavity squamous cell carcinoma', *Head and Neck*, 40(11), 2340–2346.

Lee, S., Moon, S. O., et al. (2006) 'Protective role of L-2-oxothiazolidine-4-carboxylic acid in cisplatin-induced renal injury', *Nephrology Dialysis Transplantation*, 21(8), 2085–2095.

Lee, S., Kim, W., et al. (2006) 'Rosiglitazone ameliorates cisplatin-induced renal injury in mice', *Nephrology Dialysis Transplantation*, 21(8), 2096–2105.

Levi, J. et al. (1980) 'Mechanism of cis-platinum nephrotoxicity: I. Effects of sulfhydryl groups in rat kidneys', *Journal of Pharmacology and Experimental Therapeutics*, 213(3), 545–550.

Li, J. J. et al. (2021) 'The role of microbiome in pancreatic cancer', *Cancer and Metastasis Reviews*.

Lindner, K. et al. (2018) 'Complex Epigenetic Regulation of Chemotherapy Resistance and Biohlogy in Esophageal Squamous Cell Carcinoma via MicroRNAs', *International journal of molecular sciences*, 19(2). doi: 10.3390/IJMS19020499.

Lippert, B. (1999) 'Cisplatin : chemistry and biochemistry of a leading anticancer drug', 563. 'Lobaplatin: D 19466' (2003) *Drugs in R&D*, 4(6), 369–372.

Lohan-Codeço, M. et al. (2022) 'Molecular mechanisms associated with chemoresistance in esophageal cancer', *Cellular and molecular life sciences : CMLS*, 79(2), 116.

Lu, H. and Chao, C. C. K. (2012) 'Cancer cells acquire resistance to anticancer drugs: an update', *Biomedical journal*, 35(6), 464–472.

Lu, J. et al. (2019) 'Cisplatin induces calcium ion accumulation and hearing loss by causing functional alterations in calcium channels and exocytosis.', *American journal of translational research*, 11(11), 6877–6889.

Luo, L. et al. (2021) 'VDAC1 as a target in cisplatin anti-tumor activity through promoting mitochondria fusion', *Biochemical and Biophysical Research Communications*, 560, 52–58.

Magnano, S. et al. (2021) 'Cisplatin induces autophagy-associated apoptosis in human oral squamous cell carcinoma (OSCC) mediated in part through reactive oxygen species', *Toxicology and Applied Pharmacology*, 427, 115646.

Makovec T. (2019). Cisplatin and beyond: molecular mechanisms of action and drug resistance development in cancer chemotherapy. *Radiology and oncology*, 53(2), 148–158.

Marieke J. Bloemink, † et al. (1996) 'Synthesis, Crystal Structure, Antitumor Activity, and DNA-Binding Properties of the New Active Platinum Compound (Bis(N-methylimidazol-2-yl)carbinol)dichloroplatinum(II), Lacking a NH Moiety, and of the Inactive Analog Dichloro(N1,N1'-dimethyl-2,2'-biimidazole)platinum(II)', *Inorganic Chemistry*, 35(3), 619–627.

Marullo, R. et al. (2013) 'Cisplatin induces a mitochondrial-ROS response that contributes to cytotoxicity depending on mitochondrial redox status and bioenergetic functions.', *PloS one*, 8(11), e81162.

Matesanz, A. I., Leitao, I. and Souza, (2013) 'Palladium(II) and platinum(II) bis(thiosemicarbazone) complexes of the 2,6-diacetylpyridine series with high cytotoxic activity in cisplatin resistant A2780cisR tumor cells and reduced toxicity', *Journal of Inorganic Biochemistry*, 125, 26–31.

Matsumiya, T. et al. (2001) 'Cisplatin inhibits the expression of X-chromosome-linked inhibitor of apoptosis protein in an oral carcinoma cell line', *Oral Oncology*, 37(3), 296–300.

Matthews, B. G., Bowden, N. A. and Wong-Brown, M. W. (2021) 'Epigenetic Mechanisms and Therapeutic Targets in Chemoresistant High-Grade Serous Ovarian Cancer', *Cancers*, 13(23).

McDonald, E. et al. (2005) 'Cisplatin preferentially binds to DNA in dorsal root ganglion neurons in vitro and in vivo: a potential mechanism for neurotoxicity', *Neurobiology of disease*, 18(2), 305–313.

Meijer, C. et al. (1999) 'Cisplatin-induced DNA-platination in experimental dorsal root ganglia neuronopathy', *NeuroToxicology*, 20(6), 883–887.

Mellor, D. (2002) 'The Sterochemistry of Square Complexes.', *Chemical Reviews*, 33(2), 137–183.

Miyamoto, N. et al. (2008) 'Tip60 is regulated by circadian transcription factor clock and is involved in cisplatin resistance', *The Journal of biological chemistry*, 283(26), 18218–18226.

Momburg, R. et al. (1987) 'Influence of time and chloride ions on the interaction of cisplatin with human albumin in-vitro', *Journal of Pharmacy and Pharmacology*, 39(9), 691–697.

Morcelli, S. R., Bull, É. S., et al. (2016) 'Synthesis, characterization and antitumoral activity of new cobalt(II)complexes: Effect of the ligand isomerism on the biological activity of the complexes', *Journal of Inorganic Biochemistry*, 161, 73–82.

Morcelli, S. R., Kanashiro, M. M., et al. (2016) 'Synthesis, characterization and antitumoral activity of new di-iron(III) complexes containing naphthyl groups: Effect of the isomerism on the biological activity', *Inorganic Chemistry Communications*, 67, 22–24.

Moreira, R. et al. (2019) 'Modulating the antitumoral activity by the design of new platinum(II) compounds: Synthesis, characterization, DFT, ultrastructure and mechanistic studies', *Journal of inorganic biochemistry*, 194, 200–213.

Muhammad, N. et al. (2021) 'Redirecting Cisplatin and Doxorubicin to Mitochondria Affords Highly Effective PlatinumIV Prodrug Against Triple Negative Breast Cancer', *Chemistry - An Asian Journal*, 16(16), 2276–2279.

Muir, M. M. et al. (1992) 'Synthesis and characterization of new platinum(II) complexes containing thiazole and imidazole donors III. Dichlorobis(styrylbenzazole) platinum(II) complexes', *Inorganica Chimica Acta*, 191(1), 131–139.

Mukherjea, D. et al. (2011) 'NOX3 NADPH Oxidase Couples Transient Receptor Potential Vanilloid 1 to Signal Transducer and Activator of Transcription 1-Mediated Inflammation and Hearing Loss', *Antioxidants & Redox Signaling*, 14(6), 999–1010.

Murphy, K. et al. (2021) 'Exploring the gut microbiota and cardiovascular disease', *Metabolites*, 11(8).

Murray, V. et al. (1992) 'The use of Taq DNA polymerase to determine the sequence specificity of DNA damage caused by cis-diamminedichloroplatinum(II), acridine-tethered platinum(II) diammine complexes or two analogues.', *Journal of Biological Chemistry*, 267(26), 18805–18809.

Mylonas, S. et al. (1988) 'Synthesis, molecular structure determination, and antitumor activity of platinum(II) and palladium(II) complexes of 2-substituted benzimidazole', *Journal of Inorganic Biochemistry*, 34(4), 265–275. doi: 10.1016/0162-0134(88)83004-6.

Natile, G. and Coluccia, M. (2001) 'Current status of trans-platinum compounds in cancer therapy', *Coordination Chemistry Reviews*, 216–217, 383–410.

Nishikawa, M. et al. (2001) 'Targeting superoxide dismutase to renal proximal tubule cells inhibits mitochondrial injury and renal dysfunction induced by cisplatin', *Archives of Biochemistry and Biophysics*, 387(1), 78–84.

Nowak, G. (2002) 'Protein Kinase C-α and ERK1/2 Mediate Mitochondrial Dysfunction, Decreases in Active Na+ Transport, and Cisplatin-induced Apoptosis in Renal Cells', *Journal of Biological Chemistry*, 277(45), 43377–43388.

Oh, S. Y. et al. (2013) 'Ototoxicity associated with oxaliplatin in a patient with pancreatic cancer', *JOP : Journal of the pancreas*, 14(6), 676–679.

Pai, V. B. and Nahata, M. C. (2000) 'Cardiotoxicity of chemotherapeutic agents. Incidence, treatment and prevention', *Drug Safety*, 22(4), 263–302.

Paola, E. D., Alonso, S., Giuliani, R., Calabrò, F., D'Alessio, A., Regine, G., Cerbone, L., Bianchi, L., Mancuso, A., Sperka, S., Rozencweig, M., & Sternberg, C. N. (2012). An open-label, dose-finding study of the combination of satraplatin and gemcitabine in patients with advanced solid tumors. *Frontiers in oncology*, 2, 175.

Pasetto, L. M. et al. (2006) 'The development of platinum compounds and their possible combination', *Critical Reviews in Oncology/Hematology*, 60(1), 59–75.

Peng, S. et al. (2022) 'Prevention of Oxaliplatin-Induced Peripheral Neuropathy: A Systematic Review and Meta-Analysis', *Frontiers in oncology*, 12.

Penning, T. M. et al. (2021) 'Aldo-Keto Reductases and Cancer Drug Resistance', *Pharmacological Reviews*, 73(3), 1150–1171.

Perde-Schrepler, M. et al. (2020) 'The expression of copper transporters associated with the ototoxicity induced by platinum-based chemotherapeutic agents', *Hearing research*, 388.

Pereira, V. et al. (2021) 'Epigenetics Involvement in Oxaliplatin-Induced Potassium Channel Transcriptional Downregulation and Hypersensitivity', *Molecular neurobiology*, 58(7), 3575–3587.

Peroutka, S. (1987) 'Chemotherapeutic agents do not interact with neurotransmitter receptors', *Cancer chemotherapy and pharmacology*, 19(2), 131–132.

Petruzzelli, R. and Polishchuk, R. S. (2019) 'Activity and Trafficking of Copper-Transporting ATPases in Tumor Development and Defense against Platinum-Based Drugs', *Cells 2019, Vol. 8, Page 1080*, 8(9), 1080.

Pizzo, S. V. et al. (1986) 'Further characterization of the platinum-reactive component of the α2-macroglobulin-receptor recognition site', *Biochemical Journal*, 238(1), 217–225.

Podratz, J. L. et al. (2011) 'Cisplatin induced Mitochondrial DNA damage in dorsal root ganglion neurons', *Neurobiology of Disease*, 41(3), 661–668.

Portilla, D. et al. (2002) 'Alterations of PPARα and its coactivator PGC-1 in cisplatin-induced acute renal failure', *Kidney International*, 62(4), 1208–1218.

Prieto-Vila, M. et al. (2017) 'Drug resistance driven by cancer stem cells and their niche', *International Journal of Molecular Sciences*, 18(12).

Rabo, Y. B. et al. (1996) 'Different mechanisms are responsible for c-jun mRNA induction by cisplatin and ultraviolet light', *International Journal of Cancer*, 65(6), 821–826.

Ramesh, G. and Reeves, W. (2005) 'p38 MAP kinase inhibition ameliorates cisplatin nephrotoxicity in mice', *American journal of physiology. Renal physiology*, 289(1).

Ramesh, G. and Reeves, W. B. (2002) 'TNF-α mediates chemokine and cytokine expression and renal injury in cisplatin nephrotoxicity', *Journal of Clinical Investigation*, 110(6), 835–842.

Ramesh, G. and Reeves, W. B. (2003) 'TNFR2-mediated apoptosis and necrosis in cisplatin-induced acute renal failure', *American Journal of Physiology - Renal Physiology*, 285(4 54-4).

Rebillard, A., Lagadic-Gossmann, D. and Dimanche-Boitrel, M.-T. (2008) 'Cisplatin Cytotoxicity: DNA and Plasma Membrane Targets', *Current Medicinal Chemistry*, 15(26), 2656–2663.

Reedijk, J. and Lohman, H. M. (1985) 'Cisplatin: Synthesis, antitumour activity and mechanism of action', *Pharmaceutisch Weekblad Scientific Edition*, 7(5), 173–180.

Ren, H. and Tang, L. (2021) 'HDAC3-mediated lncRNA-LOC101928316 contributes to cisplatin resistance in gastric cancer via activating the PI3K-Akt-mTOR pathway', *Neoplasma*, 68(5), 1043–1051.

Rosenberg, B. et al. (1967) 'The Inhibition of Growth or Cell Division in Escherichia coli by Different Ionic Species of Platinum(IV) Complexes', *Journal of Biological Chemistry*, 242(6), 1347–1352.

Rosenberg, B., Van Camp, L. and Krigas, T. (1965) 'Inhibition of cell division in Escherichia coli by electrolysis products from a platinum electrode [17]', *Nature*. Nature Publishing Group, 698–699.

Rosenberg, B. and VanCamp, L. (1970) 'The Successful Regression of Large Solid Sarcoma 180 Tumors by Platinum Compounds', *Cancer Research*, 30(6), 1799–1802.

Rosic, G. et al. (2016) 'The effects of N-acetylcysteine on cisplatin-induced changes of cardiodynamic parameters within coronary autoregulation range in isolated rat hearts', *Toxicology Letters*, 242, 34–46.

Salinas, E. et al. (2021) 'Bioactive compounds in food as a current therapeutic approach to maintain a healthy intestinal epithelium', *Microorganisms*, 9(8).

Sánchez-Pérez, I. et al. (2000) 'CL100/MKP-1 modulates JNK activation and apoptosis in response to cisplatin', *Oncogene*, 19(45), 5142–5152.

Sánchez-Pérez, I. et al. (2002) 'Cell stress and MEKK1-mediated c-Jun activation modulate NFκB activity and cell viability', *Molecular Biology of the Cell*, 13(8), 2933–2945.

Sánchez-Perez, I., Murguía, J. R. and Perona, R. (1998) 'Cisplatin induces a persistent activation of JNK that is related to cell death', *Oncogene*, 16(4), 533–540.

Saris, C. et al. (1996) 'In vitro formation of DNA adducts by cisplatin, lobaplatin and oxaliplatin in calf thymus DNA in solution and in cultured human cells', *Carcinogenesis*, 17(12), 2763–2769.

Schächtle, M. A. and Rosshart, S. (2021) 'The Microbiota-Gut-Brain Axis in Health and Disease and Its Implications for Translational Research.', *Frontiers in cellular neuroscience*, 15, 698172.

Schoch, S. et al. (2021) 'In Vitro Nephrotoxicity Studies of Established and Experimental Platinum-Based Compounds', *Biomedicines*, 9(8), 1033.

Shanker, M. et al. (2010) 'Drug resistance in lung cancer', *Lung Cancer: Targets and Therapy*, 1, 23–36.

Shen, D. W. et al. (2012) 'Cisplatin resistance: a cellular self-defense mechanism resulting from multiple epigenetic and genetic changes', *Pharmacological reviews*, 64(3), 706–721.

Shen, W. et al. (2021) 'Penicilliumin B Protects against Cisplatin-Induced Renal Tubular Cell Apoptosis through Activation of AMPK-Induced Autophagy and Mitochondrial Biogenesis', *Kidney Diseases*, 7(4), 278–292.

Sobhakumari, A. et al. (2012) 'Susceptibility of Human Head and Neck Cancer Cells to Combined Inhibition of Glutathione and Thioredoxin Metabolism', *PLoS ONE*, 7(10).

Spitz, D. R. et al. (1993) 'Cellular resistance to oxidative stress is accompanied by resistance to cisplatin: The significance of increased catalase activity and total glutathione in hydrogen peroxide-resistant fibroblasts', *Journal of Cellular Physiology*, 156(1), 72–79.

Steele, N. et al. (2009) 'Combined inhibition of DNA methylation and histone acetylation enhances gene re-expression and drug sensitivity in vivo', *British journal of cancer*, 100(5), 758–763.

Sternberg CN, Petrylak DP, Sartor O, Witjes JA, Demkow T, Ferrero JM, Eymard JC, Falcon S, Calabrò F, James N, et al. 2009. Multinational, double-blind, phase III study of prednisone and either satraplatin or placebo in patients with castrate-refractory prostate cancer progressing after prior chemotherapy: The SPARC trial. *J Clin Oncol,* 27: 5431–5438.

Sumkhemthong, S. et al. (2021) 'Cisplatin-induced hydroxyl radicals mediate pro-survival autophagy in human lung cancer H460 cells', *Biological Research*, 54(1).

Sykes, TR, S., Stephens-Newsham, L. and Noujaim, A. (1985) 'In vitro binding of platinum compounds to human transferrin', *Research communications in chemical pathology and pharmacology*, 50(3), 387–394.

Ta, L. E. et al. (2006) 'Neurotoxicity of oxaliplatin and cisplatin for dorsal root ganglion neurons correlates with platinum-DNA binding', *Neurotoxicology*, 27(6), 992–1002.

Takami, N., Sakamoto, H. and Yamamoto, T. (2003) 'Steroid and xenobiotic receptor (SXR) is a key system for the acquisition of cisplatin resistance in endometrial cancer cells', *Journal of International Medical Research*, 31(2), 59–68.

Tang, Q. et al. (2021) 'Cisplatin-induced ototoxicity: Updates on molecular mechanisms and otoprotective strategies', *European journal of pharmaceutics and biopharmaceutics : official journal of Arbeitsgemeinschaft fur Pharmazeutische Verfahrenstechnik e.V*, 163, 60–71.

Tchounwou, B. et al. (2021) 'Advances in Our Understanding of the Molecular Mechanisms of Action of Cisplatin in Cancer Therapy', *Journal of experimental pharmacology*, 13, 303–328.

Tkacova, E. and Kuzela, S. (1985) 'Interaction of cis-diamminedichloroplatinum(II) with mitochondrial phosphate carrier', *Neoplasma*, 32(6), 679–683.

Tomar, T. et al. (2016) 'Genome-wide methylation profiling of ovarian cancer patient-derived xenografts treated with the demethylating agent decitabine identifies novel epigenetically regulated genes and pathways', *Genome medicine*, 8(1).

Topal, İ. et al. (2018) 'The effect of rutin on cisplatin-induced oxidative cardiac damage in rats', *Anatolian Journal of Cardiology*, 20(3), 136–142.

Townsend, D. M. et al. (2009) 'Role of glutathione S-transferase Pi in cisplatin-induced nephrotoxicity', *Biomedicine and Pharmacotherapy*, 63(2), 79–85.

Treiber, D. et al. (1994) 'Cisplatin-DNA adducts are molecular decoys for the ribosomal RNA transcription factor hUBF (human upstream binding factor)', *Proceedings of the National Academy of Sciences of the United States of America*, 91(12), 5672–5676.

Uchida, M. et al. (2022) 'Renin-Angiotensin-Aldosterone System Inhibitors Prevent the Onset of Oxaliplatin-Induced Peripheral Neuropathy: A Retrospective Multicenter Study and in Vitro Evaluation', *Biological & pharmaceutical bulletin*, 45(2), 226–234.

Wang, D. and Lippard, S. J. (2005) 'Cellular processing of platinum anticancer drugs.', *Nature reviews. Drug discovery*, 4(4), 307–20.

Wang, H. et al. (2021) 'DNA methylation markers in esophageal cancer: an emerging tool for cancer surveillance and treatment.', *American journal of cancer research*, 11(11), 5644–5658.

Wang, Haifang et al. (2020) 'Enhanced histone H3 acetylation of the PD-L1 promoter via the COP1/c-Jun/HDAC3 axis is required for PD-L1 expression in drug-resistant cancer cells', *Journal of experimental & clinical cancer research : CR*, 39(1).

Ward, J. M. et al. (1977) 'Prevention of Renal Failure in Rats Receiving cis-Diamminedichloroplatinum(Il) by Administration of Furosemide', *Cancer Research*, 37(4), 1238–1240.

Ween, M. et al. (2015) 'The role of ABC transporters in ovarian cancer progression and chemoresistance', *Critical Reviews in Oncology/Hematology*, 96(2), 220–256.

Weiss, R. B. and Christian, M. C. (2012) 'New Cisplatin Analogues in Development', *Drugs 1993 46:3*, 46(3), 360–377.

Wells, W. et al. (1991) 'Interactions of platinum complexes with thioltransferase(glutaredoxin), in vitro', *Biochemical and biophysical research communications*, 180(2), 735–741.

Wheate, N. J. et al. (2010) 'The status of platinum anticancer drugs in the clinic and in clinical trials', *Dalton Transactions*, 39(35), 8113–8127.

Wu, K. et al. (2021) 'Hypoxia-induced ROS promotes mitochondrial fission and cisplatin chemosensitivity via HIF-1α/Mff regulation in head and neck squamous cell carcinoma', *Cellular oncology (Dordrecht)*.

Xing, J. J. et al. (2019) 'Supplementation of saponins from leaves of Panax quinquefolius mitigates cisplatin-evoked cardiotoxicity via inhibiting oxidative stress-associated inflammation and apoptosis in mice', *Antioxidants*, 8(9).

Yadav, A., Choudhary, R. and Bodakhe, S. H. (2018) 'Role of Nitric Oxide in the Development of Cataract Formation in CdCl2-induced Hypertensive Animals', *Current Eye Research*, 1–11.

Yan, F. et al. (2015) 'Role of platinum DNA damage-induced transcriptional inhibition in chemotherapy-induced neuronal atrophy and peripheral neurotoxicity', *Journal of Neurochemistry*, 135(6), 1099–1112.

Yang, Yanyan et al. (2021) 'Circadian clock, carcinogenesis, chronochemotherapy connections', *Journal of Biological Chemistry*, 297(3), 101068.

Yang, Yang et al. (2021) 'Targeting strategies for oxaliplatin-induced peripheral neuropathy: clinical syndrome, molecular basis, and drug development', *Journal of experimental & clinical cancer research : CR*, 40(1).

Yang, Z. et al. (2000) 'Decreased cisplatin/DNA adduct formation is associated with cisplatin resistance in human head and neck cancer lines', *Cancer Chemotherapy and Pharmacology*, 46(4), 255–262.

Yang, Z. et al. (2006) 'Cisplatin preferentially binds mitochondrial DNA and voltage-dependent anion channel protein in the mitochondrial membrane of head and neck squamous cell carcinoma: Possible role in apoptosis', *Clinical Cancer Research*, 12(19), 5817–5825.

Yoon, J.-H. et al. (2021) 'Implications of inhibition of Rev1 interaction with Y family DNA polymerases for cisplatin chemotherapy', *Genes & Development*, 35(17–18), 1256–1270.

Yu, C. et al. (2021) 'Danshensu attenuates cisplatin-induced nephrotoxicity through activation of Nrf2 pathway and inhibition of NF-κB', *Biomedicine & pharmacotherapy = Biomedecine & pharmacotherapie*, 142, 111995.

Zhai, X. et al. (1998) 'Cisplatin-DNA adducts inhibit ribosomal RNA synthesis by hijacking the transcription factor human upstream binding factor', *Biochemistry*, 37(46), 16307–16315.

Zisowsky, J. et al. (2007) 'Relevance of drug uptake and efflux for cisplatin sensitivity of tumor cells', *Biochemical Pharmacology*, 73(2), 298–307.

Zong, S. et al. (2017) 'Endoplasmic reticulum stress is involved in cochlear cell apoptosis in a cisplatin-induced ototoxicity rat model', *Audiology and Neurotology*, 22(3), 160–168.

Zunino, F. et al. (1989) 'Protective effect of reduced glutathione against cisplatin-induced renal and systemic toxicity and its influence on the therapeutic activity of the antitumor drug', *Chemico-biological interactions*, 70(1–2), 89–101.

Chapter 2

Role of Cellular Senescence in Resistance to Platinum-Based Chemotherapy

Aleksandra Olszewska[1,2,*], Monika Granica[1,3,*], Aleksandra Klemba[1,4], Claudine Kieda[1] and Halina Was[1,†]

[1]Laboratory of Molecular Oncology and Innovative Therapies, Military Institute of Medicine, Warsaw, Poland
[2]Postgraduate School of Molecular Medicine, Medical University of Warsaw, Warsaw, Poland
[3]Doctoral School of Translational Medicine, Centre of Postgraduate Medical Education, Warsaw, Poland
[4]College of Inter-Faculty Individual Studies in Mathematics and Natural Sciences, University of Warsaw, Warsaw, Poland

Abstract

Development of chemoresistance is one of the major problems related with cancer treatment. The primary goal of most anti-cancer therapies is to kill cancer cells. Although, due to different intratumoral mechanisms, the spectrum of cellular responses to chemotherapeutics may be wide - from cell death to cell proliferation. There is an additional one that is underestimated, namely cellular senescence. This is a phenomenon related to reaching the division limit known as the Hayflick limit. Of importance, in response to stressful factors, cancer cells can also undergo cellular senescence, namely Stress-Induced Premature Senescence

*Equal contribution.
†Corresponding Author's Email: hwas@wim.mil.pl.

In: Platinum-Based Chemotherapy
Editors: Kulmira Nurgali and Raquel Abalo
ISBN: 978-1-68507-972-7
© 2022 Nova Science Publishers, Inc.

(SIPS). One of the SIPS type is Therapy-Induced Senescence (TIS). TIS cells demonstrate an increased activity of the Senescence Associated β-galactosidase (SA-β-gal) and an irreversible growth arrest. A number of studies have shown that platinum derivatives, including cisplatin, oxaliplatin and carboplatin may induce TIS in different cancer types and experimental settings. Noticeably, recent data suggest that TIS cells can re-activate their proliferative potential and lead to cancer recurrence. Moreover, TIS cells exhibit an increased metabolism and so-called Senescence-Associated Secretory Phenotype (SASP). SASP is manifested by an augmented secretion of cytokines and chemokines that affect tumor microenvironment and key processes for tumor growth and metastases, including: migration, invasion, angiogenesis and immune response. Altogether, TIS cells may enhance the risk of developing chemoresistance and patient death. The following overview presents the state of the knowledge on the role of TIS cells in resistance to platinum-based drugs both *in vitro* and *in vivo.*

Keywords: cancer treatment, chemoresistance, senescence, senescence-associated secretory phenotype, therapy-induced senescence

Introduction

Cellular Senescence – The General Overview

Cellular senescence has a direct impact on the aging of the whole organism. It is based on permanent cell cycle arrest; however senescent cells remain metabolically active. This phenomenon was discovered by Hayflick and Moorhead, who observed a limited ability of human fibroblasts for divisions (Hayflick and Moorhead, 1961). This discovery allowed to overturn the previous paradigm of cell immortality in *in vitro* cultures (Carrel and Ebeling, 1921). "Hayflick limit" term described the maximum number of cell divisions before a cell undergoes apoptosis. The "Hayflick limit" theory is linked with a terminal replication and telomere erosion. A unique feature of normal, somatic, eukaryotic cells is the presence of repeated sequences, telomeres, at the end of chromosomes, that form a kind of protection for coding parts of the genetic material (Olovnikov, 1973, Olovnikov, 1996). Each cell, upon reaching its own critical telomere length, leaves the cell cycle and enters the path of cellular senescence. In most normal cells, telomerase activity, which elongates telomeres, is none or very low. In contrast, stem cells (Collins and Mitchell, 2002) or cancer cells can divide without any restrictions

(Bremermann, 1982), which is a consequence of the active telomerase (TERT) (Yuan et al., 2019). Apart from the progressive loss of the nucleotides in telomeric sequences with each division, also their structural changes may contribute to senescence (Li et al., 2003). Senescence associated with the gradual shortening ends of chromosomes and loss of stability of the telomeres is identified as replicative cellular senescence (Liu et al., 2019).

In the 1990s, Chen and Ames were the ones, who first identified a different mechanism of cellular senescence, namely stress-induced premature senescence (SIPS). They demonstrated that hydrogen peroxide inhibited the cell cycle and as a result senescence-like phenotype manifestations rapidly occurred in human fibroblasts (Chen and Ames, 1994). This type of senescence is independent of division potential and telomere shortening. SIPS is a rapid and acute response to stressful stimuli, that is observed within days or even hours. It can be activated by oxidative stress, oncogenes, DNA-damaging agents or oncogenic viruses (Tounekti et al., 1993, Lock and Stribinskiene, 1996). It seems that a direct cause of SIPS are DNA double-strand breaks (DSBs), which trigger a permanent cascade of DNA damage response signals (DDR) in the cell (Martinez et al., 2016, Rodier et al., 2005). DDR increases the expression of cell cycle inhibitors such as p16 and p21, which negatively control G1 and G2/M or S progression, respectively (Ciemerych et al., 2011).

Senescent cells (both replicative and through SIPS) present a typical phenotype based on morphological and biochemical changes, like increased cell size and granularity, enhanced production of reactive oxygen species (ROS) by dysfunctional mitochondria, increased activity of senescence-associated-β-galactosidase (SA-β-gal) and mammalian target of rapamycin (mTOR) pathway, activation of DDR signaling pathway, senescence-associated heterochromatin foci (SAHF), decreased level of lamin B1 leading to the loss of nuclear integrity and DNA damage and presence of senescence-associated secretory phenotype (SASP) (Freund et al., 2012, Pollina and Brunet, 2011, Was et al., 2017).

The occurrence of senescent cells may have both beneficial and detrimental consequences. Recent findings indicate that cellular senescence is a very important process during embryogenesis, tissue remodeling and wound healing (Calcinotto et al., 2019, Munoz-Espin et al., 2013, Demaria et al., 2014). Another advantage of cellular senescence is the protection against cancer development. Senescence could be activated in response to aberrant proliferation signals, such as oncogene activation or loss of tumor suppressors (oncogene-induced senescence, OIS). Additionally, it can turn on permanent cell cycle arrest in already proliferating cancer cells through therapy-induced senescence (TIS) (Lee and Lee, 2019). On the other hand, accumulation of high numbers of cells with a senescent phenotype in tissues plays an important role in pathological processes like cardiovascular (North and Sinclair, 2012) and neurodegenerative diseases (Kritsilis et al., 2018), muscle atrophy (Tezze et al., 2017), alterations in wound healing (Mahmoudi et al., 2019) or cancer. In the context of cancer, senescent cells often escape the control of the immune system. Their reduced proliferation makes them less resistant to conventional cancer treatments. Also, many of them are able to modify the niche of the tumor microenvironment to best suit their needs (Gonzalez et al., 2016).

Taken together, cellular senescence is a mechanism that can bring both benefits and losses. Especially, in terms of cancer initiation and progression, senescence seems to present a Janus face.

Senescence of Cancer Cells

Despite new possibilities for cancer treatment, conventional methods such as chemotherapy and radiotherapy are still used for cancer patients. These therapies mainly induce the death of cells with a high proliferation rate. An anti-cancer treatment in the early stages of the disease is often successful and prolongs survival of patients, although sometimes the treatment protocols bring short-term recovery or limited effectiveness. One of the reasons is too low concentration of chemotherapeutics, which decrease rapidly in tumor tissues (Gewirtz, 1999). As a result, tumor cells can still divide or become senescent. It should therefore be emphasized that geno- and cytotoxic drugs might induce the formation of TIS cancer cells. Senescence of cancer cells might be induced also by oncogene (OIS) or virus (virus-induced senescence, VIS). In recent years, a close connection between senescence of cancer cells and chemoresistance has been noted. The escape of tumor cells from apoptosis, in response to therapy, into a senescent phenotype, results in a decreased sensitivity to death signals and enhancement of proliferation (Prasanna et al., 2021, Fitsiou et al., 2021, Fan and Schmitt, 2017, Wu et al., 2010, Ewald et al., 2010). Such resistant cancer cells can take on stemness-like features and undergo polyploidization. Polyploid cancer cells may undertake amitotic divisions (neosis) and produce aneuploid progeny. Additionally, senescent cancer cells may have an impact on their microenvironment (e.g., non-senescent cancer cells, stromal cells, immune cells, vascular and lymphatic cells) through SASP, accelerating tumor growth and metastasis (Sundaram et al., 2004, Rajaraman et al., 2006, Rajaraman et al., 2005, Navolanic et al., 2004, Mosieniak et al., 2015, Was et al., 2017, Erenpreisa et al., 2015, Zhang et al., 2014b, Zhang et al., 2014c, Was et al., 2021) (Figure 1). Consequently, accumulation of senescent cancer cells could be associated with poor patient survival prognosis (Roberson et al., 2005, Wu et al., 2012).

Altogether, it should be remembered that the senescence occurring in cancer cells shows two sides. It acts as a possible defense mechanism to remove abnormal, damaged cells. On the other hand, the dark side of TIS increases the chemoresistance of tumor cells and its further development.

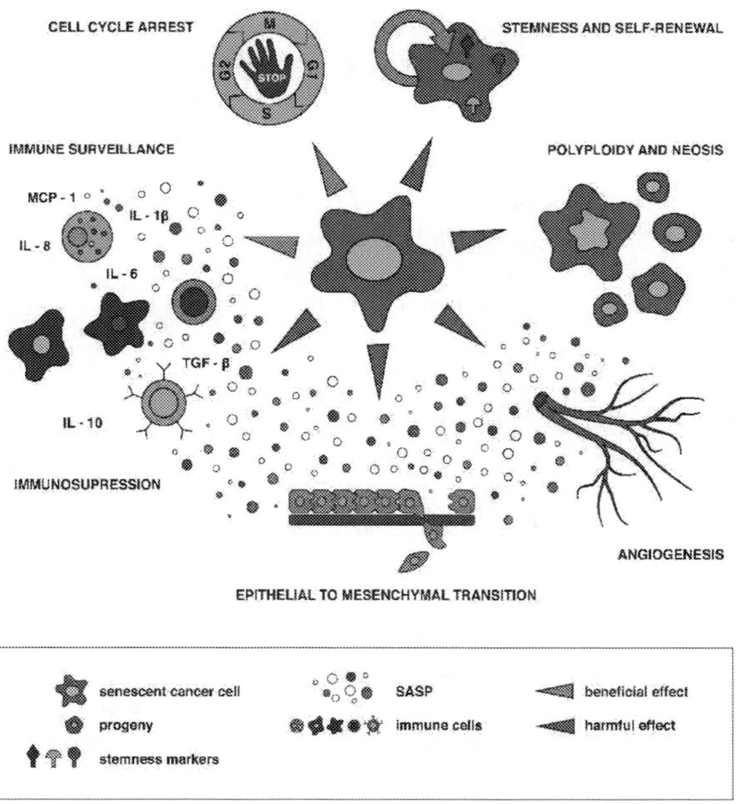

Figure 1. Beneficial and harmful effects of a senescent cancer cell. Abbreviations: IL, interleukin; MCP-1, monocyte chemotactic protein 1; SASP, Senescence-Associated Secretory Phenotype.

Polyploidy, Neosis and Stem Cells

More and more evidence suggest that some subpopulations of cancer cells escape from senescence. There are two different explanations for this problem: the first one describes the resistance of the cells to senescence (Elmore et al., 2005), the second one points to the return of growth after senescence phase (Sikora et al., 2020). In response to antineoplastic agents these cells can transform to polyploid giant cancer cells (PGCCs). PGCCs have been detected in many types of cancer (Alharbi et al., 2018, Coward and Harding, 2014) and might be responsible for therapy resistance (Was et al., 2017, Tredan et al., 2007). The pattern of polyploid cell formation may result from endoreplication, cell fusion, or cell cannibalism (Was et al., 2021). Polyploidy can be induced by ionizing radiation, hypoxia, metabolic stress, compounds that disrupt DNA structure and function and others (Amend et al., 2019). Polyploid cancer cells can divide and produce aneuploid progeny that might be even more resistant to further therapies than "maternal" cells. These differences are linked with transient stemness phenotype and immunogenicity decrease in new generations of descendants (Erenpreisa and Cragg, 2013). Amitotic divisions of senescent cells were described for the first time by Rajaraman and colleagues. They proposed that "neosis" involves polyploidization and the generation of new cells (Raju cells) by budding nuclei and asymmetric cytokinesis (Rajaraman et al., 2006). Additionally, Erenpreisa and Cragg suggested that Raju cells have stemness properties derived from the unstable genome of maternal PGGCs (Erenpreisa and Cragg, 2013). The stem cell phenotype is characterized by a unique ability to self-renew and at the same time differentiate into various cell types derived from different germ layers. The cancer stem cell (CSC) model of cancer origin claims that only a small subset of cancer cells is responsible for tumor initiation, progression and therapy resistance. The presence of CSC in hematopoietic malignancies and solid tumors has been extensively documented. The CSC hypothesis explains resistance to radio- or chemotherapy and tumor recurrence. Quiescent or slow cycling CSCs may survive therapeutic treatment and generate a relapse (Visvader and Lindeman, 2012, Batlle and Clevers, 2017, You et al., 2017). Of importance, hypoxia promotes the PGCCs and stem-like phenotype (Zhang et al., 2014c). Hypoxia is very common in solid tumors. The metabolism of tumor cells, altered by reduced oxygen content, may result in resistance to treatment. A group coordinated by Liu concluded, that PGCCs are able to self-renew their own population by endoreplication and then divide by budding or nuclear fragmentation (Niu et al., 2016). In accordance, Erenpreisa's team detected nuclear markers of stemness (octamer-binding transcription factor 4 (OCT4), homeobox protein NANOG (NANOG) and sex determining region Y-box 2 (SOX2) in rare, highly polyploid cells that produced rejuvenated descendants (Erenpreisa et al., 2011, Salmina et al., 2010). Moreover, triploid breast cancer cells, non-responsive to neoadjuvant chemotherapy were demonstrated to contain the fraction of polyploid cells exhibiting both, NANOG and a cell cycle inhibitor p16 expression (Gerashchenko et al., 2016). Also in our study, after treatment with DNA-damaging agents, a subpopulation of PGCCs with stem cell-like features, including expression of NANOG, cluster of differentiation 24 (CD24) and side population (SP) was found. Importantly, they were able to generate progeny *in vitro* as well as *in vivo* (Was et al., 2017, Was et al., 2018). Moreover, we and others found that rare polyploid cancer cells resembled blastocysts, suggesting that they may be a very early cancer-initiating cells capable of tumor re-population (Was et al., 2018, Niu et al., 2016).

To summarize, it seems that interactions between senescence, polyploidy and stemness of cells are important mechanisms that allow cancer cells to survive harmful conditions e.g., chemotherapy, and recapitulate the tumor.

Immune Response

It is commonly believed that chronic inflammation contributes to the aging process. The high levels of proinflammatory mediators such as cytokines, chemokines or proteases present in plasma (Michaud et al., 2013, Cesari et al., 2004, Fulop et al., 2017) promote the formation of pathologies like: atherosclerosis, osteoarthritis, Alzheimer's disease or cancer. It has been observed that elderly people have 2-4 fold increased levels of proinflammatory factors like: interleukin 6 (IL-6) or tumor necrosis factor alpha (TNF-α) compared to younger individuals (Bruunsgaard, 2006, Puzianowska-Kuznicka et al., 2016). There are also studies performed on centenarians, where in healthier ones the ratio between anti- and pro-inflammatory factors was higher than in frail centenarians (Franceschi et al., 2007). Such chronic activation of the immune system results in immunosenescence, leading to typical cellular anergy. It is manifested by a decrease of naive T lymphocytes and clonal expansion among T and B cells, making the organism unable to respond effectively to new antigens (McElhaney and Effros, 2009). Age-related damage to the immune system is also associated with a disruption of the ratio between the subpopulations of hematopoietic stem cells (Dorshkind et al.,

2020). The changes result in reduction of innate immune cells potential. This is almost always accompanied by an increase in proinflammatory cytokines (Qin et al., 2016).

Senescent cells may also be the source of cytokines, chemokines and other factors, as they secrete, i.e., IL-1, IL-6 or IL-8. These interleukins cause a strong recruitment of innate immune response cells (Prelog, 2006). Production of various factors by cells undergoing senescence is called SASP. It has been observed to be accompanied by a significant increase in the production of 40-80 factors, involved in the transmission of various signals in response to DDR (Coppe et al., 2010). Expression of SASP factors is controlled at the mRNA level (Coppe et al., 2008) and depends on the transcription factors nuclear factor κ-light-chain-enhancer of activated B cells (NF-κB) and CCAAT/enhancer-binding protein β (C/EBPβ) (Acosta et al., 2008). Likewise, the SASP is more often triggered by genotoxic stress than proliferation inhibition (Coppe et al., 2008). Besides, we and others indicated strong induction of many molecules in senescent cancer cells, including: granulocyte macrophage colony-stimulating factor (GM-CSF), growth regulated oncogene (GRO) α, β, γ, insulin-like growth factor binding proteins (IGFBP) -7, IL-1α, IL-7, monocyte chemotactic protein (MCP) -1,2, macrophages inflammatory protein (MIP) -1α and matrix metalloproteinases (MMP) -1, -3, -10 (Coppe et al., 2008, Acosta et al., 2008, Bavik et al., 2006, Liu and Hornsby, 2007, Was et al., 2018, Was et al., 2017). Increased p53 expression promotes MCP-1 secretion (Iannello et al., 2013, Was et al., 2018), which recruites monocytes into the inflammatory zone, foster diapedesis and transform macrophages towards the M1 phenotype (Covarrubias et al., 2020). However, T cell activation can be modulated by presenting inhibitory molecules like cytotoxic T-lymphocyte protein 4 (CTLA-4) and programmed cell death ligand 1 (PD-L1) on tumors surface (Intlekofer and Thompson, 2013). Recently, Hao and coworkers demonstrated that SASP correlated with overcoming resistance to immune checkpoint blockade (ICB) in ovarian cancer. They showed that intraperitoneal transfer of cisplatin-induced, SASP-boosted senescent cells with irinotecan sensitized ovarian tumor to anti-programed cell death protein 1 (PD-1) antibody and improved the survival of tumor-bearing mice. This correlated with the infiltration of activated $CD8^+$ T cells and dendritic cells in the tumor bed (Hao et al., 2021).

It is important to note that TIS-induced SASP might have both effects – beneficial, such as stimulation of the immune system to eliminate cancer cells - and harmful, as a source of chronic inflammation and drug resistance (Ewald et al., 2010). Thus, senescent cancer cells are able to modulate the microenvironment to best suit their needs. High plasma concentrations of certain factors play a crucial role in metastasis and tumor growth, by stimulating angiogenesis, proliferation or epithelial-mesenchymal transition (EMT) (Heidemann et al., 2003). The mechanism of SASP is not so clear. Many studies show that SASP contributes to the immune response evasion in the tumor microenvironment (TME). This is manifested by decreased expression of major histocompatibility complex (MHC) class I and tumor-specific antigens (Bujak et al., 2018). Also, in our previous experiments conducted on human colon cancer cells - HCT116, we observed an increased IL-10 secretion after senescence-inducing agents - irinotecan or 5-fluorouracil. In contrast, oxaliplatin neither activated senescence of colon cancer cells nor upregulated IL-10 (Was et al., 2018). IL-10 as well as transforming growth factor-β (TGF-β) (Fabregat et al., 2014) formed local immunosuppression, supported by regulatory T cells (Treg) and myeloid-derived suppressor cells (MDSC) (Gabrilovich, 2017). To avoid death, senescent cells present inhibitory ligands that bind to the natural killer group 2A (NKG2A) receptor on NK cells. Blocking death leads to accumulation of senescent cells in the tissue (Kale et al., 2020). Furthermore, studies on senescent thyroid cells showed that SASP triggered activation of immunosuppressive M2 phenotype of macrophages (Mazzoni et al., 2019). Polarization toward this phenotype contributes to angiogenesis through vascular endothelial growth factor (VEGF) production (He et al., 2012).

Taken together, interactions between immune cells and senescent cells depend on specificity of SASP components and ligands present on the senescent cells. Further studies should elucidate what the reason is for different SASP composition and how we can modulate it.

Angiogenesis

Rapid proliferation of cancer cells within the tumor results in an increased requirement for nutrients and oxygen. Therefore, the formation of new blood vessels is essential. It is not uncommon for their morphology and arrangement to be different compared to normal vessels (Tredan et al., 2007). It is also known that the predominance of proangiogenic components encourages angiogenic switch. After that, tumor transitions from the avascular to the vascular phase (Salavati et al., 2018). The hypoxic environment of cancer cells and the activity of the transcription factor hypoxia-inducible factor 1α (HIF-1α), responsible for overproduction of VEGF, is also crucial in tumor angiogenesis (Ribatti, 2008). The formation of tumor blood vessels can manifest in two ways. Angiogenesis is based on the use of pre-existing vessels, whereas vasculogenesis is the recruitment of progenitor cells from the bone marrow (Folkman, 1971, Ding et al., 2008). In solid tumors also vascular-like structures are developed. This phenomenon is called vascular mimicry (VM) and it involves transdifferentiation of tumor cells into cells with a phenotype similar to endothelial cells. The mechanism of VM is independent of endothelial cell proliferation and VEGF (Maniotis et al., 1999). However, it is known that there is an increase in MMPs activity (Liu et al., 2012), TME remodeling (Millimaggi et al., 2009) and expression of markers that suggest their multipotent phenotype (SOX2, TWIST-1, CD133, CD44) (Lai et al., 2012, Ricci-Vitiani et al., 2010, Wu et al., 2016, Wang et al., 2010).

Senescent cells also produce proangiogenic factors. IL-6 and VEGF seem to play a paramount role in neovascularization (Ancrile et al., 2007). They both affect proliferation and migration of endothelial cells, accompanied by the remodeling of the extracellular matrix (ECM) through MMPs (Deryugina and Quigley, 2010). In our publication, we unequivocally confirmed that VEGF, IL-8, platelet-derived growth factor (PDGF), angiogenin and vascular endothelial cadherin (VE-cadherin) secretion levels were significantly increased in human senescent colon cancer cells (HCT116), treated with doxorubicin or irinotecan (Was et al., 2018). In addition, we also observed faster tumor formation in mice implanted with HCT116 cells previously treated with chemotherapy and an autophagy inhibitor. This was accompanied by a much higher level of VEGF in sera of tumor-bearing mice and better vascularization than in control tumors. Thus, we authenticated the correlation between TIS and proangiogenic factor production (Was et al., 2017). Luo and coworkers showed that prostate cancer patients with VM had the tendency to develop bone metastasis. Interestingly, activations of cell apoptosis and senescence regulation pathways in VM structures were detected (Luo et al., 2014). Additionally, the presence of erythrocytes in the lumen of VM vessels indicated that they combine with nearby blood vessels (Maniotis et al., 1999, Kieda, 2013). Surprisingly, the source of erythrocytes in vascular-like structures might be the tumor cells themselves, showing characteristics of PGCCs (Zhang et al., 2014a, Zhang et al., 2008).

It is noteworthy that many anticancer therapies are also accompanied by drug-induced hypoxia, which drives angiogenesis and consequently cancer cell metastasis. The examples presented here suggest that paracrine SASP activity of senescent cells affect angiogenesis or vascularization that support tumor growth, survival and metastasis.

Epithelial-Mesenchymal Transition (EMT)

Recruitment to the immediate environment of TIS cancer cells is often associated with the process of EMT. It has been detected in breast (De Francesco et al., 2018), lung (Chae et al., 2018), renal (Wang et al., 2019) and prostate cancer (Odero-Marah et al., 2018). EMT is a prominent process in the organism that provides spatial and molecular tissue flexibility during embryogenesis or facilitates wound healing (Faheem et al., 2020, Dongre and Weinberg, 2019). In the context of cancer cells, the EMT process increases the potential for distant tumor formation and resistance to elimination by various therapeutic regimens (Dongre and Weinberg, 2019). The molecular mechanism of EMT transformation in cancer cells is not well understood, although it is linked to the Wnt/ β-catenin pathway and the TNF family factors. For example, TNF-α expression is decreased and correlates with an increased tumor mass and the appearance of metastases in renal cell carcinoma. It is related with a decreased expression of a characteristic epithelial cells marker - E-cadherin, and an increase in mesenchymal vimentin (Szymanski et al., 2019). Transcription factors such as Snail-1 and Zeb-1 promote the repression of the E-cadherin adhesion molecule and accumulation of N-cadherin (Hazan et al., 2000). Thus, cancer cells lose their polarity and cell-to-cell adhesion, while they gain migratory and invasive properties (Eger et al., 2005). In addition, changes in the levels of other proteins such as cytokeratin, N-cadherin, TWIST-1, zinc-finger factor Snai1 (Snail-1) and zinc finger E-box-binding homeobox 1 (Zeb-1) are also observed in the mechanism of EMT (Ansieau et al., 2008, Furuya et al., 2017, Liu et al., 2013). Besides, radiotherapy often leads to the development of distant metastases in patients with advanced stage of lung cancer. Liu and colleagues in their research observed that irradiation of A549 human lung cancer cells promotes EMT, suggesting a TIS role in disease progression (Liu et al., 2014). We also observed increased expression of the mesenchymal protein Zeb-1 in nuclei of some senescent/ polyploid colon cancer cells. At the same time, production of intercellular adhesion molecules (ICAMs) were downregulated in these cells (Was et al., 2018). Administration of bleomycin to A549 cells caused fibrosis through the crosstalk between EMT and TIS upon chemotherapy (Muthuramalingam et al., 2020). In accordance, we showed that senescent HCT116 colon cancer cells had formed small tumors with high ratio of collagen fibers. Subsequently, they underwent angiogenic switch and progressed into big and vascularized tumors (Was et al., 2017).

Taken together, senescent cells through SASP and beyond ensures their ability to continue proliferation, invasiveness, and induction of EMT.

Mechanism of Action of Platinum-Based Drugs

Cisplatin is the first metal-based chemotherapeutic agent, whose ability to inhibit cell division was established in 1965 by Barnett Rosenberg. It was accepted by the U.S. Food and Drug Administration for the treatment of bladder and testicular cancer in 1978 (Chen and Chang, 2019). Today cisplatin is used in different type of cancers, including gynecological cancers, germ cell cancer, testicular cancer, head and neck cancer, bladder cancer, lung cancer, head and neck cancer, lymphoma and melanoma (Ho et al., 2016, Ghosh, 2019). The molecular structure contains a platinum complex with two amides and two chloride ligands arranged in the cis position (Chen and Chang, 2019). Cisplatin is administered intravenously. It can bind to plasma proteins, causing its partial inactivation. However, due to the relatively high concentration of chloride ions, it is transported mainly unchanged. In contrast, during cell penetration by passive diffusion or via the copper transporter protein 1 (CTR1), chlorine ions dissociate from the cisplatin molecule. This is caused by the relatively low concentration of chloride ions in cytoplasm, resulting in the formation of a positively charged molecule capable of interacting with nucleophilic molecules in the cell, including DNA, RNA and proteins. DNA is considered the preferential binding site for platinum compounds. On the purine principles, three types of bonds can arise: monoadducts, single-strand breaks, and double-strand breaks cross-links (Rabik and Dolan, 2007, Ghosh, 2019). Cisplatin can cause oxidative stress due to its ability to cross-link purine bases in DNA, thereby damaging DNA and interfering with its repair mechanisms.

The most serious disadvantages of this drug are high toxicity and rapid degradation rate (Casares et al., 2012, Ghosh, 2019). Therefore, there was a big need to develop less toxic cisplatin derivatives. The first one was carboplatin, which was introduced into clinics for ovarian cancer in 1988 (Kenny et al., 2017). Now it is also commonly used for lung and head and neck cancers. Carboplatin has a bidentate dicarboxylate (CBDCA) ligand instead of chloride atoms, which results in its lower reactivity and a slower binding rate to DNA. It also exhibits slower kinetics with a retention half-life of 30 hours comparing to 1.5-3.6 hours for cisplatin. Therefore, carboplatin shows fewer side effects, especially nephrotoxicity (Dasari and Tchounwou,

2014). Although its administration is related with myelosuppression, which is manifested mainly by neutropenia and thrombocytopenia (Dasari and Tchounwou, 2014, Chen et al., 2017). The literature indicates another disadvantage of carboplatin comparing to cisplatin in terms of sensitization to radiation and subsequent survival benefits. However, this limitation seems to be abolished during combination therapy with other chemotherapeutics (Ho et al., 2016).

A third generation of platinum derivative is oxaliplatin. It was introduced into the clinics in France in 1996 year to overcome cisplatin and carboplatin resistance (Perego and Robert, 2016). It is used in combination with 5-fluorouracil and folinate in the treatment of cisplatin-resistant colorectal cancer. Oxaliplatin contains 1,2-diaminocyclohexane (DACH) ligand and oxalate. DACH increases the lipophilic properties of the molecule, making it easier to penetrate the cell membrane. Increased lipophilicity of oxaliplatin causes its additional penetration into the cells by organic cation transporters OCT1 and OCT2. It was demonstrated that colorectal cancer cells show increased OCT2 expression, and this may explain the higher effectiveness of oxaliplatin in that type of cancer comparing to other ones. Oxaliplatin is as effective as cisplatin. It was shown that the numbers of single and double breaks are similar for both drugs. Importantly, oxaliplatin is less toxic that cisplatin, causing less neuropathy-related side effects (Rabik and Dolan, 2007, Dilruba and Kalayda, 2016).

Additional platinum-based drugs have been introduced in Asian countries: heptaplatin (Korea), lobaplatin (China), nedaplatin and miriplatin (Japan) (Rottenberg et al., 2021, Oun et al., 2018).

A number of studies conducted on platinum derivatives have shown that therapeutic doses of these drugs can cause not only apoptosis of cancer cells, but also push them into TIS (Li et al., 2014, Qu et al., 2013a).

Mechanism of Senescence Induction After Platinum-Based Chemotherapy Exposure

There is a growing body of evidence showing that platinum-based therapy can induce senescence of cancer cells (Qu et al., 2013b, Coppe et al., 2008, Nacarelli et al., 2020). As a result of cisplatin-induced DNA damage, the p53 protein is modified, mainly it is phosphorylated by ataxia telangiectasia mutated (ATM) and ataxia telangiectasia and Rad3-related (ATR) kinases. p53 is preferentially phosphorylated by ATR kinase in response to single-stranded DNA regions, DSBs, and cross-strand DNA cross-links, while ATM kinase works mainly in response to DSBs (Murray and Mirzayans, 2020, Blackford and Jackson, 2017). Activation of p53 in the cell leads to the transcription of target genes related to DNA repair, apoptosis and senescence (Riley et al., 2008). p53 can respond to severe stress, activating proteins such as: p21, plasminogen activator inhibitor 1 (PAI1), and promyelocytic leukemia protein (PML). As a result, it leads to induction of senescence (Brady and Attardi, 2010). Cisplatin-induced cellular senescence is also associated with an increase in p16 protein, however the pathways leading to p16 induction are not fully recognized (Gire and Dulic, 2015, Veena et al., 2014). It is noteworthy, that the doses of cisplatin achievable in cancer patients, when used in *in vitro* conditions, cause mostly senescence (Eastman, 2017, Berndtsson et al., 2007).

Senescence plays a dual role in cancer. On the one hand, it can exhibit anti-tumor effects, as it prevents most cancer cells from dividing. On the other hand, it may lead to resistance to therapy and cancer recurrence, as senescent cancer cells may undergo rare, amitotic divisions and affect their microenvironment through SASP (Faheem et al., 2020). Therefore, it is crucial to understand molecular details of the process that may allow us to predict the fate of cancer cells in response to therapy and to design more effective treatments.

Beneficial Outcome of Platinum-Induced Senescence

Since the main problem in neoplastic diseases is an uncontrolled proliferation of transformed cells, cellular senescence might be a potentially beneficial phenomenon appearing in response to therapy. TIS acts as a major tumor suppressor mechanism by arresting cancer cells in cell cycle. It has been shown that chemotherapeutic agents, including platinum derivatives, can induce cellular senescence, while escaping from senescence or apoptosis leads to treatment failure (Wang et al., 2021). A number of *in vitro,* pre- and clinical studies showed a correlation between cellular senescence and chemosensitivity to platinum derivatives.

Combination of a platinum derivative and a chemotherapeutic agent from the taxane group is a standard therapy for patients with ovarian cancer. It was shown, using *in vitro* models, that carboplatin and paclitaxel combination treatment leads to induction of senescence markers such as: SA-β-gal, p16 and a decrease in laminin B. Of importance, analysis of samples from patients with

High-Grade Serous Ovarian Cancer (HGSOC) demonstrated that the decrease of laminin B and the upregulation of p16 correlated with improved patient survival, pointing to the benefits of senescence induction (Calvo et al., 2018). Furthermore, using 3D organoids obtained from cisplatin-sensitive and cisplatin-resistant ovarian cancer tissue samples, it was found that the sensitive ones showed elevated SA-β-gal activity and increased expression of genes involved in cellular senescence: p53, p21, retinoblastoma-associated protein (RB) and p16 (Sun et al., 2020). In another study, authors compared cisplatin-sensitive, A2780 and cisplatin-resistant, C13K ovarian cancer cell lines in terms of senescence and proliferation. They demonstrated that cisplatin-sensitive cells exhibited senescence phenotype, manifested by an increase in SA-β-gal, an accumulation of cells in the G2/M phase and a reduced proliferation index (Li et al., 2014).

In vitro studies on hepatocellular carcinoma cells (HCC) showed that oxaliplatin-induced senescent cells exhibited increased expression of p21 and p53 proteins. Importantly, it was also demonstrated that p53 protein inhibited the expression of forkhead box protein M1 (FoxM1). Since FoxM1 appeared to be associated with poor prognosis in HCC patients by promoting proliferation, the induction of senescence may have a positive effect on tumor suppression (Qu et al., 2013b).

Using KP mouse model of non-small-cell lung carcinoma (NSCLC) utilizing the activation of oncogenic K-ras and the loss of function of p53, Hemann group showed the effect of cisplatin-induced cellular senescence on effectiveness of therapy. They used cells with knock out of Rev7 (also known as: MAD2L2 - Mitotic Arrest Deficient 2 Like 2), which is a DNA polymerase zeta subunit involved in DNA repair. They demonstrated that Rev7 KO cells exhibited increased sensitivity to cisplatin with simultaneous induction of senescence in colony formation assay. The benefits of senescence induction were indicated also in a mouse model, where it correlated with an increase in animal survival, a decrease in tumor volume and reduced rate of proliferation (Vassel et al., 2020).

The presence of cancer stem cells could be the factor that increases chemoresistance. Therefore, their elimination may be a way to augment chemosensitization. Research on adenoid cystic carcinoma (ACC) showed a positive link between senescence induction and the reduction of CSCs in response to cisplatin and an FDA-approved histone deacetylation inhibitor (HDACi), vorinostat (Almeida et al., 2017).

Hao and coworkers pointed to the benefits of SASP in sensitizing neoplastic cells to immunotherapy. They showed that UPK10 mouse ovarian carcinoma cells underwent senescence after cisplatin treatment and exhibited a secretory phenotype. Production of SASP components was further potentiated, when cells were treated additionally with irinotecan, a chemotherapeutic agent that inhibits topoisomerase-1. Implantation of SASP-induced TIS cells into mice with ovarian cancer resulted in sensitization to anti-PD-1 therapy. This effect was associated with an increase in infiltration of activated $CD69^{+}$/ $CD4^{+}$ T and dendritic cells into the tumor. As a result, tumor mass decreased and animal survival was improved (Hao et al., 2021).

In conclusion, many *in vitro* and *in vivo* data confirm positive correlation between induction of senescence in cancer cells and increased chemosensitivity. It could be related directly with inhibition of cancer cells proliferation or indirectly with effects of senescent cells on their microenvironment.

The Influence of Platinum-Induced Senescence on Chemoresistance in Tumor Tissues

Although cellular senescence in the context of cancer has many benefits, some features of senescent cells can lead to the development of chemoresistance. The literature indicates that SASP, the development of stem cell features and polyploidy may contribute to the recurrence of therapy-resistant cancer (Figure 2).

SASP

DNA-damaging drugs such as cisplatin induce SASP, which may increase the chemoresistance of cancer cells *in vitro* and *in vivo* (Yu et al., 2020, Coppe et al., 2008, Xu et al., 2019, Chatterjee et al., 2020). Sun and coworkers demonstrated that cisplatin-induced senescence resulted in SASP induction *via* activation of p53 and p21 signaling pathways in A375 melanoma cells *in vitro*. It was manifested by elevation of IL-1α, IL-1β, IL-6, IL-8 and TNF-α, wherein IL-1α was an upstream SASP regulator. Evidence of the superior role of IL-1α in the induction of the secretory phenotype of senescent cells is its ability to induce pro-inflammatory IL-6 and IL-8. Moreover, blockade of IL-1α has been shown to reduce IL-6/IL-8 secretion of senescent cells (Orjalo et al., 2009, Olan and Narita, 2021). Of importance, SASP factors promoted the growth and survival of A375 melanoma cells. It was also proved that the presence of TIS cells promoted the proliferation of non-senescent cells in animal experiments. It was attributed to an increased IL-1α and IL-8 secretion by senescent cells (Sun et al., 2018).

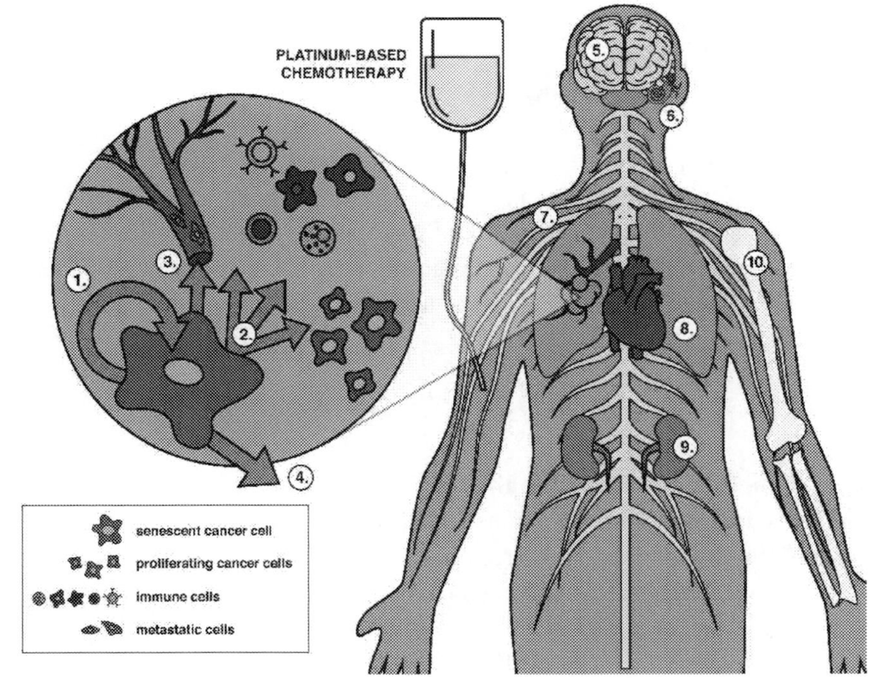

Figure 2. Effects of platinum-induced senescent cancer cell: intratumoral vs systemic perspective. 1. Self-renewal and neosis, 2. Interactions with other cellular components, 3. Epithelial-mesenchymal transition (EMT), 4. Systemic effects, 5. Central nervous system toxicity, 6. Ototoxicity, 7. Peripheral nervous system toxicity, 8. Cardiovascular toxicity, 9. Nephrotoxicity, 10. Hematotoxicity.

The Bonaldi group indicated that protein arginine methyltransferase 1 (PRMT1) may be responsible for SASP-mediated effects. PRMT1 is involved in a variety of cellular processes, including the repair of DNA double breaks. It is overexpressed in many cancers and is associated with a poor outcome of chemotherapy. In studies on SKOV3 ovarian cancer cells, PRMT1 was shown to mediate the activation of the SASP in response to cisplatin. Importantly, the inhibition of PRMT1 expression made the cells more sensitive to cisplatin treatment, as showed by decreased clonogenic survival and apoptosis induction. The above data indicate that reduction of SASP by PRMT1 inhibition makes cells more sensitive to chemotherapy (Musiani et al., 2020).

The high cancer cell metabolism requires an increase in the amount of the cofactor nicotinamide adenine dinucleotide (NAD). Nicotinamide phosphoribosyltransferase (NAMPT) is a regulator of NAD and is often overexpressed in many cancers, including breast cancer, gastric cancer, colorectal cancer, ovarian cancer, prostate cancer, well-differentiated thyroid cancer, myeloma, melanoma and astrocytomas. NAMPT is a molecular and experimental target in cancer therapies (Garten et al., 2015). Studies conducted on the human ovarian carcinoma OVCAR3 line and in a murine model showed that treatment with cisplatin increased the level of NAD, which in turn activated SASP signaling and increased production of cytokines, namely IL-1β, IL-6 and IL-8. Importantly, the inhibition of NAMPT activity delayed the recurrence of the cancer in mice, suggesting the importance of SASP reduction in improved response to therapy (Nacarelli et al., 2020).

Stemness

One of the features related with TIS-induce chemoresistance and therapy failure is stemness. Stem cells have the ability to self-renew and possess cancer-initiating properties. Moreover, they have low rate of division, which makes them insensitive to chemotherapeutic agents targeting dividing cells. Stemness is recognized as one of the key features determining tumor repopulation after treatment (Telleria, 2013).

Nacarelli and coworkers showed an increased expression of the stemness-related genes: aldehyde dehydrogenase 1 family, member A1 (ALDH1A1), Sox2, Nestin1, CD133, and CD44 in cells treated with conditioned media from cisplatin-induced senescent cells. Authors claimed that it was related with SASP, as downregulated expression of SASP component by NAMPT inhibition resulted in a reduction of the stemness phenotype (Nacarelli et al., 2020). A study conducted on an ACC demonstrated a simultaneous increase in the markers of TIS cells (SA-β-gal and gamma histone H2AX (γ-H2AX) foci) and stemness. Stem cells were identified there as cells positive for two markers: aldehyde dehydrogenase 1 (ALDH1) and CD44 expression, which increased almost to 400% after cisplatin treatment (Almeida et al., 2017).

Research conducted on the ovarian cancer cell line SKOV3 showed that DNA damage caused by a cisplatin derivative led to the development of stemness. In response to carboplatin, cells underwent senescence and expressed characteristic features: inhibition of proliferation, an increase in SA-β-gal activity, p21 expression and secretory phenotype. At the same time TIS cells displayed stemness phenotype, as expression of OCT4, CD44, CD117 and CD133 were upregulated. The authors suggested connection between TIS, stemness phenotype and the chemoresistance after carboplatin treatment (Rohnalter et al., 2015).

Summarizing, the literature data indicate that the stemness phenotype accompanying TIS can be induced by SASP factors and may contribute to the recurrence of chemoresistant cancer.

Polyploidy

Another feature related with TIS and chemoresistance might be the development of polyploidy. Polyploid neoplastic cells may undergo atypical division, which may be responsible for tumor repopulation after treatment (Telleria, 2013). Polyploidy formation in response to cisplatin treatment was observed already in the last century (Wolf et al., 1996). Also, exposure of cell lines derived from tumors with p53 mutation to carboplatin or oxaliplatin induced a cytostatic response, that might be associated with the formation of PGCCs (Murray and Mirzayans, 2020).

Polyploidy formation can be related with DNA repair disorders. Excision repair cross-complementation group 1 (ERCC1) is involved in the removal of cisplatin-induced DNA cross-links. Studies on the human non-small cell lung cancer line demonstrated that cisplatin-treated ERCC1-deficient cells exhibited impaired cytokinesis and an increased number of centrosomes, leading to polyploidy (Friboulet et al., 2013). Rohnalter and coworkers showed, using SKOV3 human ovarian carcinoma cell line, that carboplatin-induced DNA damage caused a mitotic catastrophe with a high percentage of polyploid cells and increased expression of p21 protein. Additionally, these cells displayed secretory and stemness phenotype as well as an increase in Snail-1 expression, indicating boosted potential for metastasis (Rohnalter et al., 2015).

Recent studies on the other cell line of ovarian cancer, OVCAR3, described their polyploidization after carboplatin treatment. The authors suggested the significance of checkpoint kinase 1 (CHK-1) phosphorylation in the process, which may be insufficient to arrest the cell at the G2 checkpoint following DNA damage. In turn, it might result in abnormal mitotic progression, leading to polyploidy (Yeung et al., 2019).

Studies conducted on colon cancer cells demonstrated that cells treated with cisplatin duplicated DNA without cell division. Cisplatin activated the process of endoreduplication, which led to successive degrees of polyploidization with cells being enlarged and mononuclear. Seven days after drug administration, cells returned to mitotic activity, but mitoses were often multipolar (Puig et al., 2008).

Data indicates that cells derived from PGCCs that form upon cisplatin treatment have increased resistance to cytotoxic drugs (Amend et al., 2019, Coward and Harding, 2014, Kalejs et al., 2006). Studies on cisplatin–treated B16F10 melanoma showed that giant cells with cancer stem-like cell characteristics were formed. They exhibited high expression of S100 and CD133 proteins, which may indicate their increased aggressiveness. Moreover, these giant cells had a higher capacity of drug efflux, which is directly related to chemoresistance. However, the authors noticed that the appearance of giant cells is not the same as senescence due to the low percentage of SA-β-gal positive cells (Weng et al., 2020).

Tumor Microenvironment Senescence

A growing body of evidence indicates that the components of TME can reprogram tumor response to therapies. TME includes non-malignant cells, blood vessels, lymphoid organs or lymph nodes, nerves, intercellular components, stromal cells, inflammatory cells, and metabolites located at the center, margin, or within the vicinity of the tumor lesion (Jin and Jin, 2020).

Mesenchymal stromal cells (MSCs) were demonstrated to undergo senescence in response to cisplatin treatment. Cisplatin caused changes in the expression of many kinases and an upregulated secretion of SASP components: IL-6 and IL-8. In turn, it resulted in augmented numbers of stem-like cells and enhanced chemoresistance of MDA-MB-231 breast cancer cells (Skolekova et al., 2016).

To mimic tumor 3D structure and extracellular matrix-based microenvironment, MCF-7 breast cancer cell line was cultured in the 3D-reconstituted basement membrane (3D-rBM). Cancer cells cultured in such conditions showed a significant increase in resistance to cisplatin and induction of senescence. The phenotype correlated with increased ATR-CHK-1 signaling and improved replication capacity of cisplatin-damaged DNA.

This research also showed that inhibition of ATR reversed several responses to cisplatin mediated by the 3D microenvironment (Gomes et al., 2019).

Bhargava and Vaishampayan emphasized the importance of another SASP component – amphiregulin (AREG). The authors used another cisplatin derivative, satraplatin, which has improved toxicity profiles and increased effectiveness in comparison to cisplatin (Bhargava and Vaishampayan, 2009). Satraplatin-treated stromal cells produced AREG. In turn, AREG induced expression of PD-L1 in surrounding cancer cells and created an immunosuppressive tumor microenvironment. In combination with classical chemotherapy, targeting AREG restored immunocompetence and reduced the chemoresistance of cancer cells (Xu et al., 2019).

The Influence of Platinum-Induced Senescence on Systemic Chemoresistance and Toxicity

As described in the previous chapter, senescent cancer cells may contribute to the tumor relapse at the intra-tumor level through SASP, the development of stem cell characteristics and polyploidy. In this chapter, we propose that platinum-induced senescence can affect other organs of cancer patients and lead to systemic toxicity and body failure (Figure 2).

Aging

Cellular senescence, including the one induced by cisplatin, is proven to accelerate aging and pathologically affect several human organs and body systems. It has been demonstrated to cause systemic toxicity correlated with: neurodegenerative diseases (Martinez-Cue and Rueda, 2020), peripheral neuropathy (Acklin et al., 2020), nephrotoxicity (Fang et al., 2021), ototoxicity (Skalleberg et al., 2020), cardio (vascular) toxicity (Qian et al., 2018), hematotoxicity and development of second primary cancers (Hudson et al., 2013). Risk for cancer occurrence significantly increases with age and chemotherapy activates premature aging in cancer survivors. Induction of cellular senescence seems to be one of the molecular mechanisms responsible for this phenomenon. It has been demonstrated that premature senescence could be related with earlier cancer onset and more frequent chronic diseases, like endocrinopathies, cardiac dysfunction, osteoporosis, pulmonary fibrosis, secondary cancers and frailty compared with matching untreated population (Cupit-Link et al., 2017). For example, cisplatin therapy hastens normally age-related tau pathology and loss of synaptic integrity (Chiang et al., 2019). Aging also increased risk of cisplatin-induced adverse effects of chemotherapy in kidney (Wen et al., 2015, Duan et al., 2020), however moderate aging did not seem to aggravate these effects (Sharp et al., 2019).

Neurotoxicity

Senescence of several types of central nervous system cells (e.g.: neurons, astrocytes, microglia, oligodendrocytes, neural stem cells) is involved in development of neurogenerative diseases (Martinez-Cue and Rueda, 2020). Patients with different types of cancer (testicular, lungs, etc.), receiving platinum-based chemotherapy, suffered from neurological changes and poorer cognitive performance (Chiang et al., 2019). Cisplatin-induced peripheral neuropathy (CIPN) is one of the most frequent adverse effects of cisplatin treatment (Chovanec et al., 2017). CIPN was associated with presence/accumulation of senescent cells in mouse dorsal root ganglia (DRG), which appeared upon anticancer treatment. Selective clearance of such senescent cells with the senolytic agent, ABT263, reversed CIPN (Acklin et al., 2020). In a well characterized CIPN mouse model, DRG sensory neurons expressed several senescence hallmarks (e.g., SA-β-gal, γ-H2AX and nuclear p65 protein) together with upregulation of pathways connected with DNA damage response (Calls et al., 2021).

Adult mice treated with cisplatin showed hasten development of taupathy, which was accompanied with increased amount of endogenous tau clusters, astrocyte activation and loss of synaptic integrity in the hippocampus. Altogether, it resulted in significantly impaired cognitive performance (Chiang et al., 2019). Eliminating cancer senescent cells with senolytic agents (ganciclovir, ABT-263, fisetin, dasatinib and quercetin) mitigated symptoms of neurodegeneration in mice (Sikora et al., 2019).

Metabolites of oxaliplatin are considered to contribute to induction of oxaliplatin-induced peripheral neuropathy (OIPN) that includes acute or chronic neurotoxicity (Argyriou et al., 2013). Both types of OIPN are developed in majority cancer patients during or shortly after chemotherapeutic treatment. Aqueous extract of *Forsythiae suspensa* fruits (EFSF) had neuroprotective effect in mice suffering from OIPN, as the co-treatment of EFSF with oxaliplatin completely reversed the oxaliplatin-induced neurotoxicity (including cytotoxicity and the inhibited neurite outgrowth). Forsythoside A, the EFSF component, exhibited neuroprotective effects against the oxaliplatin-induced neurotoxicity. Moreover, in the mouse peripheral neuropathy model EFSF reduced the oxaliplatin-induced mechanical allodynia and loss of intra-epidermal nerve fiber to the levels of the vehicle control (Yi et al., 2019).

Neurotoxicity is much less common in patients receiving carboplatin treatment (Go and Adjei, 1999). It can at least be partially explained by the fact, that carboplatin must be administrated in 10-fold higher concentration that cisplatin to induce similar toxicity. Moreover, both cisplatin and oxaliplatin induced elevated ROS generation and DNA 8-oxoguanine damage, but carboplatin did not (Kanat et al., 2017).

Taken together, neurotoxicity induced by cisplatin and oxaliplatin seems to be at least partially mediated via cellular senescence and targeting senescent cells might improve clinical outcome of treatment with these chemotherapeutic drugs.

Ototoxicity

Ototoxicity is also a problem during cisplatin treatment and significantly impairs patients' quality of life, affecting 20% to 75% of them (Chovanec et al., 2017, Drogemoller et al., 2019). Cisplatin is known to target several cell types in basal and middle turn of cochlea, namely: outer hair cells (OHCs), supporting cells, marginal cells of stria vascularis (SVA), spiral ligament (SL) and spiral ganglion neurons (SGN) (Sheth et al., 2019). Sheth and coworkers suggested that caffeine consumption should be limited in patients treated with cisplatin. Research on rats showed that it exacerbated cisplatin-induced ototoxicity in terms of OHCs damage. Moreover, when administrated repeatedly, it increased synaptopathy and inflammation in the cochlea (Sheth et al., 2019). Cisplatin-related hearing loss (HL) is claimed to be developing after treatment. However, high-frequency HL in first post-treatment decade did not seem to progress into later decades in testicular cancer survivors (Skalleberg et al., 2020). In the study analyzing head and neck cancer patients, only 1 in 12 developed permanent HL. Of importance, this low rate was attributed to long-term administration of low cisplatin doses accompanied by the antibiotic, fosfomycin (Sakamoto et al., 2000).

HL is also an important side effect of platinum-based treatment in pediatric patients. Factors having impact on the risk of HL include:

(maximum) dose of cisplatin, presence of additional carboplatin and age at treatment (van As et al., 2016). HL was also prevalent among childhood cancer survivors treated with antineoplastic agents including cisplatin (Hudson et al., 2013). Vulnerability to cisplatin ototoxicity seemed to have a genetic component in some cancer patients' population (Tserga et al., 2019).

The exact mechanism of whether and how cellular senescence is associated with ototoxicity remains to be investigated. However, recent data showed that damage of hair cells (sensory cells of inner ear) is responsible for HL (Wu et al., 2020). Of importance, cochlear cells treated with H_2O_2 displayed key hallmarks of senescent cells (Benkafadar et al., 2019) and ROS (reactive oxygen species) induction is a well-known mechanism of cisplatin cytotoxic action (Marullo et al., 2013). Cochlea hair cell senescence was also induced by inhibition of dynamin-related protein-1 (DRP-1)-dependent mitophagy and aggravated age-related HL in a mouse model (Lin et al., 2019).

Ototoxicity is rather an infrequent effect of carboplatin treatment (Go and Adjei, 1999).

To summarize, involvement of cellular senescence in cisplatin-induced ototoxicity seems to be related with damage of hair cells in cochlea, although the exact mechanism of that phenomenon remains to be fully investigated.

Nephrotoxicity

Nephrotoxicity is a very common side effect of cisplatin treatment in both adults and children, limiting clinical use of this therapeutic drug (Fang et al., 2021, Duan et al., 2020). Prevalence of cisplatin-induced nephrotoxicity and acute kidney injury (AKI) is higher among seniors than in younger patients (Duan et al., 2020). Mechanisms involved in the development of AKI include drug transport and metabolism, apoptosis, autophagy, DNA damage, oxidative stress, and inflammation (Fang et al., 2021). Defective recovery from AKI may result in chronic kidney disease (CKD). Increased number of senescent cells was observed in both aged and injured kidney and targeting them decreased age-related damage of this organ and improved its performance (Valentijn et al., 2018, Docherty et al., 2020).

Cisplatin-induced premature renal senescence was associated with interstitial fibrosis in a murine model. NAD-dependent protein deacetylase sirtuin-1 (SIRT1) activation and p53 deacetylation seemed to be involved, at least partially, in the process. Of importance, both senescence and fibrosis could be inhibited by an antioxidant, N-acetylcysteine (NAC) (Li et al., 2019).

Moreover, development of renal fibrosis could be mediated by inflammatory and profibrotic elements of SASP (Xu et al., 2020). Cellular senescence together with massive collagen accumulation in kidney tubules, and fibrin deposits in peritubular capillaries were also induced by high phosphate. *In vitro* high phosphate directly induced injury, EMT and H_2O_2-induced cellular senescence. These were abrogated by Klotho, an important regulator of mineral metabolism expressed, e.g., in kidneys. Klotho deficiency led to premature aging-like syndrome in mice. Its low level is also observed in patients with CKD and seems to be associated with the stage of the disease. Therefore, Klotho emerges as a potential therapeutic target (Maique et al., 2020, Donate-Correa et al., 2021).

DRP-1-depedent mitophagy also seemed to be useful a as potential renoprotective target for the treatment of cisplatin-induced AKI (Zhao et al., 2017).

Cisplatin-induced nephrotoxicity was elevated in lung cancer patients having diabetes mellitus plus ischemic heart disease (Mathe et al., 2011). Moreover, dipeptidyl peptidase-4 (DPP-4) inhibitors, frequently used to control blood glucose levels, turned out to have potency to lower the risk of cisplatin nephrotoxicity in diabetic cancer patients (Iwakura et al., 2020). Importantly, DPP-4 seemed to be useful in selective targeting of senescent cells (Kim et al., 2017).

Altogether, cellular senescence seems to play a significant role in cisplatin-induced renal toxicity and targeting this process emerges as a very promising therapeutic option to improve life quality of cancer patients.

Cardiovascular Toxicity

Cisplatin clinical use is limited due to the risk of cardiotoxic events like electrocardiographic changes, arrhythmias, angina pectoris, cardiac failure, vascular events (Qian et al., 2018). Cisplatin/carboplatin treatment was shown to elevate cardiovascular diseases risk factors, i.e., hypertension and dyslipidemia (Hudson et al., 2013). The exact mechanism of cisplatin-induced cardiac toxicity development remains to be elucidated. However, some data suggest that cellular senescence may be implicated in the process. Cisplatin-induced cardiotoxicity was at least partially mediated via extracellular signal regulated kinase (ERK) activation (that is involved in regulation of cellular senescence) in cardiomyocytes (Qian et al., 2018), but the exact mechanism of this process remains to be elucidated. Moreover, this cardiotoxicity could be inhibited by cyanidin, that effectively delayed senescence by targeting ROS (Choi et al., 2010). Of importance, senolytic agents also seemed to be effective in reducing cardiac dysfunctions in rats (Demaria et al., 2017).

Taken together, targeting cellular senescence might reduce cardiotoxic effects of cisplatin.

Hematotoxicity/Myelosuppression

Hematotoxicity is one of the adverse effects of platin-derived chemotherapy (Cheng et al., 2017, Go and Adjei, 1999). Patients receiving carboplatin chemotherapy were more prone to suffer from anemia, neutropenia, and thrombocytopenia that patients receiving non-carboplatin therapy. Gene analysis revealed that carboplatin significantly affects the development of blood cells (Cheng et al., 2017). Data on cancer patients from US show increased risk of developing therapy-related myelodysplastic syndrome or acute myeloid leukemia (tMDS/AML) following chemotherapy for most solid tumor types investigated, including treatment with cisplatin (Morton et al., 2019). There was a non-significant trend to elevated risk of leukemia/myelodysplasia following cisplatin-based chemotherapy. However, the risk of developing second primary cancers after treatment with cisplatin seems to be similar to the risk following treatment with non-cisplatin-based agents (Liang et al., 2017). The exact mechanism still needs to be precisely evaluated, but it could be related to ROS-induced senescence. Recently, the involvement of glutathione, a major antioxidant, in cisplatin-induced development of hematological changes in mice bearing lymphoma was demonstrated. Blood hemoglobin, erythrocytes, packed cell volume and leukocytes (eosinophils, basophils, and lymphocytes) were reduced along with the development of various morphological abnormalities in erythrocytes (microcytes, macrocytes, echinocytes, acanthocytes, etc.) after cisplatin treatment. Combination with cysteine (precursor for glutathione synthesis) led to an increased glutathione levels and a decrease in hematological toxicities (Khynriam and Prasad, 2001). In accordance, Demaria and coworkers showed that TIS cells were important for bone marrow suppression. They demonstrated that functions of hematopoietic precursor cells were significantly reduced by another ROS-generating drug (doxorubicin) and were rescued upon elimination of senescent cells (Demaria et al., 2017).

To summarize, eliminating senescent cells might reduce hematotoxic effects of cisplatin, although further studies are needed to elucidate the exact mechanisms.

Conclusion

Platinum-based chemotherapy is still frequently given to cancer patients. While it is often effective, it has many adverse effects, including chemoresistance and relapse after treatment. One of the mechanisms responsible for this phenomenon may be cellular senescence. We have described this process in detail above, focusing on the atypical division of senescent cells and the effects of individual components of the secretory phenotype on tumor microenvironment. Later in this chapter, we have presented the current state of research supporting the contribution of platinum-based cellular senescence to the development of chemoresistance. This applies not only to the microenvironment of the tumor itself and the interaction of various cellular elements, but it could also affect different organs of cancer patients leading to systemic failure. Importantly, recent studies with the use of senolytic compounds indicate that the elimination of senescent cells may have a beneficial therapeutic effect. However, this approach still requires an in-depth analysis and additional research with the use of comprehensive research models and long-term perspective.

In conclusion, we propose that cellular senescence should be taken into account in the diagnosis of cancer, both in the early stages of the disease and in the assessment of treatment progress and the risk of recurrence.

References

Acklin, S., Zhang, M., Du, W., Zhao, X., Plotkin, M., Chang, J., Campisi, J., Zhou, D. & Xia, F. 2020. Depletion of senescent-like neuronal cells alleviates cisplatin-induced peripheral neuropathy in mice. *Sci Rep,* 10, 14170.

Acosta, J. C., O'loghlen, A., Banito, A., Guijarro, M. V., Augert, A., Raguz, S., Fumagalli, M., Da Costa, M., Brown, C., Popov, N., Takatsu, Y., Melamed, J., D'adda Di Fagagna, F., Bernard, D., Hernando, E. & Gil, J. 2008. Chemokine signaling via the CXCR2 receptor reinforces senescence. *Cell,* 133, 1006-18.

Alharbi, A. M., De Marzo, A. M., Hicks, J. L., Lotan, T. L. & Epstein, J. I. 2018. Prostatic Adenocarcinoma With Focal Pleomorphic Giant Cell Features: A Series of 30 Cases. *Am J Surg Pathol,* 42, 1286-1296.

Almeida, L. O., Guimaraes, D. M., Martins, M. D., Martins, M. a. T., Warner, K. A., Nor, J. E., Castilho, R. M. & Squarize, C. H. 2017. Unlocking the chromatin of adenoid cystic carcinomas using HDAC inhibitors sensitize cancer stem cells to cisplatin and induces tumor senescence. *Stem Cell Res,* 21, 94-105.

Amend, S. R., Torga, G., Lin, K. C., Kostecka, L. G., De Marzo, A., Austin, R. H. & Pienta, K. J. 2019. Polyploid giant cancer cells: Unrecognized actuators of tumorigenesis, metastasis, and resistance. *Prostate,* 79, 1489-1497.

Ancrile, B., Lim, K. H. & Counter, C. M. 2007. Oncogenic Ras-induced secretion of IL6 is required for tumorigenesis. *Genes Dev,* 21, 1714-9.

Ansieau, S., Bastid, J., Doreau, A., Morel, A. P., Bouchet, B. P., Thomas, C., Fauvet, F., Puisieux, I., Doglioni, C., Piccinin, S., Maestro, R., Voeltzel, T., Selmi, A., Valsesia-Wittmann, S., Caron De Fromentel, C. & Puisieux, A. 2008. Induction of EMT by twist proteins as a collateral effect of tumor-promoting inactivation of premature senescence. *Cancer Cell,* 14, 79-89.

Argyriou, A. A., Cavaletti, G., Briani, C., Velasco, R., Bruna, J., Campagnolo, M., Alberti, P., Bergamo, F., Cortinovis, D., Cazzaniga, M., Santos, C., Papadimitriou, K. & Kalofonos, H. P. 2013. Clinical pattern and associations of oxaliplatin acute neurotoxicity: a prospective study in 170 patients with colorectal cancer. *Cancer,* 119, 438-44.

Batlle, E. & Clevers, H. 2017. Cancer stem cells revisited. *Nat Med,* 23, 1124-1134.

Bavik, C., Coleman, I., Dean, J. P., Knudsen, B., Plymate, S. & Nelson, P. S. 2006. The gene expression program of prostate fibroblast senescence modulates neoplastic epithelial cell proliferation through paracrine mechanisms. *Cancer Res,* 66, 794-802.

Benkafadar, N., Francois, F., Affortit, C., Casas, F., Ceccato, J. C., Menardo, J., Venail, F., Malfroy-Camine, B., Puel, J. L. & Wang, J. 2019. ROS-Induced Activation of DNA Damage Responses Drives Senescence-Like State in Postmitotic Cochlear Cells: Implication for Hearing Preservation. *Mol Neurobiol,* 56, 5950-5969.

Berndtsson, M., Hagg, M., Panaretakis, T., Havelka, A. M., Shoshan, M. C. & Linder, S. 2007. Acute apoptosis by cisplatin requires induction of reactive oxygen species but is not associated with damage to nuclear DNA. *Int J Cancer,* 120, 175-80.

Bhargava, A. & Vaishampayan, U. N. 2009. Satraplatin: leading the new generation of oral platinum agents. *Expert Opin Investig Drugs,* 18, 1787-97.

Blackford, A. N. & Jackson, S. P. 2017. ATM, ATR, and DNA-PK: The Trinity at the Heart of the DNA Damage Response. *Mol Cell,* 66, 801-817.

Brady, C. A. & Attardi, L. D. 2010. p53 at a glance. *J Cell Sci,* 123, 2527-32.

Bremermann, H. J. 1982. Reliability of proliferation controls. The Hayflick limit and its breakdown in cancer. *J Theor Biol,* 97, 641-62.

Bruunsgaard, H. 2006. The clinical impact of systemic low-level inflammation in elderly populations. With special reference to cardiovascular disease, dementia and mortality. *Dan Med Bull,* 53, 285-309.

Bujak, J. K., Pingwara, R., Nelson, M. H. & Majchrzak, K. 2018. Adoptive cell transfer: new perspective treatment in veterinary oncology. *Acta Vet Scand,* 60, 60.

Calcinotto, A., Kohli, J., Zagato, E., Pellegrini, L., Demaria, M. & Alimonti, A. 2019. Cellular Senescence: Aging, Cancer, and Injury. *Physiol Rev,* 99, 1047-1078.

Calls, A., Torres-Espin, A., Navarro, X., Yuste, V. J., Udina, E. & Bruna, J. 2021. Cisplatin-induced peripheral neuropathy is associated with neuronal senescence-like response. *Neuro Oncol,* 23, 88-99.

Calvo, L., Cheng, S., Skulimowski, M., Clément, I., Portelance, L., Zhan, Y., Carmona, E., Lafontaine, J., De Ladurantaye, M., Rahimi, K., Provencher, D., Mes-Masson, A.-M. & Rodier, F. 2018. Cellular senescence is a central response to cytotoxic chemotherapy in high-grade serous ovarian cancer. *bioRxiv*, 425199.

Carrel, A. & Ebeling, A. H. 1921. Age and Multiplication of Fibroblasts. *J Exp Med,* 34, 599-623.

Casares, C., Ramirez-Camacho, R., Trinidad, A., Roldan, A., Jorge, E. & Garcia-Berrocal, J. R. 2012. Reactive oxygen species in apoptosis induced by cisplatin: review of physiopathological mechanisms in animal models. *Eur Arch Otorhinolaryngol,* 269, 2455-9.

Cesari, M., Penninx, B. W., Pahor, M., Lauretani, F., Corsi, A. M., Rhys Williams, G., Guralnik, J. M. & Ferrucci, L. 2004. Inflammatory markers and physical performance in older persons: the InCHIANTI study. *J Gerontol A Biol Sci Med Sci,* 59, 242-8.

Chae, Y. K., Chang, S., Ko, T., Anker, J., Agte, S., Iams, W., Choi, W. M., Lee, K. & Cruz, M. 2018. Epithelial-mesenchymal transition (EMT) signature is inversely associated with T-cell infiltration in non-small cell lung cancer (NSCLC). *Sci Rep,* 8, 2918.

Chatterjee, N., Whitman, M. A., Harris, C. A., Min, S. M., Jonas, O., Lien, E. C., Luengo, A., Vander Heiden, M. G., Hong, J., Zhou, P., Hemann, M. T. & Walker, G. C. 2020. REV1 inhibitor JH-RE-06 enhances tumor cell response to chemotherapy by triggering senescence hallmarks. *Proc Natl Acad Sci USA,* 117, 28918-28921.

Chen, Q. & Ames, B. N. 1994. Senescence-like growth arrest induced by hydrogen peroxide in human diploid fibroblast F65 cells. *Proc Natl Acad Sci USA,* 91, 4130-4.

Chen, S. H. & Chang, J. Y. 2019. New Insights into Mechanisms of Cisplatin Resistance: From Tumor Cell to Microenvironment. *Int J Mol Sci,* 20.

Chen, X., Wang, J., Fu, Z., Zhu, B., Wang, J., Guan, S. & Hua, Z. 2017. Curcumin activates DNA repair pathway in bone marrow to improve carboplatin-induced myelosuppression. *Sci Rep,* 7, 17724.

Cheng, Y. J., Wu, R., Cheng, M. L., Du, J., Hu, X. W., Yu, L., Zhao, X. K., Yao, Y. M., Long, Q. Z., Zhu, L. L., Zhu, J. J., Huang, N. W., Liu, H. J., Hu, Y. X. & Wan, F. 2017. Carboplatin-induced hematotoxicity among patients with non-small cell lung cancer: Analysis on clinical adverse events and drug-gene interactions. *Oncotarget,* 8, 32228-32236.

Chiang, A. C. A., Huo, X., Kavelaars, A. & Heijnen, C. J. 2019. Chemotherapy accelerates age-related development of tauopathy and results in loss of synaptic integrity and cognitive impairment. *Brain Behav Immun,* 79, 319-325.

Choi, M. J., Kim, B. K., Park, K. Y., Yokozawa, T., Song, Y. O. & Cho, E. J. 2010. Anti-aging effects of cyanidin under a stress-induced premature senescence cellular system. *Biol Pharm Bull,* 33, 421-6.

Chovanec, M., Abu Zaid, M., Hanna, N., El-Kouri, N., Einhorn, L. H. & Albany, C. 2017. Long-term toxicity of cisplatin in germ-cell tumor survivors. *Ann Oncol,* 28, 2670-2679.

Ciemerych, M. A., Archacka, K., Grabowska, I. & Przewozniak, M. 2011. Cell cycle regulation during proliferation and differentiation of mammalian muscle precursor cells. *Results Probl Cell Differ,* 53, 473-527.

Collins, K. & Mitchell, J. R. 2002. Telomerase in the human organism. *Oncogene,* 21, 564-79.

Coppe, J. P., Desprez, P. Y., Krtolica, A. & Campisi, J. 2010. The senescence-associated secretory phenotype: the dark side of tumor suppression. *Annu Rev Pathol,* 5, 99-118.

Coppe, J. P., Patil, C. K., Rodier, F., Sun, Y., Munoz, D. P., Goldstein, J., Nelson, P. S., Desprez, P. Y. & Campisi, J. 2008. Senescence-associated secretory phenotypes reveal cell-nonautonomous functions of oncogenic RAS and the p53 tumor suppressor. *PLoS Biol,* 6, 2853-68.

Covarrubias, A. J., Kale, A., Perrone, R., Lopez-Dominguez, J. A., Pisco, A. O., Kasler, H. G., Schmidt, M. S., Heckenbach, I., Kwok, R., Wiley, C. D., Wong, H. S., Gibbs, E., Iyer, S. S., Basisty, N., Wu, Q., Kim, I. J., Silva, E., Vitangcol, K., Shin, K. O., Lee, Y. M., Riley, R., Ben-Sahra, I., Ott, M., Schilling, B., Scheibye-Knudsen, M., Ishihara, K., Quake, S. R., Newman, J., Brenner, C., Campisi, J. & Verdin, E. 2020. Senescent cells promote tissue NAD(+) decline during ageing via the activation of CD38(+) macrophages. *Nat Metab,* 2, 1265-1283.

Coward, J. & Harding, A. 2014. Size Does Matter: Why Polyploid Tumor Cells are Critical Drug Targets in the War on Cancer. *Front Oncol,* 4, 123.

Cupit-Link, M. C., Kirkland, J. L., Ness, K. K., Armstrong, G. T., Tchkonia, T., Lebrasseur, N. K., Armenian, S. H., Ruddy, K. J. & Hashmi, S. K. 2017. Biology of premature ageing in survivors of cancer. *ESMO Open,* 2, e000250.

Dasari, S. & Tchounwou, P. B. 2014. Cisplatin in cancer therapy: molecular mechanisms of action. *Eur J Pharmacol,* 740, 364-78.

De Francesco, E. M., Maggiolini, M. & Musti, A. M. 2018. Crosstalk between Notch, HIF-1alpha and GPER in Breast Cancer EMT. *Int J Mol Sci,* 19.

Demaria, M., O'leary, M. N., Chang, J., Shao, L., Liu, S., Alimirah, F., Koenig, K., Le, C., Mitin, N., Deal, A. M., Alston, S., Academia, E. C., Kilmarx, S., Valdovinos, A., Wang, B., De Bruin, A., Kennedy, B. K., Melov, S., Zhou, D., Sharpless, N. E., Muss, H. & Campisi, J. 2017. Cellular Senescence Promotes Adverse Effects of Chemotherapy and Cancer Relapse. *Cancer Discov,* 7, 165-176.

Demaria, M., Ohtani, N., Youssef, S. A., Rodier, F., Toussaint, W., Mitchell, J. R., Laberge, R. M., Vijg, J., Van Steeg, H., Dolle, M. E., Hoeijmakers, J. H., De Bruin, A., Hara, E. & Campisi, J. 2014. An essential role for senescent cells in optimal wound healing through secretion of PDGF-AA. *Dev Cell,* 31, 722-33.

Deryugina, E. I. & Quigley, J. P. 2010. Pleiotropic roles of matrix metalloproteinases in tumor angiogenesis: contrasting, overlapping and compensatory functions. *Biochim Biophys Acta,* 1803, 103-20.

Dilruba, S. & Kalayda, G. V. 2016. Platinum-based drugs: past, present and future. *Cancer Chemother Pharmacol,* 77, 1103-24.

Ding, Y. T., Kumar, S. & Yu, D. C. 2008. The role of endothelial progenitor cells in tumour vasculogenesis. *Pathobiology,* 75, 265-73.

Docherty, M. H., Baird, D. P., Hughes, J. & Ferenbach, D. A. 2020. Cellular Senescence and Senotherapies in the Kidney: Current Evidence and Future Directions. *Front Pharmacol,* 11, 755.

Donate-Correa, J., Ferri, C. M., Martin-Nunez, E., Perez-Delgado, N., Gonzalez-Luis, A., Mora-Fernandez, C. & Navarro-Gonzalez, J. F. 2021. Klotho as a biomarker of subclinical atherosclerosis in patients with moderate to severe chronic kidney disease. *Sci Rep,* 11, 15877.

Dongre, A. & Weinberg, R. A. 2019. New insights into the mechanisms of epithelial-mesenchymal transition and implications for cancer. *Nat Rev Mol Cell Biol,* 20, 69-84.

Dorshkind, K., Hofer, T., Montecino-Rodriguez, E., Pioli, P. D. & Rodewald, H. R. 2020. Do haematopoietic stem cells age? *Nat Rev Immunol,* 20, 196-202.

Drogemoller, B. I., Wright, G. E. B., Lo, C., Le, T., Brooks, B., Bhavsar, A. P., Rassekh, S. R., Ross, C. J. D. & Carleton, B. C. 2019. Pharmacogenomics of Cisplatin-Induced Ototoxicity: Successes, Shortcomings, and Future Avenues of Research. *Clin Pharmacol Ther,* 106, 350-359.

Duan, Z., Cai, G., Li, J. & Chen, X. 2020. Cisplatin-induced renal toxicity in elderly people. *Ther Adv Med Oncol,* 12, 1758835920923430.

Eastman, A. 2017. Improving anticancer drug development begins with cell culture: misinformation perpetrated by the misuse of cytotoxicity assays. *Oncotarget,* 8, 8854-8866.

Eger, A., Aigner, K., Sonderegger, S., Dampier, B., Oehler, S., Schreiber, M., Berx, G., Cano, A., Beug, H. & Foisner, R. 2005. DeltaEF1 is a transcriptional repressor of E-cadherin and regulates epithelial plasticity in breast cancer cells. *Oncogene,* 24, 2375-85.

Elmore, L. W., Di, X., Dumur, C., Holt, S. E. & Gewirtz, D. A. 2005. Evasion of a single-step, chemotherapy-induced senescence in breast cancer cells: implications for treatment response. *Clin Cancer Res,* 11, 2637-43.

Erenpreisa, J. & Cragg, M. S. 2013. Three steps to the immortality of cancer cells: senescence, polyploidy and self-renewal. *Cancer Cell Int,* 13, 92.

Erenpreisa, J., Salmina, K., Huna, A., Jackson, T. R., Vazquez-Martin, A. & Cragg, M. S. 2015. The " virgin birth," polyploidy, and the origin of cancer. *Oncoscience,* 2, 3-14.

Erenpreisa, J., Salmina, K., Huna, A., Kosmacek, E. A., Cragg, M. S., Ianzini, F. & Anisimov, A. P. 2011. Polyploid tumour cells elicit paradiploid progeny through depolyploidizing divisions and regulated autophagic degradation. *Cell Biol Int,* 35, 687-95.

Ewald, J. A., Desotelle, J. A., Wilding, G. & Jarrard, D. F. 2010. Therapy-induced senescence in cancer. *J Natl Cancer Inst,* 102, 1536-46.

Fabregat, I., Fernando, J., Mainez, J. & Sancho, P. 2014. TGF-beta signaling in cancer treatment. *Curr Pharm Des,* 20, 2934-47.

Faheem, M. M., Seligson, N. D., Ahmad, S. M., Rasool, R. U., Gandhi, S. G., Bhagat, M. & Goswami, A. 2020. Convergence of therapy-induced senescence (TIS) and EMT in multistep carcinogenesis: current opinions and emerging perspectives. *Cell Death Discov,* 6, 51.

Fan, D. N. & Schmitt, C. A. 2017. Detecting Markers of Therapy-Induced Senescence in Cancer Cells. *Methods Mol Biol,* 1534, 41-52.

Fang, C. Y., Lou, D. Y., Zhou, L. Q., Wang, J. C., Yang, B., He, Q. J., Wang, J. J. & Weng, Q. J. 2021. Natural products: potential treatments for cisplatin-induced nephrotoxicity. *Acta Pharmacol Sin.*

Fitsiou, E., Soto-Gamez, A. & Demaria, M. 2021. Biological functions of therapy-induced senescence in cancer. *Semin Cancer Biol.*

Folkman, J. 1971. Tumor angiogenesis: therapeutic implications. *N Engl J Med,* 285, 1182-6.

Franceschi, C., Capri, M., Monti, D., Giunta, S., Olivieri, F., Sevini, F., Panourgia, M. P., Invidia, L., Celani, L., Scurti, M., Cevenini, E., Castellani, G. C. & Salvioli, S. 2007. Inflammaging and anti-inflammaging: a systemic perspective on aging and longevity emerged from studies in humans. *Mech Ageing Dev,* 128, 92-105.

Freund, A., Laberge, R. M., Demaria, M. & Campisi, J. 2012. Lamin B1 loss is a senescence-associated biomarker. *Mol Biol Cell,* 23, 2066-75.

Friboulet, L., Postel-Vinay, S., Sourisseau, T., Adam, J., Stoclin, A., Ponsonnailles, F., Dorvault, N., Commo, F., Saulnier, P., Salome-Desmoulez, S., Pottier, G., Andre, F., Kroemer, G., Soria, J. C. & Olaussen, K. A. 2013. ERCC1 function in nuclear excision and interstrand crosslink repair pathways is mediated exclusively by the ERCC1-202 isoform. *Cell Cycle,* 12, 3298-306.

Fulop, T., Larbi, A., Dupuis, G., Le Page, A., Frost, E. H., Cohen, A. A., Witkowski, J. M. & Franceschi, C. 2017. Immunosenescence and Inflamm-Aging As Two Sides of the Same Coin: Friends or Foes? *Front Immunol,* 8, 1960.

Furuya, S., Endo, K., Takahashi, A., Miyazawa, K. & Saitoh, M. 2017. Snail suppresses cellular senescence and promotes fibroblast-led cancer cell invasion. *FEBS Open Bio,* 7, 1586-1597.

Gabrilovich, D. I. 2017. Myeloid-Derived Suppressor Cells. *Cancer Immunol Res,* 5, 3-8.

Garten, A., Schuster, S., Penke, M., Gorski, T., De Giorgis, T. & Kiess, W. 2015. Physiological and pathophysiological roles of NAMPT and NAD metabolism. *Nat Rev Endocrinol,* 11, 535-46.

Gerashchenko, B. I., Salmina, K., Eglitis, J., Huna, A., Grjunberga, V. & Erenpreisa, J. 2016. Disentangling the aneuploidy and senescence paradoxes: a study of triploid breast cancers non-responsive to neoadjuvant therapy. *Histochem Cell Biol,* 145, 497-508.

Gewirtz, D. A. 1999. A critical evaluation of the mechanisms of action proposed for the antitumor effects of the anthracycline antibiotics adriamycin and daunorubicin. *Biochem Pharmacol,* 57, 727-41.

Ghosh, S. 2019. Cisplatin: The first metal based anticancer drug. *Bioorg Chem,* 88, 102925.

Gire, V. & Dulic, V. 2015. Senescence from G2 arrest, revisited. *Cell Cycle,* 14, 297-304.

Go, R. S. & Adjei, A. A. 1999. Review of the comparative pharmacology and clinical activity of cisplatin and carboplatin. *J Clin Oncol,* 17, 409-22.

Gomes, L. R., Rocha, C. R. R., Martins, D. J., Fiore, A., Kinker, G. S., Bruni-Cardoso, A. & Menck, C. F. M. 2019. ATR mediates cisplatin resistance in 3D-cultured breast cancer cells via translesion DNA synthesis modulation. *Cell Death Dis,* 10, 459.

Gonzalez, L. C., Ghadaouia, S., Martinez, A. & Rodier, F. 2016. Premature aging/senescence in cancer cells facing therapy: good or bad? *Biogerontology,* 17, 71-87.

Hao, X., Zhao, B., Zhou, W., Liu, H., Fukumoto, T., Gabrilovich, D. & Zhang, R. 2021. Sensitization of ovarian tumor to immune checkpoint blockade by boosting senescence-associated secretory phenotype. *iScience,* 24, 102016.

Hayflick, L. & Moorhead, P. S. 1961. The serial cultivation of human diploid cell strains. *Exp Cell Res,* 25, 585-621.

Hazan, R. B., Phillips, G. R., Qiao, R. F., Norton, L. & Aaronson, S. A. 2000. Exogenous expression of N-cadherin in breast cancer cells induces cell migration, invasion, and metastasis. *J Cell Biol,* 148, 779-90.

He, H., Xu, J., Warren, C. M., Duan, D., Li, X., Wu, L. & Iruela-Arispe, M. L. 2012. Endothelial cells provide an instructive niche for the differentiation and functional polarization of M2-like macrophages. *Blood,* 120, 3152-62.

Heidemann, J., Ogawa, H., Dwinell, M. B., Rafiee, P., Maaser, C., Gockel, H. R., Otterson, M. F., Ota, D. M., Lugering, N., Domschke, W. & Binion, D. G. 2003. Angiogenic effects of interleukin 8 (CXCL8) in human intestinal microvascular endothelial cells are mediated by CXCR2. *J Biol Chem,* 278, 8508-15.

Ho, G. Y., Woodward, N. & Coward, J. I. 2016. Cisplatin versus carboplatin: comparative review of therapeutic management in solid malignancies. *Crit Rev Oncol Hematol,* 102, 37-46.

Hudson, M. M., Ness, K. K., Gurney, J. G., Mulrooney, D. A., Chemaitilly, W., Krull, K. R., Green, D. M., Armstrong, G. T., Nottage, K. A., Jones, K. E., Sklar, C. A., Srivastava, D. K. & Robison, L. L. 2013. Clinical ascertainment of health outcomes among adults treated for childhood cancer. *JAMA,* 309, 2371-2381.

Iannello, A., Thompson, T. W., Ardolino, M., Lowe, S. W. & Raulet, D. H. 2013. p53-dependent chemokine production by senescent tumor cells supports NKG2D-dependent tumor elimination by natural killer cells. *J Exp Med,* 210, 2057-69.

Intlekofer, A. M. & Thompson, C. B. 2013. At the bench: preclinical rationale for CTLA-4 and PD-1 blockade as cancer immunotherapy. *J Leukoc Biol,* 94, 25-39.

Iwakura, T., Fukasawa, H., Kitamura, A., Ishibuchi, K., Yasuda, H. & Furuya, R. 2020. Effect of dipeptidyl peptidase-4 inhibitors on cisplatin-induced acute nephrotoxicity in cancer patients with diabetes mellitus: A retrospective study. *PLoS One,* 15, e0229377.

Jin, M. Z. & Jin, W. L. 2020. The updated landscape of tumor microenvironment and drug repurposing. *Signal Transduct Target Ther,* 5, 166.

Kale, A., Sharma, A., Stolzing, A., Desprez, P. Y. & Campisi, J. 2020. Role of immune cells in the removal of deleterious senescent cells. *Immun Ageing,* 17, 16.

Kalejs, M., Ivanov, A., Plakhins, G., Cragg, M. S., Emzinsh, D., Illidge, T. M. & Erenpreisa, J. 2006. Upregulation of meiosis-specific genes in lymphoma cell lines following genotoxic insult and induction of mitotic catastrophe. *BMC Cancer,* 6, 6.

Kanat, O., Ertas, H. & Caner, B. 2017. Platinum-induced neurotoxicity: A review of possible mechanisms. *World J Clin Oncol,* 8, 329-335.

Kenny, R. G., Chuah, S. W., Crawford, A. & Marmion, C. J. 2017. Platinum(IV) Prodrugs – A Step Closer to Ehrlich's Vision? *European Journal of Inorganic Chemistry,* 2017, 1596-1612.

Khynriam, D. & Prasad, S. B. 2001. Hematotoxicity and blood glutathione levels after cisplatin treatment of tumor-bearing mice. *Cell Biol Toxicol,* 17, 357-70.

Kieda, C. 2013. Heterogeneity of endothelial cells--role in vessel specialization and cooperation in vasculogenic mimicry. *Postepy Biochem,* 59, 372-8.

Kim, K. M., Noh, J. H., Bodogai, M., Martindale, J. L., Yang, X., Indig, F. E., Basu, S. K., Ohnuma, K., Morimoto, C., Johnson, P. F., Biragyn, A., Abdelmohsen, K. & Gorospe, M. 2017. Identification of senescent cell surface targetable protein DPP4. *Genes Dev,* 31, 1529-1534.

Kritsilis, M., S, V. R., Koutsoudaki, P. N., Evangelou, K., Gorgoulis, V. G. & Papadopoulos, D. 2018. Ageing, Cellular Senescence and Neurodegenerative Disease. *Int J Mol Sci,* 19.

Lai, C. Y., Schwartz, B. E. & Hsu, M. Y. 2012. CD133+ melanoma subpopulations contribute to perivascular niche morphogenesis and tumorigenicity through vasculogenic mimicry. *Cancer Res,* 72, 5111-8.

Lee, S. & Lee, J. S. 2019. Cellular senescence: a promising strategy for cancer therapy. *BMB Rep,* 52, 35-41.

Li, C., Xie, N., Li, Y., Liu, C., Hou, F. F. & Wang, J. 2019. N-acetylcysteine ameliorates cisplatin-induced renal senescence and renal interstitial fibrosis through sirtuin1 activation and p53 deacetylation. *Free Radic Biol Med,* 130, 512-527.

Li, G. Z., Eller, M. S., Firoozabadi, R. & Gilchrest, B. A. 2003. Evidence that exposure of the telomere 3' overhang sequence induces senescence. *Proc Natl Acad Sci U S A,* 100, 527-31.

Li, W., Wang, W., Dong, H., Li, Y., Li, L., Han, L., Han, Z., Wang, S., Ma, D. & Wang, H. 2014. Cisplatin-induced senescence in ovarian cancer cells is mediated by GRP78. *Oncol Rep,* 31, 2525-34.

Liang, F., Zhang, S., Xue, H. & Chen, Q. 2017. Risk of second primary cancers in cancer patients treated with cisplatin: a systematic review and meta-analysis of randomized studies. *BMC Cancer,* 17, 871.

Lin, H., Xiong, H., Su, Z., Pang, J., Lai, L., Zhang, H., Jian, B., Zhang, W. & Zheng, Y. 2019. Inhibition of DRP-1-Dependent Mitophagy Promotes Cochlea Hair Cell Senescence and Exacerbates Age-Related Hearing Loss. *Front Cell Neurosci,* 13, 550.

Liu, D. & Hornsby, P. J. 2007. Senescent human fibroblasts increase the early growth of xenograft tumors via matrix metalloproteinase secretion. *Cancer Res,* 67, 3117-26.

Liu, J., Wang, L., Wang, Z. & Liu, J. P. 2019. Roles of Telomere Biology in Cell Senescence, Replicative and Chronological Ageing. *Cells,* 8.

Liu, R., Yang, K., Meng, C., Zhang, Z. & Xu, Y. 2012. Vasculogenic mimicry is a marker of poor prognosis in prostate cancer. *Cancer Biol Ther,* 13, 527-33.

Liu, W., Huang, Y. J., Liu, C., Yang, Y. Y., Liu, H., Cui, J. G., Cheng, Y., Gao, F., Cai, J. M. & Li, B. L. 2014. Inhibition of TBK1 attenuates radiation-induced epithelial-mesenchymal transition of A549 human lung cancer cells via activation of GSK-3beta and repression of ZEB1. *Lab Invest,* 94, 362-70.

Liu, Y., Sanchez-Tillo, E., Lu, X., Huang, L., Clem, B., Telang, S., Jenson, A. B., Cuatrecasas, M., Chesney, J., Postigo, A. & Dean, D. C. 2013. Sequential inductions of the ZEB1 transcription factor caused by mutation of Rb and then Ras proteins are required for tumor initiation and progression. *J Biol Chem,* 288, 11572-80.

Lock, R. B. & Stribinskiene, L. 1996. Dual modes of death induced by etoposide in human epithelial tumor cells allow Bcl-2 to inhibit apoptosis without affecting clonogenic survival. *Cancer Res,* 56, 4006-12.

Luo, F., Yang, K., Liu, R. L., Meng, C., Dang, R. F. & Xu, Y. 2014. Formation of vasculogenic mimicry in bone metastasis of prostate cancer: correlation with cell apoptosis and senescence regulation pathways. *Pathol Res Pract,* 210, 291-5.

Mahmoudi, S., Mancini, E., Xu, L., Moore, A., Jahanbani, F., Hebestreit, K., Srinivasan, R., Li, X., Devarajan, K., Prelot, L., Ang, C. E., Shibuya, Y., Benayoun, B. A., Chang, A. L. S., Wernig, M., Wysocka, J., Longaker, M. T., Snyder, M. P. & Brunet, A. 2019. Heterogeneity in old fibroblasts is linked to variability in reprogramming and wound healing. *Nature,* 574, 553-558.

Maique, J., Flores, B., Shi, M., Shepard, S., Zhou, Z., Yan, S., Moe, O. W. & Hu, M. C. 2020. High Phosphate Induces and Klotho Attenuates Kidney Epithelial Senescence and Fibrosis. *Front Pharmacol,* 11, 1273.

Maniotis, A. J., Folberg, R., Hess, A., Seftor, E. A., Gardner, L. M., Pe'er, J., Trent, J. M., Meltzer, P. S. & Hendrix, M. J. 1999. Vascular channel formation by human melanoma cells in vivo and in vitro: vasculogenic mimicry. *Am J Pathol,* 155, 739-52.

Martinez-Cue, C. & Rueda, N. 2020. Cellular Senescence in Neurodegenerative Diseases. *Front Cell Neurosci,* 14, 16.

Martinez, I., Garcia-Carpizo, V., Guijarro, T., Garcia-Gomez, A., Navarro, D., Aranda, A. & Zambrano, A. 2016. Induction of DNA double-strand breaks and cellular senescence by human respiratory syncytial virus. *Virulence,* 7, 427-42.

Marullo, R., Werner, E., Degtyareva, N., Moore, B., Altavilla, G., Ramalingam, S. S. & Doetsch, P. W. 2013. Cisplatin induces a mitochondrial-ROS response that contributes to cytotoxicity depending on mitochondrial redox status and bioenergetic functions. *PLoS One,* 8, e81162.

Mathe, C., Bohacs, A., Duffek, L., Lukacsovits, J., Komlosi, Z. I., Szondy, K., Horvath, I., Muller, V. & Losonczy, G. 2011. Cisplatin nephrotoxicity aggravated by cardiovascular disease and diabetes in lung cancer patients. *Eur Respir J,* 37, 888-94.

Mazzoni, M., Mauro, G., Erreni, M., Romeo, P., Minna, E., Vizioli, M. G., Belgiovine, C., Rizzetti, M. G., Pagliardini, S., Avigni, R., Anania, M. C., Allavena, P., Borrello, M. G. & Greco, A. 2019. Senescent thyrocytes and thyroid tumor cells induce M2-like macrophage polarization of human monocytes via a PGE2-dependent mechanism. *J Exp Clin Cancer Res,* 38, 208.

Mcelhaney, J. E. & Effros, R. B. 2009. Immunosenescence: what does it mean to health outcomes in older adults? *Curr Opin Immunol,* 21, 418-24.

Michaud, M., Balardy, L., Moulis, G., Gaudin, C., Peyrot, C., Vellas, B., Cesari, M. & Nourhashemi, F. 2013. Proinflammatory cytokines, aging, and age-related diseases. *J Am Med Dir Assoc,* 14, 877-82.

Millimaggi, D., Mari, M., S, D. A., Giusti, I., Pavan, A. & Dolo, V. 2009. Vasculogenic mimicry of human ovarian cancer cells: role of CD147. *Int J Oncol,* 35, 1423-8.

Morton, L. M., Dores, G. M., Schonfeld, S. J., Linet, M. S., Sigel, B. S., Lam, C. J. K., Tucker, M. A. & Curtis, R. E. 2019. Association of Chemotherapy for Solid Tumors With Development of Therapy-Related Myelodysplastic Syndrome or Acute Myeloid Leukemia in the Modern Era. *JAMA Oncol,* 5, 318-325.

Mosieniak, G., Sliwinska, M. A., Alster, O., Strzeszewska, A., Sunderland, P., Piechota, M., Was, H. & Sikora, E. 2015. Polyploidy Formation in Doxorubicin-Treated Cancer Cells Can Favor Escape from Senescence. *Neoplasia,* 17, 882-893.

Munoz-Espin, D., Canamero, M., Maraver, A., Gomez-Lopez, G., Contreras, J., Murillo-Cuesta, S., Rodriguez-Baeza, A., Varela-Nieto, I., Ruberte, J., Collado, M. & Serrano, M. 2013. Programmed cell senescence during mammalian embryonic development. *Cell,* 155, 1104-18.

Murray, D. & Mirzayans, R. 2020. Cellular Responses to Platinum-Based Anticancer Drugs and UVC: Role of p53 and Implications for Cancer Therapy. *Int J Mol Sci,* 21.

Musiani, D., Giambruno, R., Massignani, E., Ippolito, M. R., Maniaci, M., Jammula, S., Manganaro, D., Cuomo, A., Nicosia, L., Pasini, D. & Bonaldi, T. 2020. PRMT1 Is Recruited via DNA-PK to Chromatin Where It Sustains the Senescence-Associated Secretory Phenotype in Response to Cisplatin. *Cell Rep,* 30, 1208-1222 e9.

Muthuramalingam, K., Cho, M. & Kim, Y. 2020. Cellular senescence and EMT crosstalk in bleomycin-induced pathogenesis of pulmonary fibrosis-an in vitro analysis. *Cell Biol Int,* 44, 477-487.

Nacarelli, T., Fukumoto, T., Zundell, J. A., Fatkhutdinov, N., Jean, S., Cadungog, M. G., Borowsky, M. E. & Zhang, R. 2020. NAMPT Inhibition Suppresses Cancer Stem-like Cells Associated with Therapy-Induced Senescence in Ovarian Cancer. *Cancer Res,* 80, 890-900.

Navolanic, P. M., Akula, S. M. & Mccubrey, J. A. 2004. Neosis and its potential role in cancer development and chemoresistance. *Cancer Biol Ther,* 3, 219-20.

Niu, N., Zhang, J., Zhang, N., Mercado-Uribe, I., Tao, F., Han, Z., Pathak, S., Multani, A. S., Kuang, J., Yao, J., Bast, R. C., Sood, A. K., Hung, M. C. & Liu, J. 2016. Linking genomic reorganization to tumor initiation via the giant cell cycle. *Oncogenesis,* 5, e281.

North, B. J. & Sinclair, D. A. 2012. The intersection between aging and cardiovascular disease. *Circ Res,* 110, 1097-108.

Odero-Marah, V., Hawsawi, O., Henderson, V. & Sweeney, J. 2018. Epithelial-Mesenchymal Transition (EMT) and Prostate Cancer. *Adv Exp Med Biol,* 1095, 101-110.

Olan, I. & Narita, M. 2021. Putting the DOT on IL1A. *J Cell Biol,* 220.

Olovnikov, A. M. 1973. A theory of marginotomy. The incomplete copying of template margin in enzymic synthesis of polynucleotides and biological significance of the phenomenon. *J Theor Biol,* 41, 181-90.

Olovnikov, A. M. 1996. Telomeres, telomerase, and aging: origin of the theory. *Exp Gerontol,* 31, 443-8.

Orjalo, A. V., Bhaumik, D., Gengler, B. K., Scott, G. K. & Campisi, J. 2009. Cell surface-bound IL-1alpha is an upstream regulator of the senescence-associated IL-6/IL-8 cytokine network. *Proc Natl Acad Sci U S A,* 106, 17031-6.

Oun, R., Moussa, Y. E. & Wheate, N. J. 2018. The side effects of platinum-based chemotherapy drugs: a review for chemists. *Dalton Trans,* 47, 6645-6653.

Perego, P. & Robert, J. 2016. Oxaliplatin in the era of personalized medicine: from mechanistic studies to clinical efficacy. *Cancer Chemother Pharmacol,* 77, 5-18.

Pollina, E. A. & Brunet, A. 2011. Epigenetic regulation of aging stem cells. *Oncogene,* 30, 3105-26.

Prasanna, P. G., Citrin, D. E., Hildesheim, J., Ahmed, M. M., Venkatachalam, S., Riscuta, G., Xi, D., Zheng, G., Van Deursen, J., Goronzy, J., Kron, S. J., Anscher, M. S., Sharpless, N. E., Campisi, J., Brown, S. L., Niedernhofer, L. J., O'loghlen, A., Georgakilas, A. G., Paris, F., Gius, D., Gewirtz, D. A., Schmitt, C. A., Abazeed, M. E., Kirkland, J. L., Richmond, A., Romesser, P. B., Lowe, S. W., Gil, J., Mendonca, M. S., Burma, S., Zhou, D. & Coleman, C. N. 2021. Therapy-Induced Senescence: Opportunities to Improve Anti-Cancer Therapy. *J Natl Cancer Inst.*

Prelog, M. 2006. Aging of the immune system: a risk factor for autoimmunity? *Autoimmun Rev,* 5, 136-9.

Puig, P. E., Guilly, M. N., Bouchot, A., Droin, N., Cathelin, D., Bouyer, F., Favier, L., Ghiringhelli, F., Kroemer, G., Solary, E., Martin, F. & Chauffert, B. 2008. Tumor cells can escape DNA-damaging cisplatin through DNA endoreduplication and reversible polyploidy. *Cell Biol Int,* 32, 1031-43.

Puzianowska-Kuznicka, M., Owczarz, M., Wieczorowska-Tobis, K., Nadrowski, P., Chudek, J., Slusarczyk, P., Skalska, A., Jonas, M., Franek, E. & Mossakowska, M. 2016. Interleukin-6 and C-reactive protein, successful aging, and mortality: the PolSenior study. *Immun Ageing,* 13, 21.

Qian, P., Yan, L. J., Li, Y. Q., Yang, H. T., Duan, H. Y., Wu, J. T., Fan, X. W. & Wang, S. L. 2018. Cyanidin ameliorates cisplatin-induced cardiotoxicity via inhibition of ROS-mediated apoptosis. *Exp Ther Med,* 15, 1959-1965.

Qin, L., Jing, X., Qiu, Z., Cao, W., Jiao, Y., Routy, J. P. & Li, T. 2016. Aging of immune system: Immune signature from peripheral blood lymphocyte subsets in 1068 healthy adults. *Aging (Albany NY),* 8, 848-59.

Qu, K., Lin, T., Wei, J., Meng, F., Wang, Z., Huang, Z., Wan, Y., Song, S., Liu, S., Chang, H., Dong, Y. & Liu, C. 2013a. Cisplatin induces cell cycle arrest and senescence via upregulating P53 and P21 expression in HepG2 cells. *Nan Fang Yi Ke Da Xue Xue Bao,* 33, 1253-9.

Qu, K., Xu, X., Liu, C., Wu, Q., Wei, J., Meng, F., Zhou, L., Wang, Z., Lei, L. & Liu, P. 2013b. Negative regulation of transcription factor FoxM1 by p53 enhances oxaliplatin-induced senescence in hepatocellular carcinoma. *Cancer Lett,* 331, 105-14.

Rabik, C. A. & Dolan, M. E. 2007. Molecular mechanisms of resistance and toxicity associated with platinating agents. *Cancer Treat Rev,* 33, 9-23.

Rajaraman, R., Guernsey, D. L., Rajaraman, M. M. & Rajaraman, S. R. 2006. Stem cells, senescence, neosis and self-renewal in cancer. *Cancer Cell Int,* 6, 25.

Rajaraman, R., Rajaraman, M. M., Rajaraman, S. R. & Guernsey, D. L. 2005. Neosis--a paradigm of self-renewal in cancer. *Cell Biol Int,* 29, 1084-97.

Ribatti, D. 2008. Judah Folkman, a pioneer in the study of angiogenesis. *Angiogenesis,* 11, 3-10.

Ricci-Vitiani, L., Pallini, R., Biffoni, M., Todaro, M., Invernici, G., Cenci, T., Maira, G., Parati, E. A., Stassi, G., Larocca, L. M. & De Maria, R. 2010. Tumour vascularization via endothelial differentiation of glioblastoma stem-like cells. *Nature,* 468, 824-8.

Riley, T., Sontag, E., Chen, P. & Levine, A. 2008. Transcriptional control of human p53-regulated genes. *Nat Rev Mol Cell Biol,* 9, 402-12.

Roberson, R. S., Kussick, S. J., Vallieres, E., Chen, S. Y. & Wu, D. Y. 2005. Escape from therapy-induced accelerated cellular senescence in p53-null lung cancer cells and in human lung cancers. *Cancer Res,* 65, 2795-803.

Rodier, F., Kim, S. H., Nijjar, T., Yaswen, P. & Campisi, J. 2005. Cancer and aging: the importance of telomeres in genome maintenance. *Int J Biochem Cell Biol,* 37, 977-90.

Rohnalter, V., Roth, K., Finkernagel, F., Adhikary, T., Obert, J., Dorzweiler, K., Bensberg, M., Muller-Brusselbach, S. & Muller, R. 2015. A multi-stage process including transient polyploidization and EMT precedes the emergence of chemoresistent ovarian carcinoma cells with a dedifferentiated and pro-inflammatory secretory phenotype. *Oncotarget,* 6, 40005-25.

Rottenberg, S., Disler, C. & Perego, P. 2021. The rediscovery of platinum-based cancer therapy. *Nat Rev Cancer,* 21, 37-50.

Sakamoto, M., Kaga, K. & Kamio, T. 2000. Extended high-frequency ototoxicity induced by the first administration of cisplatin. *Otolaryngol Head Neck Surg,* 122, 828-33.

Salavati, H., Soltani, M. & Amanpour, S. 2018. The pivotal role of angiogenesis in a multi-scale modeling of tumor growth exhibiting the avascular and vascular phases. *Microvasc Res,* 119, 105-116.

Salmina, K., Jankevics, E., Huna, A., Perminov, D., Radovica, I., Klymenko, T., Ivanov, A., Jascenko, E., Scherthan, H., Cragg, M. & Erenpreisa, J. 2010. Up-regulation of the embryonic self-renewal network through reversible polyploidy in irradiated p53-mutant tumour cells. *Exp Cell Res,* 316, 2099-112.

Sharp, C. N., Doll, M., Dupre, T. V., Beverly, L. J. & Siskind, L. J. 2019. Moderate aging does not exacerbate cisplatin-induced kidney injury or fibrosis despite altered inflammatory cytokine expression and immune cell infiltration. *Am J Physiol Renal Physiol,* 316, F162-F172.

Sheth, S., Sheehan, K., Dhukhwa, A., Al Aameri, R. F. H., Mamillapalli, C., Mukherjea, D., Rybak, L. P. & Ramkumar, V. 2019. Oral Administration of Caffeine Exacerbates Cisplatin-Induced Hearing Loss. *Sci Rep,* 9, 9571.

Sikora, E., Bielak-Zmijewska, A. & Mosieniak, G. 2019. Targeting normal and cancer senescent cells as a strategy of senotherapy. *Ageing Res Rev,* 55, 100941.

Sikora, E., Czarnecka-Herok, J., Bojko, A. & Sunderland, P. 2020. Therapy-induced polyploidization and senescence: Coincidence or interconnection? *Semin Cancer Biol.*

Skalleberg, J., Smastuen, M. C., Oldenburg, J., Osnes, T., Fossa, S. D. & Bunne, M. 2020. The Relationship Between Cisplatin-related and Age-related Hearing Loss During an Extended Follow-up. *Laryngoscope,* 130, E515-E521.

Skolekova, S., Matuskova, M., Bohac, M., Toro, L., Durinikova, E., Tyciakova, S., Demkova, L., Gursky, J. & Kucerova, L. 2016. Cisplatin-induced mesenchymal stromal cells-mediated mechanism contributing to decreased antitumor effect in breast cancer cells. *Cell Commun Signal,* 14, 4.

Sun, H., Wang, H., Wang, X., Aoki, Y., Wang, X., Yang, Y., Cheng, X., Wang, Z. & Wang, X. 2020. Aurora-A/SOX8/FOXK1 signaling axis promotes chemoresistance via suppression of cell senescence and induction of glucose metabolism in ovarian cancer organoids and cells. *Theranostics,* 10, 6928-6945.

Sun, X., Shi, B., Zheng, H., Min, L., Yang, J., Li, X., Liao, X., Huang, W., Zhang, M., Xu, S., Zhu, Z., Cui, H. & Liu, X. 2018. Senescence-associated secretory factors induced by cisplatin in melanoma cells promote non-senescent melanoma cell growth through activation of the ERK1/2-RSK1 pathway. *Cell Death Dis,* 9, 260.

Sundaram, M., Guernsey, D. L., Rajaraman, M. M. & Rajaraman, R. 2004. Neosis: a novel type of cell division in cancer. *Cancer Biol Ther,* 3, 207-18.

Szymanski, L., Helbrecht, I., Fiedorowicz, M., Matak, D., Bartnik, E., Golik, P., Szczylik, C. & Czarnecka, A. M. 2019. Cancer stem cells in renal carcinoma. *Postepy Biochem,* 65, 95-102.

Telleria, C. M. 2013. Repopulation of ovarian cancer cells after chemotherapy. *Cancer Growth Metastasis,* 6, 15-21.

Tezze, C., Romanello, V., Desbats, M. A., Fadini, G. P., Albiero, M., Favaro, G., Ciciliot, S., Soriano, M. E., Morbidoni, V., Cerqua, C., Loefler, S., Kern, H., Franceschi, C., Salvioli, S., Conte, M., Blaauw, B., Zampieri, S., Salviati, L., Scorrano, L. & Sandri, M. 2017. Age-Associated Loss of OPA1 in Muscle Impacts Muscle Mass, Metabolic Homeostasis, Systemic Inflammation, and Epithelial Senescence. *Cell Metab,* 25, 1374-1389 e6.

Tounekti, O., Pron, G., Belehradek, J., Jr. & Mir, L. M. 1993. Bleomycin, an apoptosis-mimetic drug that induces two types of cell death depending on the number of molecules internalized. *Cancer Res,* 53, 5462-9.

Tredan, O., Galmarini, C. M., Patel, K. & Tannock, I. F. 2007. Drug resistance and the solid tumor microenvironment. *J Natl Cancer Inst,* 99, 1441-54.

Tserga, E., Nandwani, T., Edvall, N. K., Bulla, J., Patel, P., Canlon, B., Cederroth, C. R. & Baguley, D. M. 2019. The genetic vulnerability to cisplatin ototoxicity: a systematic review. *Sci Rep,* 9, 3455.

Valentijn, F. A., Falke, L. L., Nguyen, T. Q. & Goldschmeding, R. 2018. Cellular senescence in the aging and diseased kidney. *J Cell Commun Signal,* 12, 69-82.

Van As, J. W., Van Den Berg, H. & Van Dalen, E. C. 2016. Platinum-induced hearing loss after treatment for childhood cancer. *Cochrane Database Syst Rev*, CD010181.

Vassel, F. M., Bian, K., Walker, G. C. & Hemann, M. T. 2020. Rev7 loss alters cisplatin response and increases drug efficacy in chemotherapy-resistant lung cancer. *Proc Natl Acad Sci U S A,* 117, 28922-28924.

Veena, M. S., Wilken, R., Zheng, J. Y., Gholkar, A., Venkatesan, N., Vira, D., Ahmed, S., Basak, S. K., Dalgard, C. L., Ravichandran, S., Batra, R. K., Kasahara, N., Elashoff, D., Fishbein, M. C., Whitelegge, J. P., Torres, J. Z., Wang, M. B. & Srivatsan, E. S. 2014. p16 Protein and gigaxonin are associated with the ubiquitination of NFkappaB in cisplatin-induced senescence of cancer cells. *J Biol Chem,* 289, 34921-37.

Visvader, J. E. & Lindeman, G. J. 2012. Cancer stem cells: current status and evolving complexities. *Cell Stem Cell,* 10, 717-728.

Wang, G., Cheng, X., Zhang, J., Liao, Y., Jia, Y. & Qing, C. 2021. Possibility of inducing tumor cell senescence during therapy. *Oncol Lett,* 22, 496.

Wang, L., Yang, G., Zhao, D., Wang, J., Bai, Y., Peng, Q., Wang, H., Fang, R., Chen, G., Wang, Z., Wang, K., Li, G., Yang, Y., Wang, Z., Guo, P., Peng, L., Hou, D. & Xu, W. 2019. CD103-positive CSC exosome promotes EMT of clear cell renal cell carcinoma: role of remote MiR-19b-3p. *Mol Cancer,* 18, 86.

Wang, R., Chadalavada, K., Wilshire, J., Kowalik, U., Hovinga, K. E., Geber, A., Fligelman, B., Leversha, M., Brennan, C. & Tabar, V. 2010. Glioblastoma stem-like cells give rise to tumour endothelium. *Nature,* 468, 829-33.

Was, H., Barszcz, K., Czarnecka, J., Kowalczyk, A., Bernas, T., Uzarowska, E., Koza, P., Klejman, A., Piwocka, K., Kaminska, B. & Sikora, E. 2017. Bafilomycin A1 triggers proliferative potential of senescent cancer cells in vitro and in NOD/SCID mice. *Oncotarget,* 8, 9303-9322.

Was, H., Borkowska, A., Olszewska, A., Klemba, A., Marciniak, M., Synowiec, A. & Kieda, C. 2021. Polyploidy formation in cancer cells: How a Trojan horse is born. *Semin Cancer Biol.*

Was, H., Czarnecka, J., Kominek, A., Barszcz, K., Bernas, T., Piwocka, K. & Kaminska, B. 2018. Some chemotherapeutics-treated colon cancer cells display a specific phenotype being a combination of stem-like and senescent cell features. *Cancer Biol Ther,* 19, 63-75.

Wen, J., Zeng, M., Shu, Y., Guo, D., Sun, Y., Guo, Z., Wang, Y., Liu, Z., Zhou, H. & Zhang, W. 2015. Aging increases the susceptibility of cisplatin-induced nephrotoxicity. *Age (Dordr),* 37, 112.

Weng, C. H., Wu, C. S., Wu, J. C., Kung, M. L., Wu, M. H. & Tai, M. H. 2020. Cisplatin-Induced Giant Cells Formation Is Involved in Chemoresistance of Melanoma Cells. *Int J Mol Sci,* 21.

Wolf, K. W., Mentzel, M. & Mendoza, A. S. 1996. Treatment with the anti-tumor drugs, cis-platin and mafosfamide, does not affect the structure of prekinetochores in a human breast cancer cell line. An immunofluorescence study using human anti-centromere autoantibodies. *Ann Anat,* 178, 425-32.

Wu, P. C., Wang, Q., Dong, Z. M., Chu, E., Roberson, R. S., Ivanova, I. C. & Wu, D. Y. 2010. Expression of coxsackie and adenovirus receptor distinguishes transitional cancer states in therapy-induced cellular senescence. *Cell Death Dis,* 1, e70.

Wu, P. C., Wang, Q., Grobman, L., Chu, E. & Wu, D. Y. 2012. Accelerated cellular senescence in solid tumor therapy. *Exp Oncol,* 34, 298-305.

Wu, P. Z., O'malley, J. T., De Gruttola, V. & Liberman, M. C. 2020. Age-Related Hearing Loss Is Dominated by Damage to Inner Ear Sensory Cells, Not the Cellular Battery That Powers Them. *J Neurosci,* 40, 6357-6366.

Wu, Z. Z., Chen, L. S., Zhou, R., Bin, J. P., Liao, Y. L. & Liao, W. J. 2016. Metastasis-associated in colon cancer-1 in gastric cancer: Beyond metastasis. *World J Gastroenterol,* 22, 6629-37.

Xu, J., Zhou, L. & Liu, Y. 2020. Cellular Senescence in Kidney Fibrosis: Pathologic Significance and Therapeutic Strategies. *Front Pharmacol,* 11, 601325.

Xu, Q., Long, Q., Zhu, D., Fu, D., Zhang, B., Han, L., Qian, M., Guo, J., Xu, J., Cao, L., Chin, Y. E., Coppe, J. P., Lam, E. W., Campisi, J. & Sun, Y. 2019. Targeting amphiregulin (AREG) derived from senescent stromal cells diminishes cancer resistance and averts programmed cell death 1 ligand (PD-L1)-mediated immunosuppression. *Aging Cell,* 18, e13027.

Yeung, T., Fung, O., Bashkurov, M., Khandani, A., Subedar, O., Wudwud, A., Shaw, P., Clarke, B., Bartlett, J., Rottapel, R. & Kapus, A. 2019. Avoidance of apoptotic death via a hyperploid salvage survival pathway after platinum treatment in high grade serous carcinoma cell line models. *Oncotarget,* 10, 6691-6712.

Yi, J. M., Shin, S., Kim, N. S. & Bang, O. S. 2019. Ameliorative effects of aqueous extract of Forsythiae suspensa fruits on oxaliplatin-induced neurotoxicity in vitro and in vivo. *BMC Complement Altern Med,* 19, 339.

You, N., Tan, Y., Zhou, L., Huang, X., Wang, W., Wang, L., Wu, K., Mi, N., Li, J. & Zheng, L. 2017. Tg737 acts as a key driver of invasion and migration in liver cancer stem cells and correlates with poor prognosis in patients with hepatocellular carcinoma. *Exp Cell Res,* 358, 217-226.

Yu, S., Ao, Z., Wu, Y., Song, L., Zhang, P., Li, X., Liu, M., Qian, P., Zhang, R., Li, X., Chen, Y., Wang, X., Wang, X., Ruan, X., Qian, G. & Ji, F. 2020. ZNF300 promotes chemoresistance and aggressive behaviour in non-small-cell lung cancer. *Cell Prolif,* 53, e12924.

Yuan, X., Larsson, C. & Xu, D. 2019. Mechanisms underlying the activation of TERT transcription and telomerase activity in human cancer: old actors and new players. *Oncogene,* 38, 6172-6183.

Zhang, D., Sun, B., Zhao, X., Ma, Y., Ji, R., Gu, Q., Dong, X., Li, J., Liu, F., Jia, X., Leng, X., Zhang, C., Sun, R. & Chi, J. 2014a. Twist1 expression induced by sunitinib accelerates tumor cell vasculogenic mimicry by increasing the population of CD133+ cells in triple-negative breast cancer. *Mol Cancer,* 13, 207.

Zhang, S., Li, M., Gu, Y., Liu, Z., Xu, S., Cui, Y. & Sun, B. 2008. Thalidomide influences growth and vasculogenic mimicry channel formation in melanoma. *J Exp Clin Cancer Res,* 27, 60.

Zhang, S., Mercado-Uribe, I. & Liu, J. 2014b. Tumor stroma and differentiated cancer cells can be originated directly from polyploid giant cancer cells induced by paclitaxel. *Int J Cancer,* 134, 508-18.

Zhang, S., Mercado-Uribe, I., Xing, Z., Sun, B., Kuang, J. & Liu, J. 2014. Generation of cancer stem-like cells through the formation of polyploid giant cancer cells. *Oncogene,* 33, 116-28.

Zhao, C., Chen, Z., Qi, J., Duan, S., Huang, Z., Zhang, C., Wu, L., Zeng, M., Zhang, B., Wang, N., Mao, H., Zhang, A., Xing, C. & Yuan, Y. 2017. Drp1-dependent mitophagy protects against cisplatin-induced apoptosis of renal tubular epithelial cells by improving mitochondrial function. *Oncotarget,* 8, 20988-21000.

Chapter 3

Main Mechanisms Involved in Major and Minor Side Effects Triggered by Cisplatin-Based Therapy

Mauricio Burotto[1], Ignacio A. Cortés-Fuentes[2,3], Jaime Gonzalez-Montero[1,4] and Juan G. Gormaz[5,*]

[1]Bradford Hill, Clinical Research Center, Santiago, Chile
[2]Hospital Barros Luco-Trudeau, San Miguel, Santiago, Chile
[3]Departamento de Otorrinolaringología, Facultad de Medicina, Universidad de Chile, Chile
[4]Departamento de Oncología básico-clínico, Universidad de Chile, Chile
[5]Facultad de Medicina, Universidad de Chile, Chile

Abstract

Cisplatin-based chemotherapies are the mainstay of several forms of cancer treatment both in adults and children, but their use may cause a plethora of side effects. Their high capacity to generate adducts with DNA accounts for their anticancer action but also for the side effects. However, that mechanism alone is not enough to completely explain their actions, especially on non-proliferative tissues, and cell damage derived from increased reactive oxygen species (ROS) production is a key mechanism involved in adverse reactions. Major side effects of cisplatin-based treatments may account for acute morbidity and even mortality during cancer treatment. They include nephrotoxicity, myelosuppression, cardiotoxicity, and hepatotoxicity, which may also lead to suspension or decreased dosage of cisplatin, which can ultimately compromise

*Corresponding Author's Email: jgormaz@med.uchile.cl.

In: Platinum-Based Chemotherapy
Editors: Kulmira Nurgali and Raquel Abalo
ISBN: 978-1-68507-972-7

© 2022 Nova Science Publishers, Inc.

oncologic long-term survival. Minor side effects include ototoxicity, hypogonadism, infertility and gastrointestinal dysfunction, among others. These effects are not normally associated with increased mortality, but they can decrease quality of life of cancer survivors. To date there are limited options to prevent cisplatin-based side effects and most interventions have a symptomatic aim or a discrete clinical efficacy. Efforts are currently directed to 1) optimize current intervention protocols and the therapeutic approach to adverse effects, 2) the application of new generation platinum-compounds, and 3) the development of innovative prophylactic strategies, which can hopefully reduce the side effects, but clinical data is still lacking.

Keywords: cisplatin-induced side effects, nephrotoxicity, neurotoxicity, ototoxicity, hypogonadism, mucositis

Introduction

Although cisplatin-based chemotherapy has been the mainstay of treatment of several malignancies of adults and children, it is associated with numerous adverse reactions which may limit their use. Considering both major and minor side effects, a cancer patient exposed to cisplatin-based therapy can suffer any combination of more than forty specific adverse effects (Oun et al., 2018).

In this chapter we describe the most relevant and frequent side effects associated to cisplatin-based treatments and the main mechanisms involved in their occurrence. For this purpose, we sort them as major and minor side effects according to their severity. Major side effects, including nephrotoxicity, myelosuppression, cardiotoxicity, and hepatotoxicity may lead to suspension of treatment or decreased dosage, which can ultimately compromise survival. Minor side effects, including ototoxicity, gastrointestinal dysfunction, and others, although they may occur more frequently and do not alter oncologic survival, might have a considerable effect on quality-of-life among cancer survivors.

Major Side Effects

Cisplatin, more than other platinum analogues, are the cornerstone of multiple cancer treatments because they have high response rate in various types of neoplasms. This compound is used regularly in the treatment of lung, digestive, gynecological, breast, head and neck neoplasms, among many others (Dilruba & Kalayda, 2016). Its use extends both to curative (generally in radio-sensitizing doses) and palliative treatments (in monotherapy or in combination). They have a proven anti-tumor effect, but the incidence of major adverse events limits their use at high doses and/or for extended periods of time (Kelland, 2007). In general terms, cisplatin and other platinum-compounds transfer their alkyl group, generating covalent bonds to DNA, to form covalent adduct with purine DNA base. While this interaction is the basis for efficacy of cisplatin in cancer treatment, together with oxidative stress, inflammation, and others, it is also responsible of major adverse events (Ghosh, 2019; Oun et al., 2018). Cisplatin treatment has been associated to various major adverse events including nephrotoxicity, cardiotoxicity, myelosuppression, hepatotoxicity, and neurotoxicity. In the following paragraphs, general clinical and pathogenic concepts about these platinum-induced major adverse events will be discussed.

Nephrotoxicity

Nephrotoxicity is a classic major toxicity caused by cisplatin treatment. It is triggered mainly by cisplatin, although it can also be generated less frequently by the other platinum-analogues. Cisplatin-induced nephrotoxicity is a dose-limiting side effect, which is manifested by acute and/or chronic impairment of kidney function (Sarin et al., 2018). The overall incidence of cisplatin-induced nephrotoxicity in elderly patients slightly exceeds 10%. It is significantly higher than its prevalence in younger patients, which reaches only 6.5% (Duan et al., 2020). Kidney damage from cisplatin is explained by multiple mechanisms. First, the kidney is the main route of cisplatin excretion; therefore, tubular cells have a tendency to accumulate cisplatin in higher levels compared to other organs, through two main membrane transporters which move cisplatin into tubular cells (COT2 and Ctrl1) (Cao et al., 2018). Once in the kidney, cisplatin undergoes biotransformation to cysteinyl glycine conjugates and other higher thiols, which may partially explain the tubular toxicity (Zhu et al., 2015). Exposure of tubular cells to cisplatin activates signaling pathways that result in tubular cell injury and cell death (Tsuruya et al., 2003). The mechanism of cisplatin-induced nephrotoxicity could be explained similarly to that of tumor cytotoxicity, involving the formation of highly reactive equated platinum species that cross-link DNA. Tubular damage generates a robust inflammatory response, as well as injury to the renal vasculature, which results in vasoconstriction, reduced blood flow and ischemic injury, leading to acute kidney injury (AKI) (Crona et al., 2017). Another important mechanism of cisplatin-induced nephrotoxicity is reactive oxygen species (ROS) generation in tubular cells mediated by direct activation of nicotinamide adenine dinucleotide phosphate (NADPH) oxidase by cisplatin, which generates massive amounts of superoxide anion and thus tubular cell necrosis and apoptosis. Based on this, experiments using apocynin (a NADPH oxidase inhibitor) in animal models have demonstrated a capacity to attenuate kidney damage caused by cisplatin (Meng et al., 2018).

Risk factors for cisplatin-induced nephrotoxicity are the use of high doses of cisplatin, previous cancer treatments involving platinum compounds, pre-existing kidney damage and concomitant use of other nephrotoxic agents (Liu et al., 2018). Although much progress has been made in understanding the mechanisms of platinum nephrotoxicity, to date there is no optimal preventive treatment. In routine clinical practice, to prevent this damage, cisplatin is used in moderate doses, with concomitant use of intravenous fluids (1 or 2 liters of isotonic fluids during cisplatin infusion) and diuretics such as furosemide and/or mannitol (Horie et al., 2018).

Neurotoxicity

Neurotoxicity is a common toxicity induced by cisplatin, but also by oxaliplatin. It can be expressed as acute (95%) and/or chronic (15%) peripheral neuropathy (Avan et al., 2015). Neuropathy is recognized as the current major dose-limiting cisplatin toxicity (Kanat et al., 2017). There are differences between oxaliplatin and cisplatin neuropathy. Cisplatin neuropathy is exhibited as autonomic neuropathy, loss of hearing and seizures. Cisplatin-induced neurotoxicity is also dose-dependent and is common among patients with a cumulative dose over 300 mg/m^2 (Santos et al., 2020), but it can reach an incidence range between 50-85% when patients are exposed to cumulative doses higher than 500 mg/m^2 (Pellacani & Eleftheriou, 2020). On the other hand, oxaliplatin neuropathy is dose and time dependent, and appears more frequently with cumulative doses of oxaliplatin higher than 680 mg/m^2. It occurs because the oxalate group binds calcium, altering its function to activate the neuron action potential (Cersosimo, 2005).

Cisplatin-associated neuropathy is generally reversible, but it has been shown that in 30-50% of patients, neuropathy is irreversible (Avan et al., 2015). There are other more serious (but less frequent) manifestations of neurotoxicity such as encephalopathy (associated with intra-arterial use of cisplatin), reversible posterior leukoencephalopathy and Guillain-Barré syndrome (Chiorazzi et al., 2015).

There are two main mechanisms proposed to explain cisplatin-induced peripheral neuropathy: cisplatin and other platinum compounds form intrastrain adducts and interstrain crosslinks, altering tertiary DNA structure (Ta et al., 2006). This effect promotes alterations in cell-cycle kinetics, which leads to an attempt of differentiated postmitotic dorsal root ganglion neurons to re-enter the cell cycle, which induces apoptosis (Gill & Windebank, 1998). Consequently, the existence of a higher accumulation of platinum DNA adducts has been demonstrated, particularly within the dorsal root ganglion of autopsied patients after platinum chemotherapy use (Salman et al., 2015). The second mechanism proposes the involvement of ROS and mitochondrial dysfunction as the trigger of neuronal apoptosis (McDonald & Windebank, 2002). Regardless of the mechanism, apoptosis results in secondary damage to peripheral nerves.

Hepatoxicity

Cisplatin and other platinum-analogue treatments can also result in hepatotoxicity, although this type of toxicity is less frequent than renal or neurological toxicity. Transaminases elevation has been reported with the use of platinum-analogues (10% of patients), in addition to moderate increases in alkaline phosphatase (Oun et al., 2018), but liver failure is a rare event. Cisplatin is also a rare cause of steatosis at standard doses (Cavalli et al., 1978). There is at least one case report of carboplatin-induced hepatic failure and one autopsy documenting a case of hepatic sinusoidal obstruction in a patient who had received high doses of carboplatin (Hruban et al., 1991). Combinations of fluoropyrimidines and oxaliplatin are used in patients with colorectal cancer prior to the liver metastases resection. These chemotherapy regimens have been associated with hepatic vascular injury and nodular regenerative hyperplasia (Kim et al., 2011). To date, there are no guidelines determining treatment with cisplatin and other platinum compounds in patients with liver dysfunction, but studies in patients with resectable liver metastases from colorectal cancer have indicated that oxaliplatin can be used at standard doses, even in patients with severe liver dysfunction (Wakiya et al., 2017).

The mechanisms of cisplatin- (and other platinum-analogues) induced hepatotoxicity are multiple, but ROS generation might play a central role. Hence, experiments have demonstrated a lower function of liver antioxidant enzymes such as glutathione peroxidase with the use of platinum-analogues and a lower amount of reduced glutathione, in addition to an increase in liver malondialdehyde and other oxidative stress parameters (Bano & Najam, 2019; Tabassum et al., 2015). It has been shown that cisplatin hepatotoxicity might be exacerbated in patients with elevated liver expression of cytochrome P450-2E1 enzyme (Lu & Cederbaum, 2006).

Myelosuppression

Hematological toxicity is clinically evidenced by myelosuppression and is more frequent with the use of cisplatin and carboplatin, with an incidence of 20-40% at conventional doses and up to 90% at high doses (Chovanec et al., 2017). Myelosuppression is the dose-limiting toxicity of carboplatin (van der Vijgh, 1991). Accordingly, the use of carboplatin at conventional doses has been reported to result in thrombocytopenia, anemia, and neutropenia occurring in 25, 60 and 20% of patients, respectively (Grueso Cuesta et al., 2019). Myelosuppression can be more severe and prolonged in patients with renal failure, previous chemotherapy treatment, poor performance status, and aged over 65 years (Cheng et al., 2017). Myelosuppression is aggravated by combination therapy with other myelosuppressive compounds (such as taxanes or anthracyclines). It is generally reversible and is not cumulative when platinum-analogues are used as a single agent, at the recommended doses and administration frequencies (Go & Adjei, 1999). The mechanism of cisplatin-induced myelosuppression is similar to its anti-tumor effect, which occurs in bone marrow cells, and can be prevented with the concomitant use of colony-stimulating factors when platinums are used in high doses (Oshita et al., 2001).

Cardiotoxicity

Although cardiac toxicity due to cisplatin and other platinum-analogues has been described, these drugs are not oncological drugs that classically generate cardiotoxicity (such as anthracyclines or anti-HER2 agents); thus, this toxicity is an infrequent adverse event, but associated with high mortality (Hu et al., 2018). Many toxic events have been reported with cisplatin and other platinum-analogues use, which include arrhythmias, congestive heart failure, electrocardiographic changes, and myocarditis (Madeddu et al., 2016). Cisplatin-induced cardiac damage could be associated to ROS generation and lipid peroxidation of cardiac membranes. Accordingly, cisplatin has been demonstrated to possibly generate myocardial histological changes such as vacuolated cytoplasm of muscle cells, inflammation of blood vessels as well as degeneration and necrosis of cardiac muscle fiber cells, accompanied with fibrous tissue reaction (El-Awady et al., 2011). Concomitantly, cisplatin administration in high doses can cause cardiac decompensation in patients with pre-existing heart failure, due to the concomitant use of high doses of intravenous fluids for prevention of kidney failure. Consequently, cisplatin should be used with caution in these patients (Crona et al., 2017)

Minor Side Effects

Despite the fact that minor side effects normally do not compromise survival, their high prevalence make them a significant problem, even more so when in many cases they generate irreversible damage in the pediatric population. Currently, it is estimated that the minor adverse effects affect virtually all patients undergoing cisplatin-based chemotherapy, and without effective prophylactic treatments, most of the cases produce irreversible sequelae. Specifically in the pediatric population, the problem is more complex because the irreversible sequelae may not only impact in growth and development, but they will accompany patients throughout their life. From a biochemical and molecular point of view, the mechanisms that account for the minor side effects of cisplatin-based chemotherapy are very similar to those that generate the major adverse effects. The only difference to consider is that in minor side effects, the contribution of oxidative stress would be higher than DNA damage, especially in those tissues and organs without replication capacity. Clinically, minor side effects caused by cisplatin-based chemotherapy are associated with ototoxicity, reproductive system alterations, gastrointestinal problems, mucositis and neurocognitive and musculoskeletal adverse conditions. In the following paragraphs, general clinical and pathogenic concepts about these platinum-induced minor adverse events will be analyzed.

Ototoxicity

Cisplatin-based treatments may cause damage to the inner ear, which often manifests as bilateral, sensorineural hearing loss and tinnitus (Frisina et al., 2016). Ototoxicity occurs frequently during cisplatin-based treatments and several risk factors have been associated, including age, concomitant use of other ototoxic drugs such as furosemide or radiotherapy for head and neck cancers (Landier, 2016). Several mechanisms have been proposed to explain ototoxicity caused by platinum-analogues, with increased ROS production as a major contributing mechanism for inner ear injury, especially for auditory hair cells and the stria vascularis (Sheth et al., 2017). Cisplatin may trigger increased ROS production through stimulation of NADPH oxidase 3 (NOX3), an exclusive inner ear isoform of NADPH, or by direct inactivation of antioxidant defenses (Rybak et al., 2009, 2012). Furthermore, several pro-inflammatory pathways are also upregulated following cisplatin-based treatments, which interact with ROS-related production mechanisms, thus increasing inner ear damage (Tang et al., 2021). For a more comprehensive analysis regarding the mechanisms related with ototoxicity derived from cisplatin-based chemotherapy see the related chapter in this book.

Hypogonadism and Infertility

Platinum-compounds represent the essential component for testicular cancer treatments, with survival rates higher than 95% (Chovanec et al., 2017). Cisplatin and radiotherapy increase the risk of developing hypogonadism compared to orchiectomy alone (Bandak et al., 2016). Hypogonadism is associated to sexual impairment, fertility problems, muscle weakness, osteoporosis and others (Fung et al., 2018). Moreover, testicular cancer survivors experience different side effects including those mentioned in this chapter also in addition to increased cardiovascular risk and secondary malignancies several years following treatment (Chovanec et al., 2017).

Cisplatin treatment is reported to induce azoospermia and a higher cumulative dose is associated with increased infertility risk, which is also higher than the use of carboplatin (Fung et al., 2018). However, other platinum compounds such as oxaliplatin and carboplatin have shown less clinical association to hypogonadism (Falk et al., 2019; Ghezzi et al., 2016; Ruf et al., 2019).

Based on preclinical data, cisplatin damages testicular cells through its known effects in the DNA and increased ROS production. Cisplatin has been observed to trigger an increase in malondialdehyde levels, inducible nitric oxide synthase, tumor necrosis factor alpha (TNF-α) and p38-mitogen-activated protein kinase (MAPK), leading to different morphologic alterations and germ cell depletion (Sherif et al., 2014). An increased expression of the interleukin 1 beta (IL-1β) is also reported, which additionally is associated to lessening of testicular antioxidant potential (Azarbarz et al., 2020). Furthermore, cisplatin may trigger apoptosis via down-regulation of the phosphatidylinositol 3-kinase/protein kinase B/mammalian target of rapamycin (PI3K/AKT/mTOR) pathways, up-regulation of the Bad/Cyt c/caspase-9/caspase-3 pathways and also increased reticulum stress-mediated apoptosis (X. Chang et al., 2021).

In cases of symptomatic hypogonadism, those patients may benefit from testosterone replacement therapy (Chovanec et al., 2017). Current alternatives for fertility conservation include sperm cryopreservation and assisted reproduction techniques (Loren et al., 2013).

In the case of women, chemotherapy may exert toxic effects on ovarian function with subsequent hypogonadism and decreased reproductive function (Spears et al., 2019). Estrogen deficiency due to ovarian insufficiency is associated with decreased quality of life, bone function and cardiovascular risk (van Dorp et al., 2018). It has been reported that chemotherapy may damage the ovary through direct loss of primordial follicles, accelerated activation of primordial follicles, follicular atresia, stromal injury and inflammation (Spears et al., 2019).

Multi-drug treatment that includes cisplatin is associated with increased risk of ovarian failure and infertility (Maneschi et al., 1994). However, clinical data regarding cisplatin-induced ovarian toxicity is lacking. Increased ROS production and antioxidant depletion is reported in ovarian tissue following platinum-drug treatment (Barberino et al., 2017; Kulhan et al., 2019; Li et al., 2013). Cisplatin induces DNA damage in the ovary and triggers specific pathways of MAPK cascade and other kinases, which are involved in apoptosis and accelerated activation of primordial follicles (Chang et al.,

2015). The tumor-suppressor p-53 protein and related proteins play a major role in the cisplatin-induced damage reparation (Kim et al., 2019).

All these factors have led the testing of different substances including tyrosine-kinase inhibitors, melatonin, ghrelin, luteinizing hormone and antioxidants to prevent ovarian damage (Spears et al., 2019). Similar to treatment in men, hormonal replacement therapies and ovarian tissue cryopreservation as an alternative for fertility conservation represent the basic treatments for ovarian damage (Spears et al., 2019; van Dorp et al., 2018).

Gastrointestinal Toxicity

Gastrointestinal symptoms following cisplatin and other platinum-based treatments represent a frequent clinical setting. Up to 67% of patients receiving cisplatin at high doses suffer diarrhea and 80% emesis (Bearcroft et al., 1999), also in addition to delayed gastric motility, nausea, malabsorption, mucositis, weight loss and others. Gastrointestinal toxicities for other platinum compounds are less defined, but with increased risk for patients with certain genetic profiles using carboplatin (He et al., 2016). Despite the use of antiemetics, severe delayed emesis (after 24h) is a significant cause of morbidity in cancer patients and it occurs more frequently at higher doses (Mitchell, 2006).

The proliferative epithelial cells of the gastrointestinal tract are especially damaged by cisplatin (Shahid et al., 2018) and this anticancer drug may alter normal microbiota by direct antibacterial effects, thus enhancing gastrointestinal disruption (Gori et al., 2019). Cisplatin has been described to induce dose-dependent damage to the small intestine, with villous degeneration, acute necrosis and apoptosis of intestinal epithelial cells, thus decreasing total surface area for nutrient absorption (Khan et al., 2012; Shahid, Farooqui, Abidi, et al., 2017). Cisplatin stimulates enterochromaffin cells to release serotonin that stimulates vagal afferents, initiating the vomiting reflex and diarrhea (Darmani et al., 2015). Furthermore, cisplatin induces morpho-functional changes in the enteric neurons and neuroimmune interactions, thus impairing the enteric nervous system and explaining the reported dysmotility (Stojanovska et al., 2015; Vera et al., 2011).

The known effects of cisplatin on the DNA and increased ROS production have been reported to be involved in the pathogenesis of gastrointestinal injury, directly reacting with cellular proteins, lipids and others (Shahid, Farooqui, Abidi, et al., 2017a). Lipid peroxidation reactions triggered by cisplatin may increase the free forms of fatty acids in intestinal mucosal cells causing alterations in cell membranes, especially in mitochondria (Chang et al., 2002), thus leading to cytochrome C releasing and apoptosis (Shahid et al., 2018). Alterations in levels of gastrointestinal cell antioxidant defenses have also been reported. Cisplatin decreases levels of glutathione (GSH) and declines activities of major antioxidant enzymes such as superoxide dismutase (SOD) and human catalase (CAT), among others (Shahid, Farooqui, Abidi, et al., 2017a; Shahid, Farooqui, Rizwan, et al., 2017b). It is thought that the induction of pro-inflammatory pathways triggered by cisplatin would further contribute to gastrointestinal toxicity; however, it is not well-described, only reporting involvement of known pro-inflammatory molecules such as interleukins and TNF-α (Shahid et al., 2018).

Several compounds have been tested, mostly in preclinical models, to ameliorate cisplatin-induced gastrointestinal toxicity, including nutrients and vitamins, serotonin-receptor antagonists, herbal-derived substances, gastric hormones and others (Shahid et al., 2018); but clinical trials remain scarce. In the case of nausea and vomiting induced by chemotherapy, treatment options include the use of dexamethasone, olanzapine, antagonists of 5-hydroxytryptamine-3 receptor and neurokinin-1 receptor (Smith et al., 2020). Furthermore, the use of probiotics containing *Lactobacillus spp.* for prevention of chemoradiotherapy and radiotherapy-induced diarrhea in patients with pelvic malignancy and hyperbaric oxygen therapy to treat radiation-induced proctitis have also been recommended (Bowen et al., 2019b). For a more comprehensive detailed analysis of gastrointestinal side-effects derived from cisplatin-based chemotherapy, see the respective chapter in this book.

Oral Mucositis

Mucositis represents a frequent adverse reaction to cancer treatments, characterized by different degrees of inflammatory and painful, ulcerative mucous membrane lesions. It may develop along the gastrointestinal tract, but oral mucositis represents one of the most common and most-studied appearances (Bachour & Sonis, 2018; Sonis, 2013). Oral mucositis may be triggered by systemic chemotherapy, radiation therapy or a combination of both. Up to 40% of patients have been reported to develop oral mucositis when conventional doses of chemotherapy for solid tumors are used (Jones et al., 2006) and up to 80% when a high dose of chemotherapy is delivered (Vera-

Llonch et al., 2007). In patients with head and neck cancer who receive radiation or chemoradiation treatments, it occurs to different degrees in practically all patients (Vera-Llonch et al., 2006). It is also more frequent when combined with cisplatin for treatments of different malignancies (Hildebrandt et al., 2010; Nishii et al., 2020). Mucositis may significantly impair cancer patient quality of life and influence several clinical outcomes such as delays in treatments, reduction in therapy dosage, nutritional compromise, increased risk of infection and thereby represents an economic burden for health systems (Bowen et al., 2019a; Lalla et al., 2014; Rosenthal, 2007).

The development of mucositis is complex and multifactorial, and several mechanisms involved in its pathogenesis have been described (Bachour & Sonis, 2018; Lalla et al., 2014; Sonis, 2013). There is a widely accepted description of the events involved in mucositis (Bowen et al., 2019a; Sonis, 2009, 2013). It starts with the initiation phase when there is DNA injury and ROS production caused by radiotherapy or chemo-radiotherapy leading to a decreased proliferation of basal cells of the epithelium. This triggers a primary damage response that promotes the transcription of pro-inflammatory pathways resulting in epithelium-cell death, which also generate an amplification of the inflammatory response such as TNF-α and IL-1β (Barasch & Peterson, 2003; Lalla et al., 2014). The bacteria colonize ulcers and produce substances that trigger activation of macrophages in the submucosa, thus enhancing the inflammatory insult. A healing phase is achieved when signaling from the extracellular matrix of submucosa, promoting epithelial proliferation and differentiation and the oral microbiota is restored. Furthermore, several risk factors for oral mucositis have been described, including age, nutritional status, genetic factors and treatment-related variables (Bowen et al., 2019a; Sonis, 2013).

Pain relief, dietary support and the prevention of secondary infections are the main elements in patient management (Elad et al., 2020). For the specific case of pelvic malignancy, current evidence supports the use of probiotics containing *Lactobacillus spp.* for diarrhea prevention (Bowen et al., 2019a; Bowen et al., 2019b). Regarding prevention, there is evidence favoring the use of cryotherapy to reduce the severity of oral mucositis during chemotherapy administration (McGuire et al., 2013). Oral glutamine has also been used with positive results (Davy & Heathcote, 2021). One of the most studied drugs used is keratinocyte growth factor and a meta-analysis showed that it is beneficial for the prevention of oral mucositis in adults receiving head and neck radiotherapy associated to cisplatin or fluorouracil or chemotherapy alone for mixed solid and hematological cancers (Riley et al., 2017). Furthermore, there are several clinical trials testing different substances to prevent mucositis (McGuire et al., 2013), which is a well-established goal.

Neurocognitive Toxicity

Various chemotherapy drugs have been reported to possibly alter brain function, triggering dysfunction in several cognitive areas including attention, memory and others (Ongnok et al., 2020; Yamada et al., 2010). Although cisplatin and other platinum-analogues have a limited entry through the blood brain barrier, there are clinical reports that patients receiving cisplatin show decreased performance in cognitive measurements (Aotani et al., 2016; John et al., 2017). However, the mechanisms behind these neurocognitive effects are not well understood, but several pathways have been described from pre-clinical studies which involve oxidative stress generation, inflammation and others (Ongnok et al., 2020).

Conclusion

Cisplatin and other platinum-based drugs remain the primary treatment for several cancers including lung, digestive, gynecological, breast, head and neck neoplasms, among many others, but their use is associated with side effects of variable severity, in an acute or delayed setting, depending on the affected organ (Table 1).

Although clinically different side effects have specific characteristics and mechanisms involved, several share common molecular mechanisms which can form the basis for understanding how they occur and how they can be prevented or treated. Each potential, platinum-based side effect represents a clinical problem that should be addressed and managed accordingly in a multi-disciplinary setting. This is relevant for major side effects but especially important for minor side effects. Several of these can be overlooked during treatment follow-ups as the focus is centered on optimizing survival, the guiding goal of oncology. Thus, together with optimizing survival it is crucial to consider the importance of identifying and managing those platinum-based side effects that can be overlooked, which can positively impact the quality of life of millions of cancer survivors, an additionally valid oncology goal.

However, it is fundamental to consider that despite the fact that cisplatin-based treatment currently holds a deserved key position in oncology, to date there is a paucity of novel solutions to well-known side effects which carry important consequences for patients. This highlights the need to advance in a multi-disciplinary approach, considering essential preclinical data as well as the unique characteristics of each patient in clinical practice.

Table 1. Association between main major and minor effects with platinum-based chemotherapy

Side Effect		Cisplatin	Carboplatin	Oxaliplatin
Major	Nephrotoxicity	+++	+	-
	Neurotoxicity	++	+	++
	Hepatoxicity	+	-	+
	Myelosuppression	++	++	+
	Cardiotoxicity	+	-	-
Minor	Ototoxicity	+++	++	+
	Hypogonadism/infertility	++	+	+
	Gastrointestinal	+++	++	+
	Oral Mucositis	++	+	+

Key: +++: Frequent association; ++: moderate association; +: low association; -: Not associated.

References

Aotani, E., Hamano, T., Gemma, A., Takeuchi, M., Takebayashi, T., & Kobayashi, K. (2016). Identification of adverse events that have a negative impact on quality of life in a clinical trial comparing docetaxel versus S-1 with cisplatin in lung cancer. International Journal of Clinical Oncology, 21(5), 836–842. https://doi.org/10.1007/s10147-016-0960-6.

Avan, A., Postma, T. J., Ceresa, C., Avan, A., Cavaletti, G., Giovannetti, E., & Peters, G. J. (2015). Platinum-Induced Neurotoxicity and Preventive Strategies: Past, Present, and Future. *The Oncologist*, *20*(4), 411–432. https://doi.org/10.1634/theoncologist.2014-0044.

Azarbarz, N., Shafiei Seifabadi, Z., Moaiedi, M. Z., & Mansouri, E. (2020). Assessment of the effect of sodium hydrogen sulfide (hydrogen sulfide donor) on cisplatin-induced testicular toxicity in rats. *Environmental Science and Pollution Research*, *27*(8), 8119–8128. https://doi.org/10.1007/s11356-019-07266-5.

Bachour, P. C., & Sonis, S. T. (2018). Predicting mucositis risk associated with cytotoxic cancer treatment regimens: rationale, complexity, and challenges. *Current Opinion in Supportive & Palliative Care*, *12*(2), 198–210. https://doi.org/10.1097/SPC.0000000000000339.

Bandak, M., Jørgensen, N., Juul, A., Vogelius, I. R., Lauritsen, J., Kier, M. G., Mortensen, M. S., Glovinski, P., & Daugaard, G. (2016). Testosterone deficiency in testicular cancer survivors - a systematic review and meta-analysis. *Andrology*, *4*(3), 382–388. https://doi.org/10.1111/andr.12177.

Bano, N., & Najam, R. (2019). Histopathological and biochemical assessment of liver damage in albino Wistar rats treated with cytotoxic platinum compounds in combination with 5-fluorouracil. *Archives of Medical Science*, *15*(4), 1092–1103. https://doi.org/10.5114/aoms.2019.86064.

Barasch, A., & Peterson, D. E. (2003). Risk factors for ulcerative oral mucositis in cancer patients: unanswered questions. *Oral Oncology*, *39*(2), 91–100. https://doi.org/10.1016/S1368-8375(02)00033-7.

Barberino, R. S., Menezes, V. G., Ribeiro, A. E. A. S., Palheta, R. C., Jiang, X., Smitz, J. E. J., & Matos, M. H. T. (2017). Melatonin protects against cisplatin-induced ovarian damage in mice via the MT1 receptor and antioxidant activity. *Biology of Reproduction*, *96*(6), 1244–1255. https://doi.org/10.1093/biolre/iox053.

Bearcroft, C. P., Domizio, P., Mourad, F. H., André, E. A., & Farthing, M. J. G. (1999). Cisplatin impairs fluid and electrolyte absorption in rat small intestine: a role for 5-hydroxytryptamine. *Gut*, *44*(2), 174–179. https://doi.org/10.1136/gut.44.2.174.

Bowen, J., Al-Dasooqi, N., Bossi, P., Wardill, H., van Sebille, Y., Al-Azri, A., Bateman, E., Correa, M. E., Raber-Durlacher, J., Kandwal, A., Mayo, B., Nair, R. G., Stringer, A., ten Bohmer, K., Thorpe, D., Lalla, R. v., Sonis, S., Cheng, K., & Elad, S. (2019a). The pathogenesis of mucositis: updated perspectives and emerging targets. *Supportive Care in Cancer*, *27*(10), 4023–4033. https://doi.org/10.1007/s00520-019-04893-z.

Bowen, J. M., Gibson, R. J., Coller, J. K., Blijlevens, N., Bossi, P., Al-Dasooqi, N., Bateman, E. H., Chiang, K., de Mooij, C., Mayo, B., Stringer, A. M., Tissing, W., Wardill, H. R., van Sebille, Y. Z. A., Ranna, V., Vaddi, A., Keefe, D. MK., Lalla, R. V., Cheng, K. K. F., & Elad, S. (2019b). Systematic review of agents for the management of cancer treatment-related gastrointestinal mucositis and clinical practice guidelines. *Supportive Care in Cancer*, *27*(10), 4011–4022. https://doi.org/10.1007/s00520-019-04892-0.

Cao, X., Nie, X., Xiong, S., Cao, L., Wu, Z., Moore, P. K., & Bian, J.-S. (2018). Renal protective effect of polysulfide in cisplatin-induced nephrotoxicity. *Redox Biology*, *15*, 513–521. https://doi.org/10.1016/j.redox.2018.01.012.

Cavalli, F., Tschopp, L., Sonntag, R. W., & Zimmermann, A. (1978). A case of liver toxicity following cis-dichlorodiammineplatinum(II) treatment. *Cancer Treatment Reports*, *62*(12), 2125–2126. http://www.ncbi.nlm.nih.gov/pubmed/751721.

Cersosimo, R. J. (2005). Oxaliplatin-Associated Neuropathy: A Review. *Annals of Pharmacotherapy*, *39*(1), 128–135. https://doi.org/10.1345/aph.1E319.

Chang, B., Nishikawa, M., Sato, E., Utsumi, K., & Inoue, M. (2002). l-Carnitine inhibits cisplatin-induced injury of the kidney and small intestine. *Archives of Biochemistry and Biophysics*, *405*(1), 55–64. https://doi.org/10.1016/S0003-9861(02)00342-9.

Chang, E. M., Lim, E., Yoon, S., Jeong, K., Bae, S., Lee, D. R., Yoon, T. K., Choi, Y., & Lee, W. S. (2015). Cisplatin Induces Overactivation of the Dormant Primordial Follicle through PTEN/AKT/FOXO3a Pathway which Leads to Loss of Ovarian Reserve in Mice. *PLOS ONE, 10*(12), e0144245. https://doi.org/10.1371/journal.pone.0144245.

Chang, X., Tian, M., Zhang, Q., Liu, F., Gao, J., Li, S., Liu, H., Hou, X., Li, L., Li, C., & Sun, Y. (2021). Grape seed proanthocyanidin extract ameliorates cisplatin-induced testicular apoptosis via PI3K/Akt/mTOR and endoplasmic reticulum stress pathways in rats. *Journal of Food Biochemistry*. https://doi.org/10.1111/jfbc.13825.

Cheng, Y.-J., Wu, R., Cheng, M.-L., Du, J., Hu, X.-W., Yu, L., Zhao, X.-K., Yao, Y.-M., Long, Q.-Z., Zhu, L.-L., Zhu, J.-J., Huang, N.-W., Liu, H.-J., Hu, Y.-X., & Wan, F. (2017). Carboplatin-induced hematotoxicity among patients with non-small cell lung cancer: Analysis on clinical adverse events and drug-gene interactions. *Oncotarget*, *8*(19), 32228–32236. https://doi.org/10.18632/oncotarget.12951.

Chiorazzi, A., Semperboni, S., & Marmiroli, P. (2015). Current View in Platinum Drug Mechanisms of Peripheral Neurotoxicity. *Toxics*, *3*(3), 304–321. https://doi.org/10.3390/toxics3030304.

Chovanec, M., Abu Zaid, M., Hanna, N., El-Kouri, N., Einhorn, L. H., & Albany, C. (2017). Long term toxicity of cisplatin in germ-cell tumor survivors. *Annals of Oncology*, *28*(11), 2670–2679. https://doi.org/10.1093/annonc/mdx360.

Crona, D. J., Faso, A., Nishijima, T. F., McGraw, K. A., Galsky, M. D., & Milowsky, M. I. (2017). A Systematic Review of Strategies to Prevent Cisplatin-Induced Nephrotoxicity. *The Oncologist*, *22*(5), 609–619. https://doi.org/10.1634/theoncologist.2016-0319.

Darmani, N. A., Zhong, W., Chebolu, S., & Mercadante, F. (2015). Differential and additive suppressive effects of 5-HT3 (palonosetron)- and NK1 (netupitant)-receptor antagonists on cisplatin-induced vomiting and ERK1/2, PKA and PKC activation. *Pharmacology Biochemistry and Behavior*, *131*, 104–111. https://doi.org/10.1016/j.pbb.2015.02.010.

Davy, C., & Heathcote, S. (2021). A systematic review of interventions to mitigate radiotherapy-induced oral mucositis in head and neck cancer patients. *Supportive Care in Cancer*, *29*(4), 2187–2202. https://doi.org/10.1007/s00520-020-05548-0.

Dilruba, S., & Kalayda, G. v. (2016). Platinum-based drugs: past, present and future. *Cancer Chemotherapy and Pharmacology*, *77*(6), 1103–1124. https://doi.org/10.1007/s00280-016-2976-z.

Duan, Z., Cai, G., Li, J., & Chen, X. (2020). Cisplatin-induced renal toxicity in elderly people. *Therapeutic Advances in Medical Oncology*, *12*, 175883592092343. https://doi.org/10.1177/1758835920923430.

Elad, S., Cheng, K. K. F., Lalla, R. v., Yarom, N., Hong, C., Logan, R. M., Bowen, J., Gibson, R., Saunders, D. P., Zadik, Y., Ariyawardana, A., Correa, M. E., Ranna, V., Bossi, P., Arany, P., Al-Azri, A. R., Blijlevens, N., Hovan, A., Fregnani, E., Zur, E. (2020). MASCC/ISOO clinical practice guidelines for the management of mucositis secondary to cancer therapy. *Cancer*, *126*(19), 4423–4431. https://doi.org/10.1002/cncr.33100.

El-Awady, E.-S. E., Moustafa, Y. M., Abo-Elmatty, D. M., & Radwan, A. (2011). Cisplatin-induced cardiotoxicity: Mechanisms and cardioprotective strategies. *European Journal of Pharmacology*, *650*(1), 335–341. https://doi.org/10.1016/j.ejphar.2010.09.085.

Falk, P., Severin, M., Guren, M. G., Österlund, P., Hofsli, E., Giwercman, A., Eberhard, J., & Sorbye, H. (2019). Sex hormones and sperm parameters after adjuvant oxaliplatin-based treatment for colorectal cancer. *Annals of Oncology*, *30*, v210. https://doi.org/10.1093/annonc/mdz246.033.

Frisina, R. D., Wheeler, H. E., Fossa, S. D., Kerns, S. L., Fung, C., Sesso, H. D., Monahan, P. O., Feldman, D. R., Hamilton, R., Vaughn, D. J., Beard, C. J., Budnick, A., Johnson, E. M., Ardeshir-Rouhani-Fard, S., Einhorn, L. H., Lipshultz, S. E., Dolan, M. E., & Travis, L. B. (2016). Comprehensive Audiometric Analysis of Hearing Impairment and Tinnitus After Cisplatin-Based Chemotherapy in Survivors of Adult-Onset Cancer. *Journal of Clinical Oncology*, *34*(23), 2712–2720. https://doi.org/10.1200/JCO.2016.66.8822.

Fung, C., Dinh, P., Ardeshir-Rouhani-Fard, S., Schaffer, K., Fossa, S. D., & Travis, L. B. (2018). Toxicities Associated with Cisplatin-Based Chemotherapy and Radiotherapy in Long-Term Testicular Cancer Survivors. *Advances in Urology*, *2018*, 1–20. https://doi.org/10.1155/2018/8671832.

Ghezzi, M., Berretta, M., Bottacin, A., Palego, P., Sartini, B., Cosci, I., Finos, L., Selice, R., Foresta, C., & Garolla, A. (2016). Impact of Bep or Carboplatin Chemotherapy on Testicular Function and Sperm Nucleus of Subjects with Testicular Germ Cell Tumor. *Frontiers in Pharmacology*, *7*. https://doi.org/10.3389/fphar.2016.00122.

Ghosh, S. (2019). Cisplatin: The first metal based anticancer drug. *Bioorganic Chemistry*, *88*, 102925. https://doi.org/10.1016/j.bioorg.2019.102925.

Gill, J. S., & Windebank, A. J. (1998). Cisplatin-induced apoptosis in rat dorsal root ganglion neurons is associated with attempted entry into the cell cycle. *Journal of Clinical Investigation*, *101*(12), 2842–2850. https://doi.org/10.1172/JCI1130.

Go, R. S., & Adjei, A. A. (1999). Review of the comparative pharmacology and clinical activity of cisplatin and carboplatin. *Journal of Clinical Oncology : Official Journal of the American Society of Clinical Oncology*, *17*(1), 409–422. https://doi.org/10.1200/JCO.1999.17.1.409.

Gori, S., Inno, A., Belluomini, L., Bocus, P., Bisoffi, Z., Russo, A., & Arcaro, G. (2019). Gut microbiota and cancer: How gut microbiota modulates activity, efficacy and toxicity of antitumoral therapy. *Critical Reviews in Oncology/Hematology*, *143*, 139–147. https://doi.org/10.1016/j.critrevonc.2019.09.003.

Grueso Cuesta, C., Poquet Jornet, J. E., Gasent Blesa, J. M., Valdivia Perez, A., Carrera Hueso, F. J., & Moreno Royo, L. (2019). Toxicity and effectiveness of carboplatin in obese or overweight patients. *Journal of Oncology Pharmacy Practice*, *25*(6), 1328–1335. https://doi.org/10.1177/1078155218790339.

He, Y. J., Winham, S. J., Hoskins, J. M., Glass, S., Paul, J., Brown, R., Motsinger-Reif, A., & McLeod, H. L. (2016). Carboplatin/taxane-induced gastrointestinal toxicity: a pharmacogenomics study on the SCOTROC1 trial. *The Pharmacogenomics Journal*, *16*(3), 243–248. https://doi.org/10.1038/tpj.2015.52.

Hildebrandt, M. A. T., Komaki, R., Liao, Z., Gu, J., Chang, J. Y., Ye, Y., Lu, C., Stewart, D. J., Minna, J. D., Roth, J. A., Lippman, S. M., Cox, J. D., Hong, W. K., Spitz, M. R., & Wu, X. (2010). Genetic Variants in Inflammation-Related Genes Are Associated with Radiation-Induced Toxicity Following Treatment for Non-Small Cell Lung Cancer. *PLoS ONE*, *5*(8), e12402. https://doi.org/10.1371/journal.pone.0012402.

Horie, S., Oya, M., Nangaku, M., Yasuda, Y., Komatsu, Y., Yanagita, M., Kitagawa, Y., Kuwano, H., Nishiyama, H., Ishioka, C., Takaishi, H., Shimodaira, H., Mogi, A., Ando, Y., Matsumoto, K., Kadowaki, D., & Muto, S. (2018). Guidelines for treatment of renal injury during cancer chemotherapy 2016. *Clinical and Experimental Nephrology*, *22*(1), 210–244. https://doi.org/10.1007/s10157-017-1448-z.

Hruban, R. H., Sternberg, S. S., Meyers, P., Fleisher, M., Menendez-Botet, C., & Boitnott, J. K. (1991). Fatal Thrombocytopenia and Liver Failure Associated with Carboplatin Therapy. *Cancer Investigation*, *9*(3), 263–268. https://doi.org/10.3109/073579091090 21323.

Hu, Y., Sun, B., Zhao, B., Mei, D., Gu, Q., & Tian, Z. (2018). Cisplatin-induced cardiotoxicity with midrange ejection fraction: A case report and review of the literature. *Medicine*, *97*(52), e13807. https://doi.org/10.1097/MD.000000000001380 7.

John, T., Lomeli, N., & Bota, D. A. (2017). Systemic cisplatin exposure during infancy and adolescence causes impaired cognitive function in adulthood. *Behavioural Brain Research*, *319*, 200–206. https://doi.org/10.1016/j.bbr.2016.11.013.

Jones, J. A., Avritscher, E. B. C., Cooksley, C. D., Michelet, M., Bekele, B. N., & Elting, L. S. (2006). Epidemiology of treatment-associated mucosal injury after treatment with newer regimens for lymphoma, breast, lung, or colorectal cancer. *Supportive Care in Cancer*, *14*(6), 505–515. https://doi.org/10.1007/s00520-006-0055-4.

Kanat, O., Ertas, H., & Caner, B. (2017). Platinum-induced neurotoxicity: A review of possible mechanisms. *World Journal of Clinical Oncology*, *8*(4), 329. https://doi.org/ 10.5306/wjco.v8.i4.329.

Kelland, L. (2007). The resurgence of platinum-based cancer chemotherapy. *Nature Reviews. Cancer*, *7*(8), 573–584. https://doi.org/10.1038/nrc2167.

Khan, R., Khan, A. Q., Qamar, W., Lateef, A., Tahir, M., Rehman, M. U., Ali, F., & Sultana, S. (2012). Chrysin protects against cisplatin-induced colon. toxicity via amelioration of oxidative stress and apoptosis: Probable role of p38MAPK and p53. *Toxicology and Applied Pharmacology*, *258*(3), 315–329. https://doi.org/10.1016/ j.taap.2011.11.013.

Kim, H. R., Min, B. S., Kim, J. S., Shin, S. J., Ahn, J. B., Rho, J. K., Kim, N. K., & Rha, S. Y. (2011). Efficacy of Oxaliplatin-Based Chemotherapy in Curatively Resected Colorectal Cancer with Liver Metastasis. *Oncology*, *81*(3–4), 175–183. https://doi.org/ 10.1159/000333440.

Kim, S.-Y., Nair, D. M., Romero, M., Serna, V. A., Koleske, A. J., Woodruff, T. K., & Kurita, T. (2019). Transient inhibition of p53 homologs protects ovarian function from two distinct apoptotic pathways triggered by anticancer therapies. *Cell Death & Differentiation*, *26*(3), 502–515. https://doi.org/10.1038/s41418-018-0151-2.

Kulhan, N. G., Kulhan, M., Turkler, C., Ata, N., Kiremitli, T., Kiremitli, S., Cimen, F. K., Suleyman, H., & Toprak, V. (2019). Effect of lycopene on oxidative ovarian damage induced by cisplatin in rats. *General Physiology and Biophysics*, *38*(03), 253–258. https://doi.org/10.4149/gpb_2019006.

Lalla, R. v., Saunders, D. P., & Peterson, D. E. (2014). Chemotherapy or Radiation-Induced Oral Mucositis. *Dental Clinics of North America*, *58*(2), 341–349. https://doi.org/10.1016/j.cden.2013.12.005.

Landier, W. (2016). Ototoxicity and cancer therapy. *Cancer*, *122*(11), 1647–1658. https://doi.org/10.1002/cncr.29779.

Li, X., Yang, S., Lv, X., Sun, H., Weng, J., Liang, Y., & Zhou, D. (2013). The mechanism of mesna in protection from cisplatin-induced ovarian damage in female rats. *Journal of Gynecologic Oncology*, *24*(2), 177–185. https://doi.org/10.3802/jgo.2013.24.2.177.

Liu, J., Cai, G., Wang, S., Song, Y., Xia, Y., Liang, S., Wang, W., Nie, S., Feng, Z., & Chen, X. (2018). The characteristics and risk factors for cisplatin-induced acute kidney injury in the elderly. *Therapeutics and Clinical Risk Management*, *Volume 14*, 1279–1285. https://doi.org/10.2147/TCRM.S165531.

Loren, A. W., Mangu, P. B., Beck, L. N., Brennan, L., Magdalinski, A. J., Partridge, A. H., Quinn, G., Wallace, W. H., & Oktay, K. (2013). Fertility Preservation for Patients With Cancer: American Society of Clinical Oncology Clinical Practice Guideline Update. *Journal of Clinical Oncology*, *31*(19), 2500–2510. https://doi.org/10.1200/JCO.2013.49.2678.

Lu, Y., & Cederbaum, A. I. (2006). Cisplatin-Induced Hepatotoxicity Is Enhanced by Elevated Expression of Cytochrome P450 2E1. *Toxicological Sciences*, *89*(2), 515–523. https://doi.org/10.1093/toxsci/kfj031

Madeddu, C., Deidda, M., Piras, A., Cadeddu, C., Demurtas, L., Puzzoni, M., Piscopo, G., Scartozzi, M., & Mercuro, G. (2016). Pathophysiology of cardiotoxicity induced by nonanthracycline chemotherapy. *Journal of Cardiovascular Medicine (Hagerstown, Md.)*, *17 Suppl 1*, e12–e18. https://doi.org/10.2459/JCM.0000000000000376.

Maneschi, F., Benedetti-Panici, P., Scambia, G., Salerno, M. G., D'Agostino, G., & Mancuso, S. (1994). Menstrual and Hormone Patterns in Women Treated with High-Dose Cisplatin and Bleomycin. *Gynecologic Oncology*, *54*(3), 345–348. https://doi.org/10.1006/gyno.1994.1221.

McDonald, E. S., & Windebank, A. J. (2002). Cisplatin-Induced Apoptosis of DRG Neurons Involves Bax Redistribution and Cytochrome cRelease But Not fas Receptor Signaling. *Neurobiology of Disease*, *9*(2), 220–233. https://doi.org/10.1006/nbdi.2001.0468.

McGuire, D. B., Fulton, J. S., Park, J., Brown, C. G., Correa, M. E. P., Eilers, J., Elad, S., Gibson, F., Oberle-Edwards, L. K., Bowen, J., & Lalla, R. v. (2013). Systematic review of basic oral care for the management of oral mucositis in cancer patients. *Supportive Care in Cancer*, *21*(11), 3165–3177. https://doi.org/10.1007/s00520-013-1942-0.

Meng, X.-M., Ren, G.-L., Gao, L., Yang, Q., Li, H.-D., Wu, W.-F., Huang, C., Zhang, L., Lv, X., & Li, J. (2018). NADPH oxidase 4 promotes cisplatin-induced acute kidney injury via ROS-mediated programmed cell death and inflammation. *Laboratory Investigation*, *98*(1), 63–78. https://doi.org/10.1038/labinvest.2017.120.

Mitchell, E. P. (2006). Gastrointestinal Toxicity of Chemotherapeutic Agents. *Seminars in Oncology*, *33*(1), 106–120. https://doi.org/10.1053/j.seminoncol.2005.12.001.

Nishii, M., Soutome, S., Kawakita, A., Yutori, H., Iwata, E., Akashi, M., Hasegawa, T., Kojima, Y., Funahara, M., Umeda, M., & Komori, T. (2020). Factors associated with severe oral mucositis and candidiasis in patients undergoing radiotherapy for oral and oropharyngeal carcinomas: a retrospective multicenter study of 326 patients. *Supportive Care in Cancer*, *28*(3), 1069–1075. https://doi.org/10.1007/s00520-019-04885-z.

Ongnok, B., Chattipakorn, N., & Chattipakorn, S. C. (2020). Doxorubicin and cisplatin induced cognitive impairment: The possible mechanisms and interventions. *Experimental Neurology*, *324*, 113118. https://doi.org/10.1016/j.expneurol.2019.113118.

Oshita, F., Yamada, K., Nomura, I., Tanaka, G., Ikehara, M., & Noda, K. (2001). Randomized study of dose or schedule modification of granulocyte colony-stimulating factor in platinum-based chemotherapy for elderly patients with lung cancer. *Oncology Reports*, *8*(4), 861–866. https://doi.org/10.3892/or.8.4.861.

Oun, R., Moussa, Y. E., & Wheate, N. J. (2018). The side effects of platinum-based chemotherapy drugs: a review for chemists. *Dalton Transactions*, *47*(19), 6645–6653. https://doi.org/10.1039/C8DT00838H.

Pellacani, C., & Eleftheriou, G. (2020). Neurotoxicity of antineoplastic drugs: Mechanisms, susceptibility, and neuroprotective strategies. *Advances in Medical Sciences*, *65*(2), 265–285. https://doi.org/10.1016/j.advms.2020.04.001.

Riley, P., Glenny, A.-M., Hua, F., & Worthington, H. v. (2017). Pharmacological interventions for preventing dry mouth and salivary gland dysfunction following radiotherapy. *Cochrane Database of Systematic Reviews*, *7*, CD012744. https://doi.org/10.1002/14651858.CD012744.

Rosenthal, D. I. (2007). Consequences of mucositis-induced treatment breaks and dose reductions on head and neck cancer treatment outcomes. *The Journal of Supportive Oncology*, *5*(9 Suppl 4), 23–31. https://doi.org/18046995.

Ruf, C. G., Borck, S., Anheuser, P., Matthies, C., Nestler, T., Zecha, H., Isbarn, H., & Dieckmann, K.-P. (2019). Adjuvant carboplatin therapy in patients with clinical stage 1 testicular seminoma: is long-term morbidity increased? *Journal of Cancer Research and Clinical Oncology*, *145*(9), 2335–2342. https://doi.org/10.1007/s00432-019-02965-5.

Rybak, L. P., Mukherjea, D., Jajoo, S., Kaur, T., & Ramkumar, V. (2012). siRNA-mediated knock-down of NOX3: therapy for hearing loss? *Cellular and Molecular Life Sciences*, *69*(14), 2429–2434. https://doi.org/10.1007/s00018-012-1016-3.

Rybak, L. P., Mukherjea, D., Jajoo, S., & Ramkumar, V. (2009). Cisplatin Ototoxicity and Protection: Clinical and Experimental Studies. *The Tohoku Journal of Experimental Medicine*, *219*(3), 177–186. https://doi.org/10.1620/tjem.219.177.

Salman, M., Naseem, I., Hassan, I., Khan, A. A., & Alhazza, I. M. (2015). Riboflavin Arrests Cisplatin-Induced Neurotoxicity by Ameliorating Cellular Damage in Dorsal Root Ganglion Cells. *BioMed Research International*, *2015*, 1–5. https://doi.org/10.1155/2015/603543.

Santos, N. A. G. dos, Ferreira, R. S., & Santos, A. C. dos. (2020). Overview of cisplatin-induced neurotoxicity and ototoxicity, and the protective agents. *Food and Chemical Toxicology*, *136*, 111079. https://doi.org/10.1016/j.fct.2019.111079.

Sarin, N., Engel, F., Rothweiler, F., Cinatl, J., Michaelis, M., Frötschl, R., Fröhlich, H., & Kalayda, G. (2018). Key Players of Cisplatin Resistance: Towards a Systems Pharmacology Approach. *International Journal of Molecular Sciences*, *19*(3), 767. https://doi.org/10.3390/ijms19030767.

Shahid, F., Farooqui, Z., Abidi, S., Parwez, I., & Khan, F. (2017a). Oral administration of thymoquinone mitigates the effect of cisplatin on brush border membrane enzymes, energy metabolism and antioxidant system in rat intestine. *Biomedicine & Pharmacotherapy*, *94*, 1111–1120. https://doi.org/10.1016/j.biopha.2017.08.044.

Shahid, F., Farooqui, Z., & Khan, F. (2018). Cisplatin-induced gastrointestinal toxicity: An update on possible mechanisms and on available gastroprotective strategies. *European Journal of Pharmacology*, *827*, 49–57. https://doi.org/10.1016/j.ejphar.2018.03.009.

Shahid, F., Farooqui, Z., Rizwan, S., Abidi, S., Parwez, I., & Khan, F. (2017b). Oral administration of Nigella sativa oil ameliorates the effect of cisplatin on brush border membrane enzymes, carbohydrate metabolism and antioxidant system in rat intestine. *Experimental and Toxicologic Pathology*, *69*(5), 299–306. https://doi.org/10.1016/j.etp.2017.02.001.

Sherif, I. O., Abdel-Aziz, A., & Sarhan, O. M. (2014). Cisplatin-induced testicular toxicity in rats: The protective effect of arjunolic acid. *Journal of Biochemical and Molecular Toxicology*, *28*(11), 515–521. https://doi.org/10.1002/jbt.21593.

Sheth, S., Mukherjea, D., Rybak, L. P., & Ramkumar, V. (2017). Mechanisms of Cisplatin-Induced Ototoxicity and Otoprotection. *Frontiers in Cellular Neuroscience*, *11*. https://doi.org/10.3389/fncel.2017.00338.

Smith, P., Lavery, A., & Turkington, R. C. (2020). An overview of acute gastrointestinal side effects of systemic anti-cancer therapy and their management. *Best Practice & Research Clinical Gastroenterology*, *48–49*, 101691. https://doi.org/10.1016/j.bpg.2020.101691.

Sonis, S. T. (2009). Mucositis: The impact, biology and therapeutic opportunities of oral mucositis. *Oral Oncology*, *45*(12), 1015–1020. https://doi.org/10.1016/j.oraloncology.2009.08.006.

Sonis, S. T. (2013). Oral Mucositis in Head and Neck Cancer: Risk, Biology, and Management. *American Society of Clinical Oncology Educational Book*, *33*, e236–e240. https://doi.org/10.1200/EdBook_AM.2013.33.e236.

Spears, N., Lopes, F., Stefansdottir, A., Rossi, V., de Felici, M., Anderson, R. A., & Klinger, F. G. (2019). Ovarian damage from chemotherapy and current approaches to its protection. *Human Reproduction Update*, *25*(6), 673–693. https://doi.org/10.1093/humupd/dmz027.

Stojanovska, V., Sakkal, S., & Nurgali, K. (2015). Platinum-based chemotherapy: Gastrointestinal immunomodulation and enteric nervous system toxicity. In *American Journal of Physiology - Gastrointestinal and Liver Physiology* (Vol. 308, Issue 4, pp. G223–G232). American Physiological Society. https://doi.org/10.1152/ajpgi.00212.2014.

Ta, L. E., Espeset, L., Podratz, J., & Windebank, A. J. (2006). Neurotoxicity of oxaliplatin and cisplatin for dorsal root ganglion neurons correlates with platinum–DNA binding. *NeuroToxicology*, *27*(6), 992–1002. https://doi.org/10.1016/j.neuro.2006.04.010.

Tabassum, H., Waseem, M., Parvez, S., & Qureshi, M. I. (2015). Oxaliplatin-induced Oxidative Stress Provokes Toxicity in Isolated Rat Liver Mitochondria. *Archives of Medical Research*, *46*(8), 597–603. https://doi.org/10.1016/j.arcmed.2015.10.002.

Tang, Q., Wang, X., Jin, H., Mi, Y., Liu, L., Dong, M., Chen, Y., & Zou, Z. (2021). Cisplatin-induced ototoxicity: Updates on molecular mechanisms and otoprotective strategies. *European Journal of Pharmaceutics and Biopharmaceutics*, *163*, 60–71. https://doi.org/10.1016/j.ejpb.2021.03.008.

Tsuruya, K., Tokumoto, M., Ninomiya, T., Hirakawa, M., Masutani, K., Taniguchi, M., Fukuda, K., Kanai, H., Hirakata, H., & Iida, M. (2003). Antioxidant ameliorates cisplatin-induced renal tubular cell death through inhibition of death receptor-mediated pathways. *American Journal of Physiology-Renal Physiology*, *285*(2), F208–F218. https://doi.org/10.1152/ajprenal.00311.2002.

van der Vijgh, W. J. (1991). Clinical pharmacokinetics of carboplatin. *Clinical Pharmacokinetics*, *21*(4), 242–261. https://doi.org/10.2165/00003088-199121040-00002

van Dorp, W., Haupt, R., Anderson, R. A., Mulder, R. L., van den Heuvel-Eibrink, M. M., van Dulmen-den Broeder, E., Su, H. I., Winther, J. F., Hudson, M. M., Levine, J. M., & Wallace, W. H. (2018). Reproductive Function and Outcomes in Female Survivors of Childhood, Adolescent, and Young Adult Cancer: A Review. *Journal of Clinical Oncology*, *36*(21), 2169–2180. https://doi.org/10.1200/JCO.2017.76.3441.

Vera, G., Castillo, M., Cabezos, P. A., Chiarlone, A., Martín, M. I., Gori, A., Pasquinelli, G., Barbara, G., Stanghellini, V., Corinaldesi, R., de Giorgio, R., & Abalo, R. (2011). Enteric neuropathy evoked by repeated cisplatin in the rat. *Neurogastroenterology and Motility*, *23*(4), 370. https://doi.org/10.1111/j.1365-2982.2011.01674.x.

Vera-Llonch, M., Oster, G., Ford, C. M., Lu, J., & Sonis, S. (2007). Oral mucositis and outcomes of allogeneic hematopoietic stem-cell transplantation in patients with hematologic malignancies. *Supportive Care in Cancer*, *15*(5), 491–496. https://doi.org/10.1007/s00520-006-0176-9.

Vera-Llonch, M., Oster, G., Hagiwara, M., & Sonis, S. (2006). Oral mucositis in patients undergoing radiation treatment for head and neck carcinoma. *Cancer*, *106*(2), 329–336. https://doi.org/10.1002/cncr.21622.

Wakiya, T., Kudo, D., Ishido, K., Kimura, N., Yakoshi, Y., Toyoki, Y., Kijima, H., & Hakamada, K. (2017). Effect of age on the development of chemotherapy-associated liver injury in colorectal cancer liver metastasis. *Molecular and Clinical Oncology*. https://doi.org/10.3892/mco.2017.1314.

Yamada, T. H., Denburg, N. L., Beglinger, L. J., & Schultz, S. K. (2010). Neuropsychological Outcomes of Older Breast Cancer Survivors: Cognitive Features Ten or More Years After Chemotherapy. *The Journal of Neuropsychiatry and Clinical Neurosciences*, *22*(1), 48–54. https://doi.org/10.1176/jnp.2010.22.1.48.

Zhu, S., Pabla, N., Tang, C., He, L., & Dong, Z. (2015). DNA damage response in cisplatin-induced nephrotoxicity. *Archives of Toxicology*, *89*(12), 2197–2205. https://doi.org/10.1007/s00204-015-1633-3.

Chapter 4

Peripheral Neuropathy and Cognitive Impairment Caused by Platinum-Based Chemotherapy

Hannah R. Wardill[1,2,*], Ysabella Z. A. Van Sebille[3], Nadeen T. Ali[4] and Lisa B. Grech[5]

[1]School of Biomedicine, The University of Adelaide, Australia
[2] Supportive Oncology Research Group, Precision Medicine (Cancer), South Australian Health and Medical Research Institute, Australia
[3]Division of Health Sciences, University of South Australia, Australia
[4]Faculty of Pharmacy, Al-Yarmouk College, Khartoum, Sudan
[5]Medicine Monash Health, Monash University, Australia

Abstract

Platinum-based compounds are used in more than 50% of all combination chemotherapeutic treatment schedules. While highly efficacious, these agents are highly neurotoxic and induce damage to neurons in the peripheral and central nervous systems. Peripheral neuropathy is particularly problematic, causing numbness and pain in the hands and feet, however in severe circumstances symptoms can progress up towards the trunk to affect the entire limb. This increases the risk of falls, impairs mobility and severely impacts daily living. Peripheral neuropathy remains without effective intervention, with current strategies largely relying on opioids to manage neuropathic pain. As such, neuropathy is a common driver of dose reductions, delays and even complete cessation of treatment. Neurotoxicity in the central nervous system most typically presents as cognitive impairment, however, is

[*]Corresponding Author's Email: hannah.wardill@adelaide.edu.au.

In: Platinum-Based Chemotherapy
Editors: Kulmira Nurgali and Raquel Abalo
ISBN: 978-1-68507-972-7
© 2022 Nova Science Publishers, Inc.

often accompanied by a range of neuropsychological symptoms including fatigue, anxiety and depression. These, often chronic, symptoms have profound impacts on a patient's capacity to return to work after cancer, and thus is associated with significant economic burden and a profound loss in quality of life. While it is understood how platinum-based drugs damage neurons, the ability of these drugs to access the brain remains unclear, and as such, cognitive impairment and associated psychoneurological symptoms are poorly managed. This chapter provides an overview of the neurotoxic profiles of platinum-based drugs, the aetiology of both peripheral neuropathy and cognitive impairment, a summary of their risk factors, assessment tools and current evidence on emerging strategies to prevent or manage these symptoms.

Keywords: cognitive impairment, neurotoxicity, peripheral neuropathy, platinum chemotherapy, supportive care

Introduction

Platinum-based chemotherapy drugs, including cisplatin, carboplatin and oxaliplatin, are used in a range of clinical scenarios, included in almost half of all multi-drug chemotherapy regimens. While these compounds have a particularly high anti-cancer potency, especially the third-generation compound oxaliplatin, their use is challenged by their high rate of neurotoxicity (Zajaczkowska et al. 2019). Unlike other side effects, neurotoxicity appears to occur independently of the anti-tumor effects of chemotherapeutic drugs, and as such, neurotoxic mechanisms are poorly defined and symptoms inadequately managed. Subsequently, they account for prolonged infusion times and significant dose-reductions, limiting the depth of response achieved by platinum-based chemotherapy treatment and increasing tumor progression.

It remains somewhat unclear why platinum-based chemotherapy drugs cause neurotoxicity given the relatively stable and quiescent nature of neurological cell populations (i.e., non-dividing) (Carozzi, Canta & Chiorazzi 2015). What has been characterized is that these agents induce a range of cellular changes in neuronal populations, including direct DNA damage and cell death, oxidative stress, mitochondrial dysfunction and neuroinflammation. It has remained unclear which of these factors causally drive symptoms, and few have been successfully targeted to prevent or manage symptoms. The general lack of understanding of these toxic consequences of platinum-based chemotherapy is further complicated by the heterogeneous presentation of neurological symptoms which fail to be clearly linked with demographic, genetic and other risk factors (Bai & Yu 2021).

Neurotoxicity affects both the peripheral and central nervous systems. Damage to peripheral neurons results in classical symptoms of neuropathy, including pain, numbness, tingling which impacts daily function, balance and increase in the risk of falls (Argyriou et al. 2012). In the central nervous system, neurotoxicity presents as an umbrella of psychological and neurocognitive symptoms including cognitive impairment, fatigue, depression and anxiety (Bai & Yu 2021). In both cases, these symptoms can persist chronically and therefore have substantial impacts on quality of life in both the active-treatment phase and post-treatment survivorship setting. This chapter will provide an overview of these neurotoxic consequences, discussing their aetiology, risk factors, clinical presentation, assessment, prevention and management. We also discuss limitations in our current understanding as well as areas of emerging and future research.

Pharmacological Actions of Platinum-Based Chemotherapy and Their Neurotoxic Potency

Platinum-based chemotherapeutic agents are widely used in the treatment of several types of solid tumors. The major platinum-based chemotherapy drugs in current clinical use are cisplatin, carboplatin and oxaliplatin; each with similar but unique mechanisms and differing clinical consequences (Table 1). Of these agents, the understanding of the mechanisms of cisplatin have been best studied owing to its longstanding clinical use.

Cisplatin (cis-diamine chloroplatinic (II)) is administered intravenously in a high concentration saline solution (~100mM), and thus remains stable and neutral in an unaltered state (Ghosh 2019). Cisplatin enters cells via passive diffusion, activated by exchanging one of the chloride ligands with a water ligand (Fuertes et al. 2003). Reflecting the low quantity of chloride in the cytoplasm (4-20 mM), cisplatin undergoes mono- and/or di-aquation, with mono-aquated platinum considered a more potent DNA binding agent. Cisplatin's cytotoxicity (against tumours) is driven by forming complex Fas-associated death domain (FADD) and procaspade-8, which work together to produce an apoptosome complex (Florea & Busselberg 2011; Fuertes et al. 2003). This apoptosome complex triggers caspase-8, which then activates caspase-3, caspase-6, and caspase-7, resulting in the cleavage of a critical substrate and cell death. Cisplatin's primary target is genomic DNA (gDNA), however, only a small percentage (1%) of intercellular cisplatin is typically linked to gDNA (Ghosh 2019). Several proteins, including high mobility group (HMG) proteins, can quickly detect cisplatin-DNA complexes, detecting and binding to 1,2-cisplatin-DNA adducts (Imamura et al. 2001) to modulate cell death (Zamble et al. 2002). Cell death also results from cisplatin-induced cell cycle arrest (G1, S, and G2 phases) via interaction with checkpoint kinases Chk1 and Chk2 (Pabla et al. 2008). Inhibiting these arrests induces cell death by forcing cells to resume the cell cycle prematurely in the face of unrepaired DNA damage (Pabla et al. 2008; Shen et al. 2013), which accelerates cell death via the nucleotide excision repair (NER) pathway.

Table 1. Mechanism of action and neurotoxicity of platinum agents

	First generation (e.g., Cisplatin)	**Second generation** (e.g., Carboplatin)	**Third generation** (e.g., Oxaliplatin)
Mechanism of action and relative neurotoxicity	Crosslink with DNA leading to cell cycle disruption and subsequently cancer cell death.	Crosslink with DNA leading to cell cycle disruption and subsequently cancer cell death. Less cytotoxic than cisplatin	Form platinum-DNA adducts which lead to blocking DNA replication. More cytotoxic than cisplatin
Drivers of central neurotoxicity	Apoptosis, oxidative stress, mitochondrial dysfunction, synaptic loss, neuroinflammation and gliosis.	Mitochondrial dysfunction, neuroinflammation and gliosis.	Mitochondrial dysfunction, oxidative stress.
Peripheral neurotoxicity	Affect peripheral nerves and dorsal root ganglia neurons and cause apoptosis, mitochondrial dysfunction, ion channel dysfunction (channelopathy affecting Ca2+ channels but not Na+ or K+ channels) and oxidative stress.	Affect peripheral nerves and dorsal root ganglia neurons and cause apoptosis, mitochondrial dysfunction, ion channel dysfunction (channelopathy affecting Ca2+ channels but not Na+ or K+ channels) and oxidative stress.	**Acute:** dysfunction of nodal axonal voltage-gated Na+ channels, secondary to an oxalate-chelating effect of both Ca2+ and Mg2. **Chronic:** affect peripheral nerves and dorsal root ganglia neurons and cause apoptosis.

Carboplatin (1,1 cyclobutyl dicarboxylate) is a second-generation platinum agent, which is generally less neurotoxic compared to cisplatin, with a 10-fold higher dose required to induce comparable effects to cisplatin (Vermorken et al. 1993). Despite this difference in potency, carboplatin has a similar mechanism of action to cisplatin, differing only in terms of its chemical structure (de Sousa et al. 2015). Importantly, carboplatin has a bidentate dicarboxylate chelate leaving ligand, which makes the molecule less chemically reactive than cisplatin. This increased chemical stability accounts for its lesser reactivity with nucleophilic sites of DNA, which is responsible for the higher dosages required to achieve antitumor effects comparable to cisplatin.

Oxaliplatin is a third-generation platinum agent that differs in a spectrum of activity from other platinum drugs (Ali, Mohamed & Yousef 2020). Oxaliplatin inhibits DNA synthesis by working as diamino cyclohexane (DACH) carrier ligand-based platinum chemical. The primary cytotoxic lesions are intra-strand platinum-DNA adducts developed by cross-linking between activated platinum species and particular base sequences (Alian, Azmi & Mohammad 2012; Hsu et al. 2019). Oxaliplatin undergoes nonenzymatic conversion into active derivatives, which then bind preferentially to guanine and cytosine moieties of DNA. This cross-linking inhibits DNA synthesis and transcription, resulting in cell cycle arrest and apoptosis. Generally, oxaliplatin is considered to be the most neurotoxic of the platinum-based compounds due to the replacement of the two amine groups (present in cisplatin) by cyclohexyldiamine increasing its neurotoxicity (Pasetto et al. 2006).

Peripheral Neuropathy

Clinical Prevalence and Presentation

Chemotherapy-induced peripheral neuropathy (CIPN) is an increasingly important and prevalent problem in cancer care as new therapies become increasingly available, patients are surviving longer, and the importance of quality of life as an endpoint is increasingly acknowledged (Forman 2004). The Multinational Association of Supportive Care in Cancer (MASCC) has highlighted that CIPN is particularly associated with platinum agents (Chan, Hertz, et al. 2019). CIPN is defined as somatic or autonomic symptoms resulting from injury to peripheral and autonomic neurons caused by chemotherapeutic agents. Reported in 57-83% of patients undergoing taxane and platinum-based chemotherapy, CIPN is amongst the most common long-term adverse effects of cancer therapy. In fact, a recent meta-analysis in over 4000 people reported acute CIPN prevalence of 68% in adults with cancer. Similarly, in a study of more than 100 children undergoing vinca alkaloids or platinum-based chemotherapy, symptoms consistent with CIPN were reported in more than 50% survivors at 8.5 years post-treatment. These peripheral nerve disorders are occurring so often in cancer patients that reduced deep tendon reflexes are found routinely on neurologic examination (Forman 2004).

While there is considerable variability in CIPN severity between patients, and it can affect all nerve fibers, symptoms are most often sensory-predominant, characterized by pain (specifically, allodynia, hyperalgesia, dysthesia and paresthesia) (Staff et al. 2017). The characteristic manifestation of CIPN is severe episodes of neuropathic pain involving tactile and thermal allodynia, hyperalgesia and spontaneous pain largely affecting the distal limbs. CIPN symptoms usually begin in the first 2 months of cancer treatment, progressing throughout chemotherapy treatment, and stabilizing soon after treatment completion. Typically, CIPN symptoms are dose-dependent, developing after several cycles of neurotoxic chemotherapy administration, however, there are drug-specific features that have been reported including acute neurotoxicity of paclitaxel and oxaliplatin, which includes cold-induced dysesthesia, most severe in the hands, face and oral cavity, particularly from oxaliplatin (Ali, Mohamed & Yousef 2020). Cold wind on the face or cold drinks may trigger the intense pain, with symptoms typically beginning with the second or third cycle of treatment and lasting for 2 to 4 days after drug infusion. Further, the worsening for several months of neuropathy after discontinuation of cisplatin or oxaliplatin, commonly termed, 'coasting' is an important characteristic of platinum-based chemotherapy-induced (Staff et al. 2017).

While sensation of pain is associated with disturbance of sensory function associated with damage of large myelinated sensory fibers, CIPN also affects motor and autonomic functions caused by general damage of PNS (Lazic et al. 2020). Thus, CIPN is also accompanied by signs and symptoms consistent with axonopathy, including 'stocking-glove' sensory loss, weakness, hyporeflexia and deficits in manual dexterity/balance. These symptoms severely impact an individual's ability to perform daily tasks and increase the risk of falls, which together have a significant and negative impact on the quality of life of people living with or beyond cancer. Further, the neurotoxic effects on peripheral nerves that cause CIPN often result in discontinuation or reduction of cancer therapy, affecting efficacy of treatment and quality of life (Carozzi, Canta & Chiorazzi 2015; Lazic et al. 2020; Miltenburg & Boogerd 2014). In addition to the significant impact on patient quality of life and survival, CIPN also significantly increases the annual costs of health care (Pike et al. 2012).

Risk Factors

Patient-Related Factors

Demographics and Biological Factors

Age and weight have been suggested to modulate the risk of platinum agent induced peripheral neuropathy (PN), with older, obese patients (body surface area > 2.0) more likely to develop symptoms (Staff et al. 2017; Timmins et al. 2021; Zajaczkowska et al. 2019). While other factors, including physical activity and diet have also been suggested as risk factors, it is largely unclear what demographic factors related to the patient make them more or less susceptible (Chan, Hertz, et al. 2019). Biological factors have also been shown to influence the risk of PN, with low magnesium, hemoglobin, and albumin levels (Argyriou et al. 2017; Argyriou et al. 2012; Staff et al. 2017), or low creatinine clearance associated with a higher risk of severe PN (Colvin 2019).

Comorbidities

Comorbid medical conditions such as diabetes (Colvin 2019), inherited neurotoxicity such as Charcot-Marie-tooth disease (Chan, Hertz, et al. 2019; Staff et al. 2017) and history of previous neurological disease all associated with a greater risk of CIPN (Argyriou et al. 2017). Importantly, the severity of previous CIPN events and the development of acute neurotoxic symptoms has also been reported to increase the risk of chronic CIPN. In fact, individuals with a history of neurotoxicity are more than eight times more likely to acquire CIPN, primarily affecting motor function (Molassiotis, Cheng, et al. 2019).

Genetic Factors

A number of single-nucleotide polymorphisms (SNPs) have been linked to CIPN in numerous studies, although the effect sizes of these studies are lacking (Molassiotis, Cheng, et al. 2019). Generally, the SNPs associated with

CIPN risk are associated with DNA repair systems, drug transport and metabolism, brain development and repair, microtubule systems, which therefore result in individuals differentially metabolizing neurotoxic drugs, clearing them at differing rates or being more susceptible to their cytotoxic properties (Avan et al. 2015; Chan, Hertz, et al. 2019; Chan, Yeo, et al. 2019; Tchounwou et al. 2021). DNA repair genes ERCC2 and XRCC1 have been identified as possible SNPs linked with CIPN in patients treated with platinum agents (Staff et al. 2017), as well as variations in glutathione-S-transferase genes P1 (GSTP1); glutathione-S-transferase genes M1 (GSTM1); and voltage-gated sodium channel genes SCN4A, SCN9A and SCN10A (Zajaczkowska et al. 2019).

Treatment-Related Factors

As outlined in this chapter, platinum compounds are particularly neurotoxic, and thus, their inclusion in multimodal cancer therapy is associated with an increased risk of neuropathy (Avan et al. 2015). Neuropathy caused by platinum compounds, namely cisplatin, has been linked to cumulative dosage rather than single doses (Jongen, Broijl & Sonneveld 2015), however, it is important to note that CIPN is high variable (Zajaczkowska et al. 2019). Neurotoxicity occurs at cumulative doses of more than 350 mg/m2 for cisplatin (Park et al. 2013) and at the cumulative dose of 500-600 mg/m2, the incidence of acute neuropathy is 92% with 5-20% still symptomatic 12 months post-therapy (Zajaczkowska et al. 2019). While oxaliplatin is considered more cytotoxic than cisplatin, the dose of oxaliplatin required to induce peripheral chronic neuropathic symptoms is 780 mg/m2 (Ali, Mohamed & Yousef 2020), and 85 to 130 mg/m2 up to 5-7 days for acute symptoms. In both cases, as the number of treatment cycles increases, the severity of peripheral neurotoxicity will also increase (Ali, Mohamed & Yousef 2020; Park et al. 2013). Carboplatin seems to be less toxic, with neuropathy observed in 13–42% of patients (Colvin 2019; Hausheer et al. 2006).

Using platinum agents in combination therapy is considered a contributing factor for peripheral neuropathy (Jongen, Broijl & Sonneveld 2015). The combination of cisplatin or carboplatin with taxanes has been associated with an increased risk of peripheral neuropathy (Argyriou et al. 2017). Some studies indicate that using FOLFOX (oxaliplatin in combination with 5-fluorouracil and leucovorin) is associated with a higher incidence of chronic oxaliplatin neurotoxicity as compared to XELOX (oxaliplatin in a combination regimen with capecitabine), while others found the reverse (Ali, Mohamed & Yousef 2020; Murono et al. 2019). The safety of other drug combinations with platinum-based therapies has also been investigated. For example, paclitaxel combined with 5-FU, folinic acid, oxaliplatin and bevacizumab (mFOLFOX6-bevacizimab) was compared to paclitaxel with capecitabine, oxaliplatin and bevacizumab (CapeOX-bevacizumab) in Phase I trial of people with colorectal cancer. Although the study population was small (N = 6), peripheral neuropathy was observed in all patients, however there were no differences in its incidence compared to oxaliplatin alone (Murono et al. 2019). While investigating adverse effects is best approached in the clinical setting, animal models offer a highly controlled environment to investigate side effects, including neuropathy. A recent study investigated oxaliplatin (i.e., 10 mg/kg cumulative), paclitaxel (i.e., 4 mg/kg cumulative) and combined oxaliplatin and paclitaxel in male Wistar rats (Paniagua et al. 2021). Neuropathy was assessed using the Von Frey test (specifically assessed tactile allodynia), acetone test (specifically assessed cold allodynia), PAM test (specifically assessed mechanical hyperalgesia) and behavioral analyses (for pain-like behavior). All agents induced chronic, painful neuropathy in the hind legs and orofacial regions. There was no additional burden when these drugs were applied in combination, underscoring the fact that combination therapy does not pose additional safety concerns related to peripheral neuropathy.

Pathobiology

Our understanding of the pathophysiological mechanisms of peripheral neuropathy has accelerated greatly over the past decade. It is generally understood that most CIPN symptoms observed arise from damage to the dorsal root ganglion neurons and and/or their axons following cancer treatment. Neuropathy, including sensory neuronopathy, length-dependent sensorimotor neuropathy, or small fiber neuropathies, are hypothesized to be based on anatomical changes including distal axonal degeneration or on physiological changes (Chan, Hertz, et al. 2019). PNS neuronal cells exposed to chemotherapy drugs accumulate the same molecular damage as do cancer cells, including damage to the genomic DNA (Lazic et al. 2020). The damage seen in peripheral neurons includes oxidative stress, change of calcium homeostasis, axon degeneration and membrane remodeling, all caused by neuroinflammation and triggering of apoptotic pathways (Staff et al. 2017). The main cause of apoptosis observed in these neurons is considered to be due to DNA damage (Carozzi, Canta & Chiorazzi 2015; Carozzi, Marmiroli &

Cavaletti 2010; Lazic et al. 2020). The inflammation noted in CIPN includes increased macrophages and inflammatory markers such as CCL2, IL-1β, and TNF-α in the Dorsal root ganglion cells (DRG) which can cause neuronal hyperexcitability by suppressing GABA production and glutamate clearance (Omran et al. 2021). There is also innate immune system involvement, with toll-like receptor 4 (TLR4) activated in the spinal cord following chemotherapy treatment (Byrd-Leifer et al. 2001). This is further evidenced as CIPN symptoms are reduced when the TLR4 pathway is blocked, either through an antagonist or genetic knock out (Li et al. 2015; Li et al. 2014).

Neuropathic pain is likely amplified by both peripheral nerve hyperexcitability through altered bioenergetics and ion channel expression and through central sensitization (Staff et al. 2017). For example, the changes in ion channels that can cause hyperactivity are demonstrated with oxaliplatin causing prolonged opening of sodium channels, down regulation of potassium channels in peripheral nerves and DRGs, increased calcium channel expression in DRGs following paclitaxel, and calcium channel antagonists reducing CIPN symptoms in rodents (Omran et al. 2021). Mitochondrial dysfunction has also been observed in CIPN, with platinum compounds causing swollen and vacuolated mitochondria with a reduction in respiration and ATP production in sensory nerves and DRGs (Omran et al. 2021). Reactive oxygen species (ROS) and reactive nitrogen species (RNS) impact neuronal excitability, with studies showing that ROS scavengers reduce CIPN symptoms (Fidanboylu, Griffiths & Flatters 2011; Janes et al. 2013; Kim et al. 2010). This oxidative stress is another hypothesis of the development of CIPN, as mitochondria and other cellular components are key sources of ROS and RNS. However, important to note is that these studies have primarily been done with taxanes not platinum compounds. The differences seen in CIPN such as the 'dying back' neuropathy of axonal degeneration at the most distal extent of the axon, which is most common, versus the sensory neuropathy observed in platinum compounds is likely related to the permeability of the blood-nerve barrier at the level of the DRG (Staff et al. 2017).

In addition to the direct damage to the neuron, there is some evidence for the role of non-neuronal cells in the development of CIPN, however more research in this area is needed. It has been suggested that there is a link between platinum compound-induced neuropathy and glial activation (Di Cesare Mannelli et al. 2013; Di Cesare Mannelli et al. 2014). Di Cesare Mennelli et al., (2014) showed in a rodent model of oxaliplatin-induced peripheral neuropathy that transient activation of microglia and astrocytes in the spinal cord and supraspinal areas involved with pain modulation was associated with a decrease in pain thresholds following oxaliplatin administration. When microglial inhibitor, minocycline, and astrocyte specific metabolic inhibitor, fluorocitrate were co-administered with oxaliplatin, tolerance to painful insults was increased. However, neither minocycline nor fluorocitrate prevented oxaliplatin-dependent morphological alterations in DRG neurons. Further, the role of other non-neuronal cells such as Schwann cells in CIPN is not well understood and requires further investigation.

While most of the research on CIPN mechanisms has focused on PNS changes, there is emerging research to suggest that the CNS may play a role in the pathogenesis of CIPN (Omran et al. 2021). Similar to the reorganization and compensation seen in other peripheral nerve damage conditions such as phantom limb pain, it is hypothesized that the brain may play a role in CIPN despite the obvious peripheral pathology that underpins CIPN. The hypothesis is supported by the fact that duloxetine, one of the only proven treatments for CIPN, is a serotonin-norepinephrine reuptake inhibitor that acts in the brain (Smith, EM et al. 2013; Smith, T & Nicholson 2007). The hypothesis of brain involvement in CIPN has been studied in humans (Boland et al. 2014; Dougherty 2016; Kleckner et al. 2018; Nudelman et al. 2016; Prinsloo et al. 2017; Weng, Cordella & Dougherty 2003) and rodents (Ferris et al. 2019; Thibault et al. 2012), and the synthesis of these studies, and subsequent presentation of the hypothesis, is outlined by Orman and colleagues (2021). Briefly, to support this hypothesis they first show that CIPN is associated with hyperactivity and hyperexcitability in the periaqueductal gray, thalamus, anterior cingulate cortex, secondary somatosensory cortex, and insula brain regions. This is unsurprising given these regions are part of a well-known circuitry related to pain sensation and perception. Secondly, they present that reduced GABAergic inhibition in the brain is associated with CIPN which changes excitatory and inhibitory balance, creating a molecular environment that promotes neuronal hyperactivity. In addition, they showed that activating GABA receptors or increasing GABA levels reduced the symptoms of CIPN. Thirdly, consistent with previous findings of oxaliplatin activating astrocytes in the anterior cingulate cortex in mice (Masocha 2016), and that neuroinflammation increases neural excitability (Leung & Cahill 2010), they presented that brain regions exhibited a pro-inflammatory state, and that blocking key inflammatory pathways in the brain restores GABA levels, reduces neuronal excitability and reduces CIPN (Omran et al. 2021). Fourth, changes in transcription and neuroinflammation caused by G protein coupled receptors (GPCR) and mitogen-activated protein kinase (MAPK) phosphorylation pathways which are implicated in CIPN are presented; with

GPCR pathway manipulation reducing protein kinase C (PKC) or MAPK phosphorylation in the brain, subsequently reducing CIPN symptoms. Finally, the link between CIPN and monoamines including serotonin, norepinephrine and dopamine, along with oxidative stress, acetylcholine receptor expression, and ion channel expression (reduced voltage-gated K^+ and increased voltage gated Ca^{2+} channel activity) in the CNS is also discussed (Omran et al. 2021). Together, this presents a strong argument for the involvement of the CNS in CIPN, supported when considering the focus on peripheral nerve damage alone has not been fruitful in producing advances in prevention or treatment, and this therefore warrants further research.

Assessment and Diagnosis

Detecting CIPN early is crucial for adequate management, and baseline and ongoing clinical examination at every cycle is critical (Jordan et al. 2020). This ongoing assessment would enable identification of potential or pre-existing symptoms before the neuropathy becomes irreversible. Before diagnosing CIPN, it is important to consider causes of neuropathy other than chemotherapy, including metabolic and endocrine-related neuropathies. For example, considering pre-existing conditions that may put a patient at greater risk of developing CIPN, such as diabetes mellitus can assist in the diagnosis of CIPN (Fallon et al. 2015). Currently, there are no recommended biomarkers for routine practice, however, serum neurofilament light determination is currently in development and appears to be promising (Khalil et al. 2018). Nevertheless, this is not currently recommended for routine assessment, and instead assessment is dependent on clinical and practical tests.

The European Society of Medical Oncology clinical practice guidelines outline considerations and methods of the assessment of CIPN (Jordan et al. 2020). Firstly, the clinical pattern is assessed with a range of questions. The most common presentation being a predominant sensory axonal neuropathy with occasional motor and autonomic involvement. Symptoms generally occur during the first 2 months of treatment, progress during active treatment and then typically stabilize soon after treatment is completed. However, in platinum-based treatment, a coasting phenomenon of worsening neuropathy after cessation of treatment is also seen. Platinum compounds also see cell bodies in the DRG be more vulnerable to neurotoxic damage that is often irreversible, due to less protection by the blood nerve barrier leading to sensory neuropathy. This may present asymmetrically and predominantly involves proprioception sense but does not exclude the motor system. The dying back axonopathy of CIPN affects large sensory nerves in a symmetrical length-dependent manner. Clinically, this presents as a sensory symptom that includes neuropathic '*plus*' features such as acral pain and paraesthesia (tingling pins and needles), accompanied by dysaesthesia, allodynia and hyperalgesia. Sensory loss from CIPN presents as a '*glove and stocking type*' disturbance that leads to numbness in hands and feet, including impaired perception of light touch, vibration sense, hypoalgesia and proprioception in clinical examination.

The European Society for Medical Oncology (ESMO) guidelines for assessment of CIPN have a practical guide for translating the clinical presentation discussed above, categorised into key questions to ask for sensory, motor and autonomic symptoms, and tests to conduct to assess sensory symptoms (Jordan et al. 2020) (Table 2).

In addition to these ESMO recommended steps in assessing CIPN (Jordan et al. 2020), there are some tests that may provide complementary information to clinical assessment. For example, neurophysiological methods including electromyography with nerve conduction studies may identify pre-existing, and/or subclinical neuropathy as separate risk factors for CIPN (Jordan et al. 2020). However, these measures are often reported to not reflect symptoms and are thus not suitable for monitoring CIPN severity during therapy. This is demonstrated in that despite patients' symptomatic clinical and functional recovery, neurophysiologic assessment will only show modest improvement. Other assessments such as somatosensory potentials could clarify if proximal sensitive nerves are affected or if there is presence of comorbidities in rare cases (Jordan et al. 2020).

While the American Society of Clinical Oncology (ASCO) does not have direct guidance on the assessment of CIPN in their most recent clinical practice guidelines, they do discuss considerations in presentation that may be helpful when diagnosing CIPN in patients receiving oxaliplatin (Loprinzi, CL et al. 2020). While in taxane based chemotherapy, like paclitaxel, chronic neuropathy symptoms are more prominent in the lower extremities, oxaliplatin neuropathy are more prominent in the upper extremities and these should therefore be considered in assessment. Further, the neuropathy improves faster in the hands than the feet in the '*coasting*' phenomenon. This is seen in platinum-based chemotherapy with a worsening of symptoms 2-3 months after cessation of treatment, with improvements beginning after approximately 3 months (Pachman et al. 2015). Diagnosis of more chronic peripheral neuropathy can be made by clinical history.

Table 2. ESMO's Approach to CIPN Assessment (adapted from (Jordan et al. 2020))

Initial assessment	• What are the individual risk factors, including comorbidities? • Are the potential neurotoxicities of an acute or chronic nature (including reversibility or not)? • Is an increase of the symptoms expected with the therapy continuation? • Is an increase of the symptoms expected after therapy has stopped (coasting phenomenon)?		
	Sensory	Motor	Autonomic
Ask	Plus symptoms: • Signature question: for tingling, pins and needles, permanent burning, jabbing pain in fingers and toes (hands and feet) • If a blanket causes discomfort on feet at night • For unusual temperature sensation on hands and feet while having a shower Minus symptoms: • Signature question: numbness in hand and feet, clumsiness while doing manual work/using cutlery • Foot pain in shoes including unobserved wounds • Difficulty walking in the dark or with eyes closed	Plus symptoms: • For having muscle cramps Minus symptoms: • Walking on heels and toes, climbing one flight of stairs	• For constipation, feeling dizzy or blurred vision after changing to vertical position (postural hypotension, reduced heart rate variability), bladder disturbances, skin changes, delayed gastric emptying
Test	Plus symptoms: • Toothpick (pin-prick hyperalgesia), cotton applicator moving on skin causing discomfort (allodynia) Minus symptoms: • Vibration sense with tuning fork at the case of the toe (impaired if <8/8; in patients >60 years, impaired if <6/8); proprioception (recognising direction of moving fingers and toes) • Sensation on hands and feet with cotton applicator (decrease in symmetrical stocking glove pattern) • Romberg test for approximately 20 seconds (standing stable with eyes closed), walking with eyes closed.	Minus symptoms: ankle jerk and ask to walk on heels and toes.	

In oncology clinical trials, CIPN measures typically encompass sensory, motor and functional components, such as quality of life. Due to inconsistent measurement methods historically used to characterise neuropathy, it has been challenging to compare and adequately characterizse neuropathy caused by different chemotherapeutics (Loprinzi, CL et al. 2020). However, more recently, the same validated neuropathy measurement tools have been used in several clinical studies, allowing for a more detailed comparison and understanding of neuropathy (Loprinzi et al. 2011; Pachman et al. 2015; Reeves et al. 2012). Most commonly used tools to measure CIPN are the National Cancer Institute Common Terminology Criteria (NCI-CTCAE) (Griffith et al. 2014; Trotti et al. 2003), the Eastern Cooperative Group (Oken et al. 1982), and the World Health Organization criteria (Miller et al. 1981). A limitation of these scales is their inability to detect incremental changes in impairment as the scales range from just 0 (asymptomatic) to 4-5 (paralysis or death) (Griffith et al. 2014). Due to the delay in time of CIPN becoming clinically identified due to the lack of standardisation and inadequate measurement of CIPN, sensory nerve fiber damage can become irreversible (Wolf et al. 2008).

The Multinational Association of Supportive Care in Cancer (MASCC), a leading international body in supportive oncology conducted an evaluation of current perception threshold (CPT), a test that uses painless electrical impulse to stimulate and measure sensory nerve functional integrity by determining the amount of current required to stimulate a sensation perceived by the patient (Griffith et al. 2014). Their preliminary findings suggested that CPT at 2,000 Htz could present as a beneficial clinical opportunity as increased CPT readings can indicate impending reduction in quality of life (QoL), thus serving as a red flag for clinicians as they plan treatment that may further reduce performance of daily activities. While these early results show promise for a non-invasive objective tool to measure the integrity of selected nerve fibers, there were a number of limitations with the study, including a small sample size and heterogeneity in both the patient population and anti-cancer treatment used. Other considerations in assisting in the diagnosis of CIPN includes considering pre-existing conditions that may put a patient at greater risk of developing CIPN, such as diabetes mellitus (Molassiotis, Cheng, et al. 2019).

Prevention and Management

The prevention and management of CIPN remains a significant challenge and an area of continued research. Currently, clinical practice is informed by the European Society of Medical Oncology (ESMO)/European Oncology Nursing Society (EONS)/European Association of Neuro-Oncology (EANO) (from here forth, shortened to ESMO only) and the American Society of Clinical

Oncology (ASCO) clinical practice guidelines (Jordan et al. 2020; Loprinzi, CL et al. 2020). While these guidelines are gold-standard for the prevention and management of CIPN, it must be noted that they have been developed for a range of treatment modalities and are not specific to platinum-based chemotherapies.

Prevention

Preventative Strategies not Recommended for CIPN Prevention

While no clinical guidelines can be made for agents to prevent CIPN, ASCO *strongly* recommends *against* the use of acetyl-l-carnitine (high evidence, no benefit, high harm). This recommendation is based on two large trials, one of which reported no benefit in people treated with sagopilone (Campone et al. 2013), and the other which reported worsened CIPN in patients receiving docetaxel assessed over a 2-year period (Hershman et al. 2018). ASCO also recommends (with moderate strength, intermediate evidence, low benefit, low harm) *against* the use of Acetylcysteine citing more evidence for harm (i.e., worsened symptoms) than benefit (Loprinzi, CL et al. 2020). Similarly, ASCO suggests clinicians *should not* recommend the use of several other approaches for CIPN prevention, citing a lack of clear/consistent data. These include all-trans retinoic acid, amifostine, amitriptyline, calcium magnesium, calmangafodipir, cannabinoids, carbamazepine, l-carnosine, diethyldithio-carbamate, gabapentin/pregabalin, glutamate, glutathione, goshajinkigan, metformin, minocycline, N-acetylcysteine, nimodipine, omega-3 fatty acids, org 2766, oxcarbazepine, recombinant human leukemia inhibitory factor, venlafaxine, vitamin B and vitamin E (Loprinzi, CL et al. 2020).

In agreement, ESMO does not currently recommend any pharmacological or non-pharmacological strategy to prevent CIPN. They do however state that the available evidence *discourages* the use of acupuncture to prevent CIPN, with one randomised trial (N = 48) showing acupuncture has no significant effect on the severity of PN in women with breast cancer, and actually delayed recovery in the months after treatment (Greenlee et al. 2016). The unclear evidence on acupuncture is also supported by a large Cochrane review (Ju et al. 2017).

Recommendations with Emerging Evidence

Although lacking strong and consistent evidence to support their use, available data suggest exercise, cryotherapy and compression therapy may prevent CIPN symptoms, and appear to be safe (Jordan et al. 2020; Loprinzi, CL et al.

2020). Patients and clinicians should however be aware of the risk of frostbite with cryotherapy. It is of interest that ganglioside-monosialic acid has shown efficacy in prevention of taxane-induced CIPN (Su et al. 2020). However, this was only observed in Chinese patients, and as such, this must be confirmed in different ethnic groups.

Exercise

Both ASCO and ESMO highlight the potential of exercise to minimise CIPN severity (ESMO Level II evidence, ASCO no recommendation, low evidence, low benefits, moderate harm). Three RCTs were identified for exercise in the prevention of CIPN (Courneya et al. 2014; Kleckner et al. 2018; Zimmer et al. 2018), the largest in N = 355 people treated with platinum-, taxane- and vinca alkaloid-based chemotherapy (EXCAP) (Kleckner et al. 2018). While fatigue was the primary outcome, secondary analyses of CIPN indicated a significant benefit of a 6-week home-based, moderate-intensity exercise intervention compared to controls. Similar benefits have been shown, albeit in smaller cohorts, with an 8-week supervised exercise program (Zimmer et al. 2018) showing benefits for neuropathy symptoms, muscle strength and balance. The CARE trial, performed in N = 301 women with breast cancer also showed comparable benefits for CIPN-related pain, and suggested that patients in younger (premenopausal) women in a healthy weight range and with higher baseline fitness were more likely to respond from high-dose exercise interventions (Courneya et al. 2014).

Cryotherapy

Cryotherapy has been suggested as possible way of reducing blood flow to the hands and feet, thus limiting the distribution of chemotherapy to areas at risk of neurotoxicity. ESMO currently supports the use of cryotherapy, however only with Level II evidence, for the prevention of CIPN. ASCO do not provide a recommendation for cryotherapy, stating low evidence, low benefit and moderate risk of harm. Cryotherapy, usually with frozen socks or gloves, has shown some benefit in small studies however these have not translated to larger cohorts. The largest Phase III Randomized Clinical Trial (RCT) (N = 180) (Beijers et al. 2020) showed no difference in CIPN subscales. Importantly, they reported significant discontinuation in treatment due to discomfort, hence ASCO's moderate harm classification.

Compression Therapy

Surgical gloves provide an accessible method of constructing blood flow to the extremities, limiting distribution of chemotherapy to the hands and feet and thus reducing the risk of neurotoxic injury. ESMO currently supports compression therapy, albeit only with Level III evidence. ASCO does not recommend its use, due to limited available evidence, however, recognize its potential as a relatively safe preventative strategy. In a relatively small study, where patients acted as their own control (i.e., glove on one hand, no glove on the other), less neuropathy was observed in the gloved hand (assessed by peripheral neuropathy questionnaire) (Tsuyuki et al. 2016). While promising, this study was ultimately flawed by the unblinded nature of its design, undermining the validity of these findings. In contrast, another study showed no effect of compression therapy in nab-paclitaxel-induced CIPN (Kanbayashi et al. 2020).

Treatment and Management

Recommended Strategies for Management/Treatment of CIPN (After Treatment Completion)

Both ASCO and ESMO do not provide any recommendations against the use of pharmacological or non-pharmacological interventions for CIPN management/treatment. However, their guidelines do differ in what strategies are recommended.

ASCO provides only a single recommendation for the management/ treatment of CIPN in patients that have finished active therapy, with a moderate recommendation for the use of duloxetine, stating it demonstrates (with intermediate evidence) moderate benefits (with low harm) for CIPN symptoms. Duloxetine was supported in ASCO's previous CIPN guideline document and was further strengthened by the addition of two new studies (Farshchian et al. 2018; Hirayama et al. 2015). In these studies, duloxetine outperformed venlaflaxine and placebo, demonstrating a beneficial effect on numbness and pain. Of note, ESMO reports that duloxetine at 30 mg/day for 1 week followed by 60 mg/kg reduced neuropathic pain with the best results observed in cisplatin-treated patients (Level I Evidence) (Smith, EM et al. 2013).

The remaining recommendations from ESMO have Level II and above evidence, indicating a lack of consistent or robust data. This is in accordance with ASCO's lack of recommendations for any other strategy. Outside of clinical trial, ASCO is unable to make recommendations for exercise, acupuncture, scrambler therapy, topical gel containing baclofen, amitriptyline HCL +/- ketamine, opioids, capsaicin-containing patches, tricyclic anti-depressants and oral cannabinoids. They do however recognise that preliminary evidence suggests a potential benefit for these interventions, larger definitive studies are needed to confirm efficacy and clarify risks.

Exercise

Both ASCO and ESMO discuss the potential benefits of exercise in CIPN management, with current evidence indicating exercise is feasible and safe, and confers some benefits in controlling symptoms of CIPN. Exercise, delivered as a 10-week home-based, muscle strengthening and balancing program, has been shown to reduce neuropathic pain scores and improve quality of life (Dhawan et al. 2020). The strength of this evidence was limited by the lack of active control. ESMO's guidelines also reiterate the challenges of generating robust evidence on the potential benefits of exercise, with exercise often integrated in a multimodal care setting. Exercise serves to improve coordination, sensory symptoms and fine motor skills, and in this manner should be implemented at the first onset of CIPN symptoms, or as early as feasibly possible (Level II Evidence).

Acupuncture

A 2017 Cochrane review highlighted insufficient data to support a recommendation for or against the use of acupuncture in the management of CIPN symptoms (Su et al. 2020). Following this review, there have been a number of smaller studies evaluating acupuncture (Phase II) which have reported benefits for CIPN symptoms. ASCO identified 5 studies in their clinical practice guidelines, with acupuncture assessed in a range of cohorts of varying sizes (N = 33-98), acupuncture strategies (e.g. electro-acupuncture and in combination with methylcobalamin) with heterogeneous treatment specifications (D'Alessandro et al. 2019; Han et al. 2017; Lu et al. 2020; Molassiotis, Suen, et al. 2019; Rostock et al. 2013). Four of the 5 studies reported positive findings, including improved pain (Han et al. 2017) and neurotoxicity-related symptoms (Molassiotis, Suen, et al. 2019), sensory symptoms (Lu et al. 2020), physical function (D'Alessandro et al. 2019) and overall quality of life. However, there was a negative study which reported no significant benefit of electro-acupuncture compared to placebo (Rostock et al. 2013). Given the high degree of variability across these studies, no clinical guideline has been made by ASCO, while ESMO suggests it may be considered in select patients.

Scrambler Therapy

This non-invasive cutaneous electrostimulation has been reported with Level II evidence by ESMO for the control of CIPN symptoms, however due to the lack of robust benefit, ESMO does not recommend its use. ASCO reports on two randomised trials evaluating scrambler therapy in two cohorts of N = 33 (Loprinzi, C et al. 2020) and N = 46 (Smith, TJ et al. 2020). In N = 33 patients, where scrambler therapy was applied for 30 min, no significant benefit was observed compared to sham treatment. The second, larger study, investigated scrambler therapy compared to transcutaneous electric nerve stimulation. Both strategies appeared to be safe, however scrambler therapy showed a more substantial benefit for pain, tingling and numbness, and recipients were more likely to recommend that treatment to other patients.

Topical Treatments

There is currently limited evidence to support the use of topical treatments for CIPN. In a RCT of N = 462 patients, topical preparations containing amitriptyline and ketamine did not have any significant impact on pain, numbness or tingling. Another study in N = 208 patients showed a similar preparation containing amitriptyline, ketamine and baclofen had no benefit on sensory symptoms, but did have an effect on motor symptoms in secondary analyses (Gewandter et al. 2014). As such, both ESMO and ASCO are unable to recommend the use of these products. Topical agents with menthol cream (1%) had a significant benefit in CIPN symptoms, however, this study (Fallon et al. 2015) was not randomised and had no control arm, thus only Level III Evidence was provided by ESMO.

Other/Miscellaneous

In addition to the recommended/emerging therapeutic options for CIPN symptoms, there are several other strategies that have been investigated. Anticonvulsants (including gabapentin, pregabalin and lamotrigine) have shown efficacy in other forms of neuropathic pain, but their use in CIPN remains questionable with limited data to indicate benefits (Loprinzi, CL et al. 2020). Opioids can be considered as a salvage option in certain circumstances to relieve neuropathic pain based on its efficacy in other forms of neuropathic pain. Glutamine showed modest efficacy in children (Sands et al. 2017), but no recommendation can be made for adults. Oral cannabinoids are increasingly recognised for their capacity to modulate and improve pain and are increasingly investigated in cancer-related pain, including CIPN (Waissengrin et al. 2021), however there remains limited prospective evidence. ASCO highlight evidence from a small, cross over study in N = 18 participants, reporting no benefit for nabiximols, an oral cannabinoid spray (Lynch, Cesar-Rittenberg & Hohmann 2014). They also highlight the potential adverse effects associated with this approach including dry mouth and fatigue.

Clinical Approaches to CIPN Considering Limited Interventions Available

The prevention and management of CIPN remains challenging, with both ASCO and ESMO unable to provide clear recommendations or clinical guidelines. Given the lack of effective agents for the prevention of CIPN and the limited effective therapy for treating established CIPN, it is recommended that the risks and benefits of agents known to cause CIPN in patients with underlying neuropathy or predisposing comorbidities, including diabetes, is assessed prior to starting treatment.

For patients presenting with CIPN symptoms during active treatment, clinicians should assess and discuss with their patient the appropriateness of dose reductions, breaks and delays. Stopping treatment entirely, or moving to a less neurotoxic drug, should also be considered if patients develop intolerable neuropathy and/or functional nerve impairment. In any case, this is a very unique and personalized decision that will differ depending on the circumstances of the patient and the severity of their disease.

The Multinational Association for Supportive Care in Cancer (MASCC) have developed a patient-centric decision framework for treatment alteration decisions to help guide dose-reductions and changes in treatment protocols (Hertz et al. 2021). This model can be used by clinicians *throughout neurotoxic chemotherapy treatment* to help determine whether their patient should continue, delay, decrease, or discontinue treatment. They recommend that a patient's CIPN symptom severity should be assessed at each dose or cycle (please see section 3.4). In the case of platinum drugs, MASCC emphasizes that the current severity should include an expectation that symptoms will continue to worsen on the current trajectory for approximately 3 months to account for coasting. They also underscore that a patient's current CIPN should be compared with some determination of the maximum tolerable CIPN severity. This determination should be made assuming no CIPN resolution post-treatment, as it is not possible to predict how much resolution a patient will experience. The determination of maximum tolerable CIPN should be individualized through consideration of their CIPN tolerance and chemotherapy efficacy, each of which have several contributing factors (e.g., lifestyle factors, acceptance of reduced function capacity, psychological factors, acceptance of reduced efficacy, benefit of neurotoxic treatment, efficacy of alternative treatment). Given some patients are reluctant to report CIPN symptoms due to concerns about treatment alteration (Salgado et al. 2020), surveys indicate that risk of persistent CIPN is a top factor influencing treatment preference (Spaich et al. 2018), as such, clinicians must adopt strategies to proactively discuss CIPN and its impact with patients, particularly those treated with platinum-based chemotherapy.

Cognitive Impairment

Clinical Prevalence and Presentation

Neurotoxicity in the central nervous system most commonly presents as an umbrella of psycho-neurological symptoms affecting cognition and mood. Chemotherapy-induced cognitive impairment (CICI) has been identified across a wide range of tumor types reported to occur pre, during and post-treatment. Research has shown that during chemotherapy 50-75% of people with cancer experience a degree of cognitive impairment (Janelsins et al. 2014). While cancer itself is associated with some decline in cognitive impairment, data indicate an exacerbatory effect of chemotherapy on cognition (Ahles et al. 2014). A study in women with breast cancer assessed high-dose, standard-dose chemotherapy, no-dose and controls and found the high-dose treatment group, but not the other two groups showed significantly poorer cognitive performance than controls 6-months post-treatment, proposing a dose relationship with persistent deficits (Schagen et al. 2006). This is in contrast to a study that found cognitive deficits at the time of treatment resolved at 6-months post-treatment (Jansen et al. 2011). Each of these studies had relatively small samples and differing methodologies, and as such, further longitudinal research is required in larger samples and in other tumor streams. Perceived cognitive impairment in cancer survivors has been reported to be as high as between 44.2-57.6% across tumor types (Schmidt et al. 2016). There is little correlation between objective and self-reported cognitive impairments, with the latter correlating higher with psychological outcomes.

The presentation of cognitive deficits due to neurotoxicity follows a subcortical pattern. Meta-analyses of adult cancer patients, primarily with breast and testicular cancer, showed a relationship with treatment and deficits in immediate recall, delayed memory, verbal memory and delayed memory, including recognition memory, selective attention, and attentional capacity, executive function and verbal fluency (Hodgson et al. 2013; Lindner et al. 2014). However, the importance of assessment at the individual level was shown by a study that assessed patients with breast cancer treated with adjuvant chemotherapy. The investigators found non-significant results for cognitive impairment at the group level, but when individual patients were analyzed, they found some people had a significantly reduced cognitive performance (Wefel, JS et al. 2004; Wefel, JSP et al. 2011). Given cognitive deficits vary in presence, severity and duration, and mechanism of risk is likely multifactorial, impacted by therapeutic agents and patient-related factors which render some patients more vulnerable to treatment related cognitive impairment than others, there is a need to assess patients at the individual level. This is consistent with National Comprehensive Cancer Network (NCCN) Survivorship Guidelines developed to support clinicians in the identification and management of cancer related cognitive impairment.

The assessment of CICI continues to rely on tools designed to detect severe cognitive impairment. These approaches lack appropriate sensitivity and specificity, and as such, cancer survivors with CICI perform at the lower end of the normal range, but not in the pathological range (Nelson & Suls 2013). This subtlety, together with the reliance on tests designed to detect more severe, localized deficits such as traumatic brain injury, strokes, and Alzheimer's disease, means that these cognitive changes are often undetected or underestimated by clinicians (Horowitz, Suls & Trevino 2018). This leads people living with or beyond cancer to question the existence and significance of their symptoms. Accordingly, cognitive impairment is associated with poorer psychosocial wellbeing and a higher rate of depression and anxiety. Functional magnetic resonance imaging (fMRI) studies have also revealed important insights on the impact of cognitive impairment, identifying increased activation in the frontal and temporal cortices, the cerebellum, and the right thalamus - areas typically affected by central neurotoxicity. It has been proposed that this may be a compensatory mechanism and suggest people living with CICI need to utilize more mental resources that then become quickly depleted (Ferguson et al. 2007; Menning et al. 2017). As such, CICI is often associated with fatigue. These co-occurring symptoms underscore the phenomenon of neuro-psychological symptom clusters that have a more pronounced impact on quality of life compared to single symptoms.

Risk Factors

Patient-Related Factors

Demographics

Cognitive abilities are influenced by age and gender (Ahles et al. 2010). Older patients acquired cognitive impairment at a higher rate than younger patients, underpinning the observation that CICI is more prevalent in older populations (Lange et al. 2014). However, it is also important to note that this may reflect the baseline cognitive reserve in older populations being generally lower than that of younger population, with pre-treatment cognitive reserve predictive of future cognitive decline (Pendergrass, Targum & Harrison 2018). A study done by Ahles et al., (2010) reported that elderly patients had poorer pre-treatment cognitive reserve and performed worse on processing speed tests when subjected to chemotherapy (Ahles et al. 2010). CICI is also more commonly reported in females compared to males (Vannorsdall 2017). It is however unclear if this is a truly biological phenomenon, or simply reflects the tendency to study CICI in women with breast cancer or the types of chemotherapy used to treat female-dominant cancers. Race, ethnicity and socioeconomic status also appear to contribute to CICI; however, data is heterogeneous preventing any clear conclusions to be drawn (Vannorsdall 2017).

Comorbidities

Understanding patient history is crucial for evaluating the impact of co-morbidities and related therapies, and knowledge of these factors can assist anticipate cognitive deficits and identify the relevance of changes in circulating components in cancer patients throughout treatment (Castel et al. 2017). Diabetes, hypertension, renal diseases and liver failure, are medical disorders that can alter the vasculature and may have a role in the development of CICI (Bai & Yu 2021). Moreover, chemotherapy-induced anaemia, dehydration, malnutrition and electrolyte imbalances, can arise as a result of severe illness and treatment effects and can impair cognitive function (Ahles et al. 2010; Mayo et al. 2021). It's also conceivable that psychological elements contribute to CICI, with anxiety, depression, sleep disturbances, and fatigue each clustering with CICI. These variables are frequently linked with subjective cognitive assessments in people undergoing cancer therapy (Mayo et al. 2021; van Dam et al. 1998), however, the causal interplay between these conditions remains unclear.

Genetic Factors

Apolipoprotein E (APOE, which is related to a variety of cognitive disorders and is the strongest single genetic risk factor for Alzheimer's disease), Catechol-O-methyltransferase (COMT) that has link to dopamine levels in the prefrontal cortex and cognitive abilities, Brain-derived Neurotrophic Factor (BDNF), and pro-inflammatory cytokine (IL-6 and TNF-α) genes are all genetic variables that have been linked with the development and risk of CICI (Mayo et al. 2021; Vannorsdall 2017). According to Amindi et al., (2017) individuals with testicular cancer who are ε 4 allele carriers had worsened general cognitive function (Amidi, Agerbaek, et al. 2017; Amidi, Hosseini, et al. 2017). Furthermore, DNA methyltransferases, which influence methylation of DNA have also been reported to modulate the risk of CICI, however these data require further replication and validation (Chan, Yeo, et al. 2019).

Treatment-Related Factors

Many aspects of cancer and its treatment are postulated to drive CICI, however, dissecting which factors regulate risk most has been a major challenge. This reflects the complex and multi-dimensional nature of CICI, which manifests from the psychological and emotional reaction to a cancer diagnosis, the psychological burden of treatment and the neurotoxic properties of the agents used to treat cancer (Mayo et al. 2021).

Surgery is an essential therapy option for solid tumors and is a cause of significant stress. It has been suggested that this, combined with the emotional toll of diagnosis, can drive cognitive symptoms prior to the start of systemic cancer therapy (Reid-Arndt & Cox 2012). This may also be responsible for the finding of increased cognitive dysfunction in older patients, who are reported to have a more profound inflammatory response after surgery, increasing the risk of neurological symptoms (Mayo et al. 2021). While surgery has been linked with cognitive impairment, evidence shows a heightened risk when chemotherapy and radiotherapy are used, and this appears to be dose-dependent (Tanguturi & Alexander 2018). Cognitive impairment has been reported to range from months to years following radiotherapy. However, short-term memory impairment caused by radiation is significantly related to elevated plasma IL-6 levels (Bai & Yu 2021). Zheng Y et al. found that patients who did not get adjuvant radiotherapy had better cognitive functioning at 18- and 36-months following diagnosis (Zheng et al. 2014).

Hematopoietic stem cell transplantation (HSCT) recipients are at a particularly high risk of CICI due to the high doses of chemotherapy used prior to HSCT as well as complete body irradiation, lengthy durations of myelosuppression, immunosuppressive treatments, and significant consequences such as graft versus host disease (Mayo et al. 2021). Although some studies have shown that cognitive functioning should be expected to return to pre-transplant levels on average over time, persistent impairment has been observed in a subset of patients up to 5 years after treatment, particularly those treated with allogeneic (vs. autologous) stem cell transplant.

While the intensity of HSCT is high, the duration of treatment is relatively low when compared to cyclic chemotherapy regimens used for the treatment of solid tumors. As such, the inclusion of both chemotherapy and radiotherapy are also recognized risk factors for cognitive impairment (Tanguturi & Alexander 2018). As discussed, platinum-based compounds are considered to be particularly neurotoxic, and thus associated with a high rate of CICI. Taxanes are also considered to be particularly neurotoxic and associated with cognitive impairment (Bray, Dhillon & Vardy 2018; Hodgson et al. 2013; Janelsins et al. 2014).

Despite recognising these factors are associated with a higher rate of CICI, it remains impossible to predict who is at risk of developing these symptoms. New approaches that combine multiple risk factors to build a multi-input predictive model is likely required given the breadth of interacting factors that ultimately dictate its occurrence.

Pathobiology

While cancer itself is also known to cause cognitive impairment, the use of non-chemotherapy treated patients as controls separates cancer-related cognitive impairment from CICI. These suggest that cognitive impairment has a biological basis related to the cytotoxic properties of chemotherapeutic agents, rather than being purely psychological or driven by the systemic impacts of the tumor.

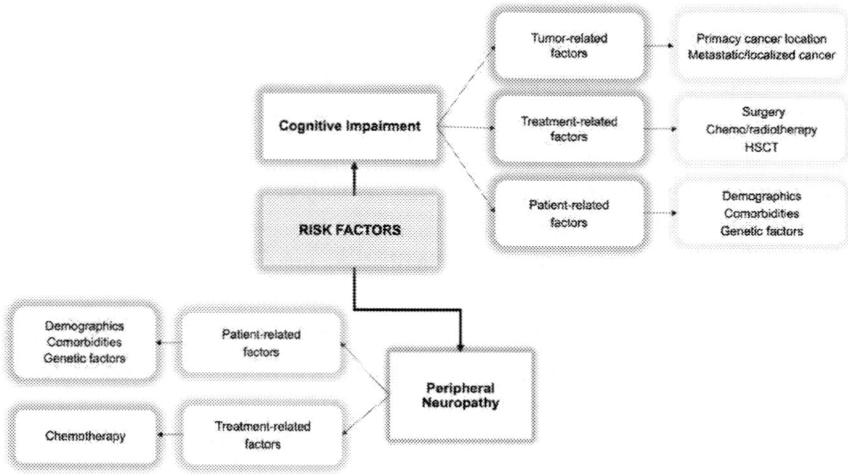

Figure 1. Risk factors of peripheral neuropathy and cognitive impairment.

The mechanisms by which chemotherapy, including platinum-based compounds, impact the central nervous system remains an area of intense interest and debate particularly given long-standing consensus that these compounds do not cross the blood brain barrier (BBB). Despite their inability to cross the BBB, evidence of central neurotoxicity has been observed in vivo (outlined below), suggesting these are driven by indirect mechanisms, or there is a level of BBB dysfunction that permit entrance of systemically administered compounds into the brain (Wardill et al. 2016). Of note, peripheral inflammation and microbial dysbiosis – both of which are seen after chemotherapy (Bowen et al. 2019) - are known to cause BBB fragility and hyper-permeability (Huang, Hussain & Chang 2021; Tang et al. 2020). As such, it is not implausible that BBB dysfunction is a critical component of CICI's pathobiology.

As described (please see section 2.0), platinum-based chemotherapeutic drugs act as DNA chelators, binding to purine residues leading to DNA damage and inducing apoptosis (Dasari & Tchounwou 2014; Tchounwou et al. 2021). This mechanism is central to the ability of these drugs to induce cell death in rapidly dividing tumor cells, however, also underpins and likely initiates the range of side effects with which they are associated. While this mechanism has been well-established to drive toxicities affecting highly proliferative cell populations, it has been more challenging to understand its relevance to CICI as most neurons are non-dividing, post-mitotic cells.

Despite challenging logic, a substantive body of evidence shows that platinum-based chemotherapy drugs induce direct injury to neurons, including telomere shortening and distorted DNA helix structure, ultimately initiating a range of downstream neuropathologies that impair their functional capacity (Tchounwou et al. 2021). Anatomical changes in the brain have been identified following chemotherapy, with neuroimaging studies identifying hippocampal alterations, reduced white matter volume, decrease grey matter density and impairments in the corpus callosum, supporting direct damage to these important brain structures (Umfress et al. 2021).

Evidence of direct cytotoxic injury to neurons has been largely evaluated in an in vitro setting, where exposure of neurons to platinum-based compounds has been shown to increase cleaved caspase-3/9 and mitochondrial dysfunction, impair cellular respiration and decrease neurogenesis (Dasari & Tchounwou 2014). This has also been observed in vivo, where evidence of direct apoptosis and loss of neuronal populations is shown by increased cleaved capsase-3 and the number of terminal deoxynucleotidyl transferase dUPT nick end labeling positive (TUNEL+) cells in key regions of the hippocampus known to regulate cognition and memory (CA1, CA3, SGZ) (Andres et al. 2014). Conversely, decreased expression of the anti-apoptotic mediator Bcl2a1, the proliferative marker Ki67 and DCX+ neural progenitor indicates reduced proliferative capacity, either induced by apoptosis or cellular quiescence (Manohar, Jamesdaniel & Salvi 2014).

Due to their affinity for mitochondrial DNA, platinum-based compounds are often accompanied by mitochondrial dysfunction. Evidence shows increased p53 accumulation, morphological changes (swelling, abnormal cistae), decreased respiration, degradation and vacuolization of neuronal mitochondria following cisplatin and oxaliplatin, hypothesized to contribute to altered cognitive function via impaired synaptic integrity. These changes appear similar to those that occur in the PNS, however, there have been no attempts to directly compare these changes. In a compensatory attempt to restore mitochondrial health, neurons have been reported to repopulate neuronal mitochondria, however, this can result in the accumulation of dysfunctional mitochondria in axons which impair synaptic function. Evidence of impaired synaptic function has been widely indicated by reduced expression of synaptophysin, post-synaptic dendritic protein 95 and dendritic spine density in a time- and dose-dependent manner (Huo et al. 2018; Lomeli et al. 2017). Of interest, a recent study showed impaired synaptic integrity in the prefrontal cortex which was normalized by the intranasal application of mesenchymal stem cells (Alexander et al. 2021).

Neuronal and mitochondrial damage in the brain have been linked with decreased expression of antioxidant genes and enzymes, suggesting secondary mechanisms related to oxidative stress. In vivo evidence shows increases in malondialdehyde, H_2O_2, acetylcholinesterase activity, reactive oxygen species, nitrite and iNOS in key regions of the brain, including the rat hippocampus after cisplatin therapy (Lomeli et al. 2017). Importantly, this oxidative stress not only impairs acute functioning, but also triggers inflammatory cascades, characterized by activation of both microglia and astrocytes (Cauli 2021); although there are inconsistent reports on the activation and lack thereof of these cell populations. The upregulation in inflammatory cytokines, including interleukin (IL)-1, IL-6, tumor necrosis factor (TNF), and interferon gamma is more readily reported, with their expression shown to identify patients with functional cognitive deficits. In a recent prospective evaluation of women with breast cancer, inflammatory cytokines mirrored the trajectory of cognitive impairment and showed an inverse correlation with brain-derived neurotrophic factor (BDNF) (Yap et al. 2021). Loss of this essential neuropeptide, which supports intracellular signaling and neurogenesis, has also been shown to occur in a time- and dose-dependent manner after cisplatin treatment in vitro (Andres et al. 2014). The persistent and irreversible loss of BDNF has been hypothesised to drive dendritic spine loss; a characteristic feature of neurotoxicity induced by cisplatin (Andres et al. 2014; Yap et al. 2021).

The observation of direct DNA damage not only challenges the long-standing concept of chemotherapeutics only targeting highly proliferative cell populations, but also the historical consensus that most chemotherapeutic drugs are not able to cross the blood brain barrier (BBB). The BBB is an important physical barrier that prevents entry of noxious substances into the brain, limiting their neurotoxic potential. For many CNS malignancies, chemotherapeutic agents lack anti-tumor efficacy, suggesting their inability to passively cross the BBB (Subramaniam et al. 2020; Wardill et al. 2016). Importantly, free diffusion of molecules across the BBB requires both lipophilicity and a molecular mass smaller than 0.5 kDa. Chemotherapy drugs are generally more than 150 kDa large, hydrophilic, and often protein-bound molecules, therefore unable to penetrate an intact BBB (Walbert & Gilbert 2009). The passage of doxorubin and cisplatin across the BBB is restricted, however, some studies have shown that these drugs exert anti-tumor effects against some brain tumors and detectable levels of these drugs after systemic administration. These data support the concept that these drugs can in fact access the CNS and implies a level of BBB permeability that has not been previously appreciated. The factors that drive BBB dysfunction remain unclear but may include direct injury by platinum-based agents, with evidence for oxaliplatin-induced BBB breakdown, or weakening of endothelial tight junctions driven by systemic inflammation (Branca et al. 2018; Wardill et al. 2016).

Assessment and Diagnosis

Clinical Assessment

Identification of cognitive impairment in people with cancer is a critical first step to providing appropriate support and is recommended as an item for standard care clinical symptom screening.

History Taking

The first essential step in identification of CICI, and CRCI more broadly, is through focused history-taking to characterise the onset and nature of the impairment, such as whether the onset of the perceived impairment as acute or gradual, is sustained or fluctuating, specific to one or more cognitive domains and how it impacts the person's functioning. This characterisation should then be considered within the context of cancer treatment history and other patient related demographic (age, education attainment), disease (symptom burden, cancer location and psychological factors). Undertaking a thorough history is of particular relevance to identifying potentially treatable contributing factors, such as emotional distress, pain or sleep disturbance. Table 3 provides an overview of components of the clinical assessment that are required when patients with cancer present with concerns about cognitive impairments, adapted from National Comprehensive Cancer Network (NCCN) Survivorship Guidelines.

Patient Reported

Use of self-reported symptom and problem lists, or patient reported outcome measures (PROMs) in routine clinical practice enables identification whether the patient perceives cognitive difficulties. For example, the NCCN Distress Thermometer and Problem List has been developed by the National Comprehensive Cancer Network (NCCN) in the US and provides a single item asking whether the person has experienced problems with memory/ concentration in the last week, this tool supports implementation of NCCN guidelines, which provide suggested follow-up questions if cognitive difficulties are suspected or reported (Network 2021; Ownby 2019; Parsons & Dietrich 2019). Similarly, commonly used PROM that measures quality of life is the European Organisation for Research and Treatment of Cancer Quality of Life Questionnaire, which includes 2-items that assess perceived memory and attention difficulties (Aaronson et al. 1993). While these options assess cognition among a range of potential problems, there are alternatives that have been developed to assess perceived cognitive function specifically. The Functional Assessment of Cancer Therapy-Cognition (Fact-cog) scale is one such example with 37-items (van Dyk et al. 2020; Wagner et al. 2009) that measure domains of perceived cognitive impairment, cognitive ability, noticeability of cognitive impairment by others and impact on quality of life (Wagner et al. 2009). A small study of breast cancer survivors that assessed the ability of the Fact-cog to detect cognitive impairment showed that the 20-items from the perceived cognitive impairment domain with a cut-score of 60 provided 79% sensitivity and 92% specificity when assessed using a self-reported functional assessment as the reference (van Dyk et al. 2020). While perceived cognitive impairment is an important measure for cancer care and warrants further investigation, a recent systematic review of the relationship between self-reported cognitive impairment found that of 45 studies that assessed this, 31 did not find an association between the two. In studies that did find an association, the cognitive domains most often represented included: verbal memory, processing speed and attention. It is noteworthy that all but one of 44 studies that assessed the relationship between self-reported cognitive impairment and other Patient Reported Outcome Measures (PROMs), including measures of depression, fatigue and distress, found moderate-to-strong associations (Bray, Dhillon & Vardy 2018), a finding shown across diseases, including multiple sclerosis and schizophrenia, for example (Raffard et al. 2020; van der Hiele et al. 2012).

Objective Assessment

There are several commonly used cognitive screening tools available. Examples include the Mini Mental State Examination, which is probably the most widely used, the Mini-Cog and Addenbrook's Cognitive Examination – Third Edition (ACE-III). While these and other screening tools are helpful in detecting more severe cognitive deficits, their sensitivity to detect subtle subcortical deficits can be limited despite the often-severe functional impact deficits may have. The ACE-III assesses the broadest range of cognitive domains, although resultingly it takes the longest time to administer. None of the screens assess information processing speed, which is a limitation given this is one of the frequently impaired cognitive domains in Cancer-related cognitive impairment (CRCI). Computerised cognitive screening assessments, such as Cogstate show preliminary evidence of detecting subcortical cognitive difficulties. For example, one study showed an ability to screen for working memory difficulties that correlated with more traditional clinician administered neuropsychological assessment in women with breast cancer (Patel et al. 2017). However, Cogstate did not detect cognitive impairment in men with testicular cancer (Patel et al. 2017). Similarly, in childhood cancer the use of Cogstate showed good specificity but poor sensitivity in detecting impairment (Balsamo et al. 2019).

Neurocognitive Assessment

A neurocognitive assessment with a trained clinical neuropsychologist is the gold standard approach to assessing and supporting cognitive impairments and is of value for patients experiencing substantial distress or functional impact. Such an assessment is likely warranted when perceived cognitive deficits have not resolved following treatment to assess and manage residual long-term impairments. A thorough neurocognitive assessment includes consideration of the person's history, including developmental and educational attainment, as well as tests selected to assess the person's presenting difficulties within the context of their cancer diagnosis. In the case of CRCI and neurotoxicity related to cancer treatment this will include tests targeting subcortical abilities, including information processing, attention, working memory and executive function, but may include assessments of other domains depending on the information gathered from history taking and the subjective difficult reported by the patient. As a guide to the type of tasks this may include, the International Cognition and Cancer Task Force have published recommendations on a core battery of cognitive tests that are useful to assess cancer related cognitive impairment (Wefel, JSP et al. 2011). Tests to assess learning and memory, information processing and executive function are recommended, including the Hopkins Verbal Learning Test-Revised, Trail Making Test and the Controlled Oral Word Association test. While they did not recommend specific working memory or attention tests, the Task Force noted that assessments of both should be added to the assessment battery (Wefel, JSP et al. 2011).

Indeed, the benefit of a neurocognitive assessment is the ability for professional feedback and provision of supportive strategies to minimize the impact of identified deficits. While the report detailing outcomes from the neurocognitive assessment may list useful strategies to manage the impact of deficits, patients experiencing substantial distress or functional impact are likely to require further input from professionals, including neuropsychologists, counsellors, occupational therapists and social workers to assist with the implementation of strategies and modifications to minimize deficits, as well as to manage the loss of ability caused by them.

Prevention and Management

While guidelines exist relating to the detection and treatment of CRCI, such as those developed by NCCN as a component of their Survivorship Guidelines (Network 2021), there are currently no guidelines specific to prevention, detection or treatment of CICI. This is likely in part due to limited evidence to determine a difference between CRCI and CICI, although this does not account for the absence of guidelines specifying when assessment for CICI should be undertaken. For example, pre-treatment baseline assessment has been recommended, so that objective cognitive decline can be evaluated over time (Parsons & Dietrich 2019). Further, guidelines about the type of assessment to be undertaken pre-and post-treatment to control for improvements related to repeated measures learning effects or at what point assessment post-treatment is warranted. Referring to NCCN guidelines, when patients with cancer reports cognitive difficulties, this should trigger focused history taking to characterise the perceived cognitive difficulties and understand potential contributing medical and psychosocial factors, as well as referral for further investigation and intervention as determined by initial assessment (Network 2021).

Prevention

There is currently no strong evidence to support preventative therapies for CICI, although a few areas require research to support or refute benefits. These include non-pharmacological and pharmacological preventative mechanisms, such as nutrition and exercise, pharmacological and complementary compounds and therapeutic interventions.

Table 3. NCCN Survivorship Guidelines for Assessing and Managing Cognitive Function (adapted from (National Comprehensive Cancer Network 2021))

History taking
• Is the neurological impairment focal, the disease metastatic or brain primary?
• Characterise onset of impairment, whether fluctuating and trajectory over time
• Cancer treatment history
• Current prescription and over the counter medications/supplements
• Medical history that may impact cognitive function
• Person's age and education attainment
Questions to clarify the nature of the impairment
• Do you have difficulty paying attention? Multitasking?
• Do you frequently leave tasks incomplete?
• Do you have difficulty finding words?
• Do you have difficulty remembering things?
• Do you need more prompts like notes or reminders than you used to?
Questions to clarify the nature of the impairment
• Does it take you longer to think through problems? Does your thinking seem slower?
• Do you notice an impact on functional performance? Job performance?
Assess for contributing/reversible factors
• Medications/side-effects
• Emotional distress: depression/anxiety
• Symptom burden: pain/fatigue/sleep disturbance
• Comorbidities
• Use of alcohol and other agents that alter cognition
• Vitamin deficiencies and endocrinopathies
Management strategies
• Provide education about cognitive difficulties associated with cancer treatment
• Teach organisation skills
• Schedule cognitive demanding tasks when energy levels are highest
• Provide relaxation/stress management skills
• Recommend physical activity
• Recommend limiting alcohol and other agents that interfere with cognitive function
• Consider meditation, yoga, mindfulness-based stress reduction and brain training.
• Optimise management of depression, fatigue, sleep disturbance, contributing symptoms and medical comorbidities
• Refer for neuropsychological assessment, cognitive rehabilitation, psychotherapy

Knowledge that micronutrients, including vitamins: B, C and D, and minerals: calcium, magnesium, iron and zinc, have an impact on cognitive performance proposes that patients undergoing cancer treatment may benefit from nutritional interventions that prevent risk of their depletion (Huskisson, Maggini & Ruf 2007; Jáuregui-Lobera 2014). One small study that assessed elderly patients undergoing treatment for lung cancer showed an association between anemia and cognitive impairment (Mancuso et al. 2006). Although, studies that have assessed the use of erythropoietin to treat anemia in cancer patients have shown inconsistent results. As such, the cardiovascular and tumor growth risks outweigh the benefit of erythropoietin administration (Mayo et al. 2021). Future research into the role of micronutrient monitoring and supplementation of cognitive function would be beneficial.

There has been mixed evidence for the protective effects of gingko biloba on cognitive decline in mild cognitive impairment and Alzheimer's disease. In cancer, a study of N = 106 women with breast cancer who received adjuvant chemotherapy found no evidence that 60mg of gingko biloba twice daily prevented CICI related cognitive changes (Barton et al. 2013).

Treatment and Management

Whether cognitive impairment is objective or subjective, it requires appropriate management to maximize the person's quality of life. Management of cognitive impairment, or cognitive rehabilitation, is a component of neuropsychological rehabilitation. It is focused on improvement of deficits in cognitive processes, including remediation and strategies to minimize the impact of impairments. Given that impairments may present differently across patients and have differing functional impacts, results of cognitive rehabilitation studies are usually presented for cognitive domains, such as for memory, attention, planning, reasoning and perception (Hodgson et al. 2013). Remediation strategies generally focus on computer-based training or 'brain-training' to improve cognitive ability by engaging in computerised tasks targeting one or more cognitive domains, while strategy-based training, focused on functional adaptation to support the implementation of compensatory strategies that utilize intact cognitive skills or reduce the reliance on impaired cognitive skills. Psychosocial management is an additionally important component in the management of cognitive impairment because the cognitive deficit/s may cause distress and impact on personal or social wellbeing, but also because psychological distress as a result of the diagnosis and associated implications of cancer may cause or exacerbate cognitive impairments, or the person's perception of impairments and their impact. Consistent with this, cognitive rehabilitation programs may encompass psychoeducation, emotional regulation and stress reduction, and social support skill development and measure improvements to cognitive domains and of patient function and quality of life (Wefel, JSP et al. 2011; Wilson et al. 2017).

Education

Patient education is important to normalise the experience of cognitive deficits related cancer generally, and as a potential side-effect due to the neurotoxic effects of cancer treatment specifically. Education about these effects should commence prior to cancer treatment, so the patient is informed of the evidence, including what is understood about prevalence, severity and potential long-term impact when risk factors of treatment side-effects are discussed.

When patients are objectively assessed for cognitive deficits and provided with impact about the outcome of results, it is imperative that this is undertaken by a trained psychologist or neuropsychologist who is able to support the person's questions and provide information about how to minimise the impact of these deficits.

Remediation Strategies

Cognitive remediation aims to improve cognitive ability through repetitive practice of cognitive tasks that engage the targeted cognitive domain, most often delivered by computer. For example, tasks aimed at improving speed of information processing will usually require the person to undertake timed computer-based tasks to either improve their performance within a specific time or to improve the time taken to complete a specific task. Training outcomes are often assessed by intermediate measures, such as cognitive test scores. While some studies have shown improvements in targeted cognitive domains when measured using cognitive tests, evidence about whether intermediate gains transfer to real-world outcomes being limited (Fernandes, Richard & Edelstein 2019), and even more so in CRCI. A recent review reporting only two CRCI rehabilitation studies that assessed real-life tasks, both with no improvement (Fernandes, Richard & Edelstein 2019). While there is likely minimal harm to patients engaging in the many commercially available cheap brain training apps, many of which have a free component, goal-directed treatment planning should be focused on evidence-based cognitive rehabilitation (van Heugten 2017).

Functional Support Strategies

Despite the limitations of cognitive training aimed at remedying cognitive deficits, cognitive rehabilitation targeting functional deficits has shown positive effects in the absence of improvements on standardised cognitive test performance (Wilson et al. 2017). This is because the aim of these strategies is to support the impact of the cognitive deficit by implementing strategies that utilise other cognitive abilities, routines and external aids. For example, strategies to assist with memory limitations may include calendar prompts, creation of routines or a home memory corner to place important items such as keys, phone and wallet to reduce misplaced items. The use of chunking and mnemonic techniques can assist to memorise important information (Wilson 2007). While patients may have developed some of their own compensation strategies, referral to neuropsychologists, psychologists or occupational therapists for specialist assistance with the development of adaptive strategies that support functioning is warranted for patients who express difficulties or distress due to cognitive limitations (Mayo et al. 2021).

Psychosocial and Lifestyle Interventions

Psychosocial support is important because of the impact cognitive deficits may have on employment and relationships, but also because cognitive deficits may be exacerbated by the psychological distress of cancer diagnosis, treatment and concerns of recurrence (Gehring et al. 2020). The importance is emphasised by the relationship between psychosocial outcomes and subjectively measured cognitive function. While there is limited evidence of a relationship between subjective and objective cognitive functioning in cancer patients, there is a strong relationship between subjective cognition and psychosocial outcomes (Bray, Dhillon & Vardy 2018). Given this, it is important that assessment for psychological distress is undertaken as a component of assessment when patients with cancer perceive cognitive difficulties so that appropriate psychological referral and/or treatment can be provided.

The type of psychosocial support accessed with depend on each person's individual preferences, but may include individual or group therapy, accessing support groups or other wellbeing initiatives, such as relaxation or art therapy, scheduling pleasant 'restorative' activities. Two studies assessed a restorative activity intervention on attention in people with breast cancer and found a significant improvement in the intervention group compared to controls (Cimprich 1993).

Exercise

The effect of exercise has shown improvements in self-reported cognitive impairments during and after cancer treatment. A recent review of randomised controlled trials found that 12 of 28 studies (43%), showed statistically significant improvements across a range of exercise modalities, including aerobic, resistance and mind-body (e.g., yoga, tai chi). Of the 9 studies that included objective assessments, 3 (33%; all breast cancer) reported cognitive improvements in exercise interventions that were either aerobic or a combination of aerobic and resistance. Most objective studies that examined cognitive function were reported as poor quality and undertaken as a secondary analysis (Campbell et al. 2020), highlighting the need for high quality studies to expand knowledge about the benefits exercise may have to prevention and management of CICI.

Mindfulness and Meditation

A recent review assessed the effects of mindfulness-based studies on improved cognition in breast cancer patients. Only one included study assessed cognition objectively, which did not show an effect; the remaining using subjectively reported measures (Cifu et al. 2018). The authors found two studies that showed cognitive benefits, sustained at 2- and 6- months, two that showed immediate benefits that were not sustained at 2-month follow-up and two studies that did not show cognitive improvements. The authors of the review noted that the studies were heterogeneous in cognitive domains and assessment tools (Cifu et al. 2018). Another small study assessing the effect of meditation on cognition in women with breast cancer found that a trend towards significance for verbal learning, short-term memory and processing speed, suggesting the study was underpowered rather than an absence of an effect (Milbury et al. 2013).

Pharmacotherapy and Supplements

Stimulants

Both methylphenidate and modifinil have been assessed for their ability to improve cognitive function in people with cancer. Methylpenidate, approved for treatment of attention deficit hyperactivity disorder, has shown improvements in cognitive flexibility, attention and processing speed in children with CNS tumours. In adults, results in both CNS and non-CNS cancer patients have been inconclusive (Karschnia, Parsons & Dietrich 2019).

Modifinil is approved for use in sleep disorders, such as narcolepsy, although it is used off label for its cognitive enhancing effects. A review of studies assessing its efficacy in healthy non-sleep deprived individuals has shown enhancements in attention, executive function and learning (Battleday & Brem 2015). A study that assessed modifinil in patients with CNS tumours showed significant improvements in processing speed and executive function, although this small study (n = 24) did not use a control group so cannot rule out improvements due to practice effects. Another study assessed 68 breast cancer patients post chemotherapy or radiation treatment with found a small but statistically significant improvement speed of processing, episodic memory and sustained attention for the group administered modifinil compared to placebo (Kohli et al. 2009).

Anti-Dementia

Donepezil and memantine come from the anti-dementia therapeutics that show promise for CICI. Donepezil is an acetylcholinesterase inhibitor and is approved by the US Food and Drug Administration for its ability to delay cognitive decline in Alzheimer's disease. In studies in CNS and non-CNS cancer it has consistently shown improvements on learning and memory tests, with some evidence of benefit to other cognitive domains, including executive function (Karschnia, Parsons & Dietrich 2019). The evidence for memantine, an N-methyl-D-aspartate receptor antagonist is less compelling at this time, with only one CNS cancer study having investigated it. Nonetheless, this well powered trial (N = 508) showed promising results, with a potential protective value of significantly longer time till cognitive decline. Executive function, processing speed and delayed memory recall were all favoured in the memantine group compared to placebo (Brown et al. 2013). There are two other trials assessing memantine for CICI in CNS cancers that are currently ongoing (Karschnia, Parsons & Dietrich 2019).

Antidepressants

The role of antidepressants in the treatment of CRCI has been mainly investigated pre-clinically but is worthy of attention because of commonalities in inflammatory mechanisms of depression and cancer, as well as the similarities in type of cognitive impairments resultant of both (Das et al. 2020). Further, the relationship between psychosocial difficulties and self-reported CRCI is noteworthy for the ability of antidepressants to improve perceived cognitive difficulties (Bray, Dhillon & Vardy 2018). A study of people with stage III or IV cancer that assessed people with depression against people without. The group experiencing depression were treated with sertraline and an improvement in executive function was shown for this group, as well as improvements in depression and quality of life measures. Unfortunately, the group that was not experiencing depression were not treated with sertraline, limiting conclusions about whether improvements in executive function were due to administration of the drug or reduction of depression symptoms (Li et al. 2014) Another study that assessed paroxetine in N = 781 patients with breast cancer found improvements in attention and memory for the group administered paroxetine compared to placebo (Jean-Pierre et a. 2009).

Vitamin E

Investigation of alpha-tocopherol (Vitamin E) to improve cognitive function has been undertaken in one small study (N = 29) specific to cognitive effects of temporal lobe radionecrosis that may occur as a result of radiotherapy to treat nasopharyngeal carcinoma. Following 1-year of supplementation the treatment arm showed significant improvement in global cognition, verbal and visual memory, and executive function, with not between group differences in attention or language.

Conclusions and Future Directions

The neurotoxic properties of platinum-based chemotherapy agents remain a clinical challenge and place significant burden on patients. As outlined in this chapter, while the macroscopic and microscopic characteristics of neurotoxicity in the peripheral and central nervous systems are relatively well documented, the factors that causally drive symptoms are unclear. This has significantly hampered efforts to develop effective preventative strategies. This is further compounded by the overlap in mechanisms that drive neurotoxicity and treatment efficacy, thus the challenge remains to identify targetable mechanisms that are mutually exclusive.

Currently, there are limited strategies for the prevention or treatment of CIPN, with the most common treatment for pain from CIPN being opioids. This underscores the fact that the molecular effects of platinum-based chemotherapies on DRG neurons are insufficiently studied, and identification of validated predictors of neuropathy could play an important role in treatment decisions in the future. However, the complications associated with these therapies are different and drug specific and thus the underlying mechanisms are different for the different treatments. Consequently, it is unlikely there is a universal approach to mitigate these side effects. Further, platinum compounds injure all components of neuronal cells, including gene expression and mitochondrial homeostasis, cytoskeleton components, and subcellular structures and membranes. Given the profound impact platinum compounds have on all of these neuronal cell functions, it is therefore near impossible to treat these endpoints individually. Instead, understanding what the key initiators of these chain of events are, or broad mediators of clinical symptoms, will be more helpful in finding effective treatments.

In addition to understanding common underlying mechanisms of neurotoxicity, it is important to consider effective management, which begins with first gaining an accurate picture of prevalence and severity of neurological symptoms. For example, the Common Terminology Criteria for Adverse Events (CTCAE), which is used in most clinical trials for anti-cancer agents, is not sensitive for measuring neuropathy and fails to appropriately acknowledge painful neuropathy. Similarly, traditional tools to assess cognition lack the sensitivity to detect the often subtle but still impactful symptoms of CICI. Together, these highlight that current estimates of prevalence may not be reliable and may in fact underestimate the prevalence of burden. Furthermore, it has been reported that health care professionals often underestimate symptoms experienced by patients, and there is discordance in patients' and health care professionals' perceptions of CIPN. Therefore, efforts to develop improved evaluation tools for patient reported- and clinician reported- outcomes for assessing neurotoxicity are mounting. For example, the European Organization for Research and Treatment of Cancer developed the QLQ-CIPN20 resource, which is a 20-item quality of life questionnaire that quantifies symptoms and impairments of sensory, motor, and autonomic neuropathy (Le-Rademacher et al. 2017). Further, Rasch analysis was used to develop the CIPN-R-ODS, an overall disability scale that provides linear measurement of CIPN-related disability (Binda et al. 2013). Given the heavy reliance on patient reported outcomes (PROs) in assessment of neurological symptoms, ensuring the PRO data collected is reliable and accurate is paramount. This is further emphasised when we recognise that patients' and health care professionals' perspectives regarding symptoms can be meaningfully different (Cirillo et al. 2009). This may reflect the tendency for many patients to experience symptoms in an out-patient setting, i.e., at home between treatments or after the completion of treatment. Therefore, using electronic PRO (ePRO) assessment systems such as apps that allow for efficient standardised assessments, decreased response burden, increased satisfaction, improved ease of use (especially outside of clinic visits), and fewer missing data points may be beneficial in the assessment of CIPN, as they have consistently shown to enhance PRO collection (Riis et al. 2021). Further, patients with CIPN who often suffer pain in their hands see electronic reporting as superior to writing or turning pages for capturing their PROs. In addition to PROs, clinical trial outcomes should also incorporate quantitative neurological examinations and neurophysiology, such as those seen in the Total Neuropathy Score clinical version (TNSc).

In the setting of CICI, there is a clear need for research to better delineate between factors of cognitive impairment related to cancer itself and those related to treatment effects and guidelines to specific to detection and monitoring of CICI, particularly with regards to understanding the point that detailed post-treatment assessment might be undertaken if residual cognitive concerns remain. This is important from a perspective of long-term management, but also to provide the patient with information about whether the impairment is likely to be ongoing or improve. Guidelines are required to consider management of CICI and CRCI more broadly for the subset of people with cancer who present with more severe and persistent impairments, or a high level of distress due to the impairment.

An important focus of research and guidelines related to potential use of pharmacotherapies is related to whom and when patients should be treated. As clinical trials provide greater evidence about the efficacy of these compounds are needed to better understand the benefits related to patient risk factors and timing of administration. For example, is the efficacy warranted for preventative use in based on a patient risk profile or does the evidence only warrant use for more severe and persistent cognitive difficulties. Indeed, further research is required into promising pharmacotherapeutics, with a particular focus on targeting specific cognitive domains.

Considering these suggestions, the neurotoxic properties of platinum compounds remain a significant challenge and our approach to better management must start with increased visibility and clinical appreciation for the resulting symptoms. This must begin with cooperative approaches to identify risk predictors and standardised methods of assessment. These assessments, when used clinically and experimentally, will enable more consistent data to be generated in larger cohorts, accelerating the move towards evidence-based prevention and management in those deemed high risk.

References

Aaronson, N, Ahmedzai, S, Bergman, B, Bullinger, M, Cull, A, Duez, N, Filiberti, A, Flechtner, H, Fleishman, S, de Haes, J, Kaasa, S, Klee, M, Osoba, D, Razavi, D, Rofe, P, Schraub, S, Sneeuw, K, Sullivan, M & Takeda, F (1993). The European Organisation for Research and Treatment of Cancer QLQ-C30: A quality-of-life instrument for use in international clinical trials in oncology. *Journal of the National Cancer Institute*, vol. 85, 365-337.

Ahles, TA, Li, Y, McDonald, BC, Schwartz, GN, Kaufman, PA, Tsongalis, GJ, Moore, JH & Saykin, AJ (2014). Longitudinal assessment of cognitive changes associated with adjuvant treatment for breast cancer: the impact of APOE and smoking, *Psychooncology*, vol. 23, no. 12, 1382-1390.

Ahles, TA, Saykin, AJ, McDonald, BC, Li, Y, Furstenberg, CT, Hanscom, BS, Mulrooney, TJ, Schwartz, GN & Kaufman, PA (2010). Longitudinal assessment of cognitive changes associated with adjuvant treatment for breast cancer: impact of age and cognitive reserve, *J Clin Oncol*, vol. 28, no. 29, 4434-4440.

Alexander, JF, Seua, AV, Arroyo, LD, Ray, PR, Wangzhou, A, Heibeta-Luckemann, L, Schedlowski, M, Price, TJ, Kavelaars, A & Heijnen, CJ (2021). Nasal administration of mitochondria reverses chemotherapy-induced cognitive deficits. *Theranostics*, vol. 11, no. 7, 3109-3130.

Ali, NT, Mohamed, AA & Yousef, BA (2020). The Incidence of Oxaliplatin-Induced Peripheral Neurotoxicity at Khartoum Oncology Hospital: A Cross-Sectional Survey, *Asia Pac J Oncol Nurs*, vol. 7, no. 3, 266-272.

Alian, OM, Azmi, AS & Mohammad, RM (2012). Network insights on oxaliplatin anti-cancer mechanisms, *Clin Transl Med*, vol. 1, no. 1, 26.

Amidi, A, Agerbaek, M, Wu, LM, Pedersen, AD, Mehlsen, M, Clausen, CR, Demontis, D, Borglum, AD, Harboll, A & Zachariae, R (2017). Changes in cognitive functions and cerebral grey matter and their associations with inflammatory markers, endocrine markers, and APOE genotypes in testicular cancer patients undergoing treatment, *Brain Imaging Behav*, vol. 11, no. 3, 769-783.

Amidi, A, Hosseini, SMH, Leemans, A, Kesler, SR, Agerbaek, M, Wu, LM & Zachariae, R (2017). Changes in Brain Structural Networks and Cognitive Functions in Testicular Cancer Patients Receiving Cisplatin-Based Chemotherapy, *J Natl Cancer Inst*, vol. 109, no. 12.

Andres, AL, Gong, X, Di, K & Bota, DA (2014). Low-doses of cisplatin injure hippocampal synapses: a mechanism for chemo brain?, *Exp Neurol*, vol. 255, 137-144.

Argyriou, AA, Bruna, J, Genazzani, AA & Cavaletti, G (2017). Chemotherapy-induced peripheral neurotoxicity: management informed by pharmacogenetics, *Nat Rev Neurol*, vol. 13, no. 8, 492-504.

Argyriou, AA, Bruna, J, Marmiroli, P & Cavaletti, G (2012). Chemotherapy-induced peripheral neurotoxicity (CIPN): an update, *Crit Rev Oncol Hematol*, vol. 82, no. 1, 51-77.

Avan, A, Postma, TJ, Ceresa, C, Avan, A, Cavaletti, G, Giovannetti, E & Peters, GJ (2015). Platinum-induced neurotoxicity and preventive strategies: past, present, and future, *Oncologist*, vol. 20, no. 4, 411-432.

Bai, L & Yu. (E 2021). A narrative review of risk factors and interventions for cancer-related cognitive impairment, *Ann Transl Med*, vol. 9, no. 1, 72.

Balsamo, LM, Mitchell, H-R, Ross, W, Metayer, C, Hardy, KK & Kadan-Lottick, NS (2019). Monitoring neurocognitive functioning in childhood cancer survivors: evaluation of CogState computerized assessment and the Behavior Rating Inventory of Executive Function (BRIEF), *BMC Psychology*, vol. 7, no. 1, 26.

Barton, DL, Burger, K, Novotny, PJ, Fitch, TR, Kohli, S, Soori, G, Wilwerding, MB, Sloan, JA, Kottschade, LA, Rowland, KM, Jr., Dakhil, SR, Nikcevich, DA & Loprinzi, CL (2013). The use of ginkgo biloba for the prevention of chemotherapy-related cognitive dysfunction in women receiving adjuvant treatment for breast cancer, N00C9, *Supportive Care in Cancer*, vol. 21, no. 4, 1185-1192.

Battleday, RM & Brem, AK (2015). Modafinil for cognitive neuroenhancement in healthy non-sleep-deprived subjects: A systematic review, *European Neuropsychopharmacology*, vol. 25, no. 11, 1865-1881.

Beijers, AJM, Bonhof, CS, Mols, F, Ophorst, J, de Vos-Geelen, J, Jacobs, EMG, van de Poll-Franse, LV & Vreugdenhil, G (2020). Multicenter randomized controlled trial to evaluate the efficacy and tolerability of frozen gloves for the prevention of chemotherapy-induced peripheral neuropathy, *Ann Oncol*, vol. 31, no. 1, 131-136.

Binda, D, Vanhoutte, EK, Cavaletti, G, Cornblath, DR, Postma, TJ, Frigeni, B, Alberti, P, Bruna, J, Velasco, R, Argyriou, AA, Kalofonos, HP, Psimaras, D, Ricard, D, Pace, A, Galie, E, Briani, C, Dalla Torre, C, Lalisang, RI, Boogerd, W, Brandsma, D, Koeppen, S, Hense, J, Storey, D, Kerrigan, S, Schenone, A, Fabbri, S, Rossi, E, Valsecchi, MG, Faber, CG, Merkies, IS, group, CI-Ps, Galimberti, S, Lanzani, F, Mattavelli, L, Piatti, ML, Bidoli, P, Cazzaniga, M, Cortinovis, D, Lucchetta, M, Campagnolo, M, Bakkers, M, Brouwer, B, Boogerd, W, Grant, R, Reni, L, Piras, B, Pessino, A, Padua, L, Granata, G, Leandri, M, Ghignotti, I, Plasmati, R, Pastorelli, F, Heimans, JJ, Eurelings, M, Meijer, RJ, Grisold, W, Lindeck Pozza, E, Mazzeo, A, Toscano, A, Russo, M, Tomasello, C, Altavilla, G, Penas Prado, M, Dominguez Gonzalez, C & Dorsey, SG (2013). Rasch-built Overall Disability Scale for patients with chemotherapy-induced peripheral neuropathy (CIPN-R-ODS), *Eur J Cancer*, vol. 49, no. 13, 2910-2918.

Boland, EG, Selvarajah, D, Hunter, M, Ezaydi, Y, Tesfaye, S, Ahmedzai, SH, Snowden, JA & Wilkinson, ID (2014). Central pain processing in chronic chemotherapy-induced peripheral neuropathy: a functional magnetic resonance imaging study, *PLoS One*, vol. 9, no. 5, p. e96474.

Bowen, J, Al-Dasooqi, N, Bossi, P, Wardill, H, Van Sebille, Y, Al-Azri, A, Bateman, E, Correa, ME, Raber-Durlacher, J, Kandwal, A, Mayo, B, Nair, RG, Stringer, A, Ten Bohmer, K, Thorpe, D, Lalla, RV, Sonis, S, Cheng, K, Elad, S & Mucositis Study Group of the Multinational Association of Supportive Care in Cancer/International Society of Oral, O (2019). The pathogenesis of mucositis: updated perspectives and emerging targets, *Support Care Cancer*, vol. 27, no. 10, 4023-4033.

Branca, JJV, Maresca, M, Morucci, G, Becatti, M, Paternostro, F, Gulisano, M, Ghelardini, C, Salvemini, D, Di Cesare Mannelli, L & Pacini, A (2018). Oxaliplatin-induced blood brain barrier loosening: a new point of view on chemotherapy-induced neurotoxicity, *Oncotarget*, vol. 9, no. 34, 23426-23438.

Bray, VJ, Dhillon, HM & Vardy, JL (2018). Systematic review of self-reported cognitive function in cancer patients following chemotherapy treatment, *J Cancer Surviv*, vol. 12, no. 4, 537-559.

Brown, PD, Pugh, S, Laack, NN, Wefel, JS, Khuntia, D, Meyers, C, Choucair, A, Fox, S, Suh, JH, Roberge, D, Kavadi, V, Bentzen, SM, Mehta, MP, Watkins-Bruner, D & Radiation Therapy Oncology, G (2013). Memantine for the prevention of cognitive dysfunction in patients receiving whole-brain radiotherapy: a randomized, double-blind, placebo-controlled trial, *Neuro Oncol*, vol. 15, no. 10, 1429-1437.

Byrd-Leifer, CA, Block, EF, Takeda, K, Akira, S & Ding, A (2001). The role of MyD88 and TLR4 in the LPS-mimetic activity of Taxol, *Eur J Immunol*, vol. 31, no. 8, 2448-2457.

Campbell, KL, Zadravec, K, Bland, KA, Chesley, E, Wolf, F & Janelsins, MC (2020). The effect of exercise on cancer-related cognitive impairment and applications for physical therapy: systematic review of randomized controlled trials, *Phys Ther*, vol. 100, no. 3, Mar 10, 523-542.

Campone, M, Berton-Rigaud, D, Joly-Lobbedez, F, Baurain, JF, Rolland, F, Stenzl, A, Fabbro, M, van Dijk, M, Pinkert, J, Schmelter, T, de Bont, N & Pautier. (P 2013). A double-blind, randomized phase II study to evaluate the safety and efficacy of acetyl-L-carnitine in the prevention of sagopilone-induced peripheral neuropathy, *Oncologist*, vol. 18, no. 11, 1190-1191.

Carozzi, VA, Canta, A & Chiorazzi, A (2015). Chemotherapy-induced peripheral neuropathy: What do we know about mechanisms?, *Neurosci Lett*, vol. 596, 90-107.

Carozzi, VA, Marmiroli, P & Cavaletti, G (2010). The role of oxidative stress and anti-oxidant treatment in platinum-induced peripheral neurotoxicity, *Curr Cancer Drug Targets*, vol. 10, no. 7, 670-682.

Castel, H, Denouel, A, Lange, M, Tonon, MC, Dubois, M & Joly, F (2017). Biomarkers Associated with Cognitive Impairment in Treated Cancer Patients: Potential Predisposition and Risk Factors, *Front Pharmacol*, vol. 8, p. 138.

Cauli, O (2021). Oxidative Stress and Cognitive Alterations Induced by Cancer Chemotherapy Drugs: A Scoping Review, *Antioxidants (Basel)*, vol. 10, no. 7.

Chan, A, Hertz, DL, Morales, M, Adams, EJ, Gordon, S, Tan, CJ, Staff, NP, Kamath, J, Oh, J, Shinde, S, Pon, D, Dixit, N, DOlimpio, J, Dumitrescu, C, Gobbo, M, Kober, K, Mayo, S, Pang, L, Subbiah, I, Beutler, AS, Peters, KB, Loprinzi, C & Lustberg. (MB 2019). Biological predictors of chemotherapy-induced peripheral neuropathy (CIPN): MASCC neurological complications working group overview, *Support Care Cancer*, vol. 27, no. 10, 3729-3737.

Chan, A, Yeo, A, Shwe, M, Tan, CJ, Foo, KM, Chu, P, Khor, CC & Ho, HK (2019). An Evaluation of DNA Methyltransferase 1 (DNMT1) Single Nucleotide Polymorphisms and Chemotherapy-Associated Cognitive Impairment: A Prospective, Longitudinal Study, *Sci Rep*, vol. 9, no. 1, 14570.

Cifu, G, Power, MC, Shomstein, S & Arem. (H 2018). Mindfulness-based interventions and cognitive function among breast cancer survivors: a systematic review, *BMC Cancer*, vol. 18, no. 1, 1163.

Cimprich, B (1993). Development of an intervention to restore attention in cancer patients, *Cancer Nurs*, vol. 16, no. 2, 83-92.

Cirillo, M, Venturini, M, Ciccarelli, L, Coati, F, Bortolami, O & Verlato, G (2009). Clinician versus nurse symptom reporting using the National Cancer Institute-Common Terminology Criteria for Adverse Events during chemotherapy: results of a comparison based on patients self-reported questionnaire, *Ann Oncol*, vol. 20, no. 12, 1929-1935.

Colvin, LA (2019). Chemotherapy-induced peripheral neuropathy: where are we now?, *Pain*, vol. 160 Suppl 1, S1-S10.

Courneya, KS, McKenzie, DC, Mackey, JR, Gelmon, K, Friedenreich, CM, Yasui, Y, Reid, RD, Vallerand, JR, Adams, SC, Proulx, C, Dolan, LB, Wooding, E & Segal, RJ (2014). Subgroup effects in a randomised trial of different types and doses of exercise during breast cancer chemotherapy, *Br J Cancer*, vol. 111, no. 9, 1718-1725.

DAlessandro, EG, Nebuloni Nagy, DR, de Brito, CMM, Almeida, EPM, Battistella, LR & Cecatto, RB (2019). Acupuncture for chemotherapy-induced peripheral neuropathy: a randomised controlled pilot study, *BMJ Support Palliat Care*.

Das, A, Ranadive, N, Kinra, M, Nampoothiri, M, Arora, D & Mudgal, J (2020). An Overview on Chemotherapy-induced Cognitive Impairment and Potential Role of Antidepressants, *Curr Neuropharmacol*, vol. 18, no. 9, 838-851.

Dasari, S & Tchounwou, PB (2014). Cisplatin in cancer therapy: molecular mechanisms of action, *Eur J Pharmacol*, vol. 740, 364-378.

de Sousa, GF, Lima Mde, A, Custodio, DF, Freitas, VM & Monteiro, G (2015). Chemogenomic Study of Carboplatin in Saccharomyces cerevisiae: Inhibition of the NEDDylation Process Overcomes Cellular Resistance Mediated by HuR and Cullin Proteins, *PLoS One*, vol. 10, no. 12, e0145377.

Dhawan, S, Andrews, R, Kumar, L, Wadhwa, S & Shukla, G (2020). A Randomized Controlled Trial to Assess the Effectiveness of Muscle Strengthening and Balancing Exercises on Chemotherapy-Induced Peripheral Neuropathic Pain and Quality of Life Among Cancer Patients, *Cancer Nurs*, vol. 43, no. 4, 269-280.

Di Cesare Mannelli, L, Pacini, A, Bonaccini, L, Zanardelli, M, Mello, T & Ghelardini, C (2013). Morphologic features and glial activation in rat oxaliplatin-dependent neuropathic pain, *J Pain*, vol. 14, no. 12, 1585-1600.

Di Cesare Mannelli, L, Pacini, A, Micheli, L, Tani, A, Zanardelli, M & Ghelardini, C (2014). Glial role in oxaliplatin-induced neuropathic pain, *Exp Neurol*, vol. 261, 22-33.

Dougherty, PM (2016). Is Chemotherapy-induced Peripheral Neuropathy More Than Just a Peripheral Nervous System Disorder?, *Anesthesiology*, vol. 124, no. 5, 992-993.

Fallon, MT, Storey, DJ, Krishan, A, Weir, CJ, Mitchell, R, Fleetwood-Walker, SM, Scott, AC & Colvin, LA (2015). Cancer treatment-related neuropathic pain: proof of concept study with menthol--a TRPM8 agonist, *Support Care Cancer*, vol. 23, no. 9, 2769-2777.

Farshchian, N, Alavi, A, Heydarheydari, S & Moradian, N (2018). Comparative study of the effects of venlafaxine and duloxetine on chemotherapy-induced peripheral neuropathy, *Cancer Chemother Pharmacol*, vol. 82, no. 5, 787-793.

Ferguson, RJ, McDonald, BC, Saykin, AJ & Ahles, TA (2007). Brain structure and function differences in monozygotic twins: possible effects of breast cancer chemotherapy, *J Clin Oncol*, vol. 25, no. 25, 3866-3870.

Fernandes, HA, Richard, NM & Edelstein, K (2019). Cognitive rehabilitation for cancer-related cognitive dysfunction: a systematic review, *Support Care Cancer*, vol. 27, no. 9, 3253-3279.

Ferris, CF, Nodine, S, Pottala, T, Cai, X, Knox, TM, Fofana, FH, Kim, S, Kulkarni, P, Crystal, JD & Hohmann, AG (2019). Alterations in brain neurocircuitry following treatment with the chemotherapeutic agent paclitaxel in rats, *Neurobiol Pain*, vol. 6, 100034.

Fidanboylu, M, Griffiths, LA & Flatters, SJ (2011). Global inhibition of reactive oxygen species (ROS) inhibits paclitaxel-induced painful peripheral neuropathy, *PLoS One*, vol. 6, no. 9, e25212.

Florea, AM & Busselberg, D (2011). Cisplatin as an anti-tumor drug: cellular mechanisms of activity, drug resistance and induced side effects, *Cancers (Basel)*, vol. 3, no. 1, 1351-1371.

Forman, AD (2004). Peripheral neuropathy and cancer, *Curr Oncol Rep*, vol. 6, no. 1, 20-25.

Fuertes, MA, Castilla, J, Alonso, C & Perez, JM (2003). Cisplatin biochemical mechanism of action: from cytotoxicity to induction of cell death through interconnections between apoptotic and necrotic pathways, *Curr Med Chem*, vol. 10, no. 3, 257-266.

Gehring, K, Klaver, K, Edwards, M, Kesler, SR, Wefel, JS & Schagen, SB (2020). Cognitive rehabilitaiton in patients with non-central nervous System Cancers and Brain Tumors., in *Cognitive Rehabilitation and Neuroimaging: Examining the Evidence from Brain to Behavior.*

Gewandter, JS, Mohile, SG, Heckler, CE, Ryan, JL, Kirshner, JJ, Flynn, PJ, Hopkins, JO & Morrow, GR (2014). A phase III randomized, placebo-controlled study of topical amitriptyline and ketamine for chemotherapy-induced peripheral neuropathy (CIPN): a University of Rochester CCOP study of 462 cancer survivors, *Support Care Cancer*, vol. 22, no. 7, 1807-1814.

Ghosh. (S 2019). Cisplatin: The first metal based anticancer drug, *Bioorg Chem*, vol. 88, 102925.

Greenlee, H, Crew, KD, Capodice, J, Awad, D, Buono, D, Shi, Z, Jeffres, A, Wyse, S, Whitman, W, Trivedi, MS, Kalinsky, K & Hershman, DL (2016). Randomized sham-controlled pilot trial of weekly electro-acupuncture for the prevention of taxane-induced peripheral neuropathy in women with early stage breast cancer, *Breast Cancer Res Treat*, vol. 156, no. 3, 453-464.

Griffith, KA, Couture, DJ, Zhu, S, Pandya, N, Johantgen, ME, Cavaletti, G, Davenport, JM, Tanguay, LJ, Choflet, A, Milliron, T, Glass, E, Gambill, N, Renn, CL & Dorsey, SG (2014). Evaluation of chemotherapy-induced peripheral neuropathy using current perception threshold and clinical evaluations, *Support Care Cancer*, vol. 22, no. 5, 1161-1169.

Han, X, Wang, L, Shi, H, Zheng, G, He, J, Wu, W, Shi, J, Wei, G, Zheng, W, Sun, J, Huang, H & Cai, Z (2017). Acupuncture combined with methylcobalamin for the treatment of chemotherapy-induced peripheral neuropathy in patients with multiple myeloma, *BMC Cancer*, vol. 17, no. 1, 40.

Hausheer, FH, Schilsky, RL, Bain, S, Berghorn, EJ & Lieberman, F (2006). Diagnosis, management, and evaluation of chemotherapy-induced peripheral neuropathy, *Semin Oncol*, vol. 33, no. 1, 15-49.

Hershman, DL, Unger, JM, Crew, KD, Till, C, Greenlee, H, Minasian, LM, Moinpour, CM, Lew, DL, Fehrenbacher, L, Wade, JL, 3rd, Wong, SF, Fisch, MJ, Lynn Henry, N & Albain, KS (2018). Two-Year Trends of Taxane-Induced Neuropathy in Women

Enrolled in a Randomized Trial of Acetyl-L-Carnitine (SWOG S0715), *J Natl Cancer Inst*, vol. 110, no. 6, 669-676.

Hertz, DL, Childs, DS, Park, SB, Faithfull, S, Ke, Y, Ali, NT, McGlown, SM, Chan, A, Grech, LB, Loprinzi, CL, Ruddy, KJ & Lustberg, M (2021). Patient-centric decision framework for treatment alterations in patients with Chemotherapy-induced Peripheral Neuropathy (CIPN), *Cancer Treat Rev*, vol. 99, 102241.

Hirayama, Y, Ishitani, K, Sato, Y, Iyama, S, Takada, K, Murase, K, Kuroda, H, Nagamachi, Y, Konuma, Y, Fujimi, A, Sagawa, T, Ono, K, Horiguchi, H, Terui, T, Koike, K, Kusakabe, T, Sato, T, Takimoto, R, Kobune, M & Kato, J (2015). Effect of duloxetine in Japanese patients with chemotherapy-induced peripheral neuropathy: a pilot randomized trial, *Int J Clin Oncol*, vol. 20, no. 5, 866-871.

Hodgson, KD, Hutchinson, AD, Wilson, CJ & Nettelbeck, T (2013). A meta-analysis of the effects of chemotherapy on cognition in patients with cancer, *Cancer Treatment Reviews*, vol. 39, no. 3, 297-304.

Horowitz, TS, Suls, J & Trevino, M (2018). A Call for a Neuroscience Approach to Cancer-Related Cognitive Impairment, *Trends Neurosci*, vol. 41, no. 8, 493-496.

Hsu, SY, Huang, WS, Lee, SH, Chu, TP, Lin, YC, Lu, CH, Beaton, RD & Jane, SW (2019). Incidence, severity, longitudinal trends and predictors of acute and chronic oxaliplatin-induced peripheral neuropathy in Taiwanese patients with colorectal cancer, *Eur J Cancer Care (Engl)*, vol. 28, no. 2, e12976.

Huang, X, Hussain, B & Chang, J (2021). Peripheral inflammation and blood-brain barrier disruption: effects and mechanisms, *CNS Neurosci Ther*, vol. 27, no. 1, 36-47.

Huo, X, Reyes, TM, Heijnen, CJ & Kavelaars, A (2018). Cisplatin treatment induces attention deficits and impairs synaptic integrity in the prefrontal cortex in mice, *Sci Rep*, vol. 8, no. 1, 17400.

Huskisson, E, Maggini, S & Ruf, M (2007). The influence of micronutrients on cognitive function and performance, *Journal of International Medical Research*, vol. 35, no. 1, 1-19.

Imamura, T, Izumi, H, Nagatani, G, Ise, T, Nomoto, M, Iwamoto, Y & Kohno, K (2001). Interaction with p53 enhances binding of cisplatin-modified DNA by high mobility group 1 protein, *J Biol Chem*, vol. 276, no. 10, 7534-7540.

Janelsins, MC, Kesler, SR, Ahles, TA & Morrow, GR (2014). Prevalence, mechanisms, and management of cancer-related cognitive impairment, *International Review of Psychiatry*, vol. 26, no. 1, 102-113.

Janes, K, Doyle, T, Bryant, L, Esposito, E, Cuzzocrea, S, Ryerse, J, Bennett, GJ & Salvemini, D (2013). Bioenergetic deficits in peripheral nerve sensory axons during chemotherapy-induced neuropathic pain resulting from peroxynitrite-mediated post-translational nitration of mitochondrial superoxide dismutase, *Pain*, vol. 154, no. 11, 2432-2440.

Jansen, CE, Cooper, BA, Dodd, MJ & Miaskowski, CA (2011). A prospective longitudinal study of chemotherapy-induced cognitive changes in breast cancer patients, *Supportive Care in Cancer*, vol. 19, no. 10, 1647-1656.

Jáuregui-Lobera, I (2014). Iron deficiency and cognitive functions, *Neuropsychiatric disease and treatment*, vol. 10, 2087-2095.

Jean-Pierre, P, Mohile, S, Morrow, G, Figueroa-Moseley, C, Berenberg, J, Atkins, J, Weiss, M. (2019). Neuroprotective effect of SSRIamong 781 cancer patients receiving chemotherapy: A URCC CCOP Study, *J. Clin. Oncol*, vol. 27, 9512.

Jongen, JL, Broijl, A & Sonneveld, P (2015). Chemotherapy-induced peripheral neuropathies in hematological malignancies, *J Neurooncol*, vol. 121, no. 2, 229-237.

Jordan, B, Margulies, A, Cardoso, F, Cavaletti, G, Haugnes, HS, Jahn, P, Le Rhun, E, Preusser, M, Scotte, F, Taphoorn, MJB, Jordan, K, EGCEa, EEWGEa. EGCEa (2020). Systemic anticancer therapy-induced peripheral and central neurotoxicity: ESMO-EONS-EANO Clinical Practice Guidelines for diagnosis, prevention, treatment and follow-up, *Ann Oncol*, vol. 31, no. 10, 1306-1319.

Ju, ZY, Wang, K, Cui, HS, Yao, Y, Liu, SM, Zhou, J, Chen, TY & Xia, J (2017). Acupuncture for neuropathic pain in adults, *Cochrane Database Syst Rev*, vol. 12, CD012057.

Kanbayashi, Y, Sakaguchi, K, Ishikawa, T, Ouchi, Y, Nakatsukasa, K, Tabuchi, Y, Kanehisa, F, Hiramatsu, M, Takagi, R, Yokota, I, Katoh, N & Taguchi, T (2020). Comparison of the efficacy of cryotherapy and compression therapy for preventing nanoparticle albumin-bound paclitaxel-induced peripheral neuropathy: A prospective self-controlled trial, *Breast*, vol. 49, 219-224.

Karschnia, P, Parsons, MW & Dietrich, J (2019). Pharmacologic management of cognitive impairment induced by cancer therapy, *Lancet Oncol*, vol. 20, no. 2, e92-e102.

Khalil, M, Teunissen, CE, Otto, M, Piehl, F, Sormani, MP, Gattringer, T, Barro, C, Kappos, L, Comabella, M, Fazekas, F, Petzold, A, Blennow, K, Zetterberg, H & Kuhle, J (2018). Neurofilaments as biomarkers in neurological disorders, *Nat Rev Neurol*, vol. 14, no. 10, 577-589.

Kim, HK, Zhang, YP, Gwak, YS & Abdi, S (2010). Phenyl N-tert-butylnitrone, a free radical scavenger, reduces mechanical allodynia in chemotherapy-induced neuropathic pain in rats, *Anesthesiology*, vol. 112, no. 2, 432-439.

Kleckner, IR, Kamen, C, Gewandter, JS, Mohile, NA, Heckler, CE, Culakova, E, Fung, C, Janelsins, MC, Asare, M, Lin, PJ, Reddy, PS, Giguere, J, Berenberg, J, Kesler, SR & Mustian, KM 2018, Effects of exercise during chemotherapy on chemotherapy-induced peripheral neuropathy: a multicenter, randomized controlled trial, *Support Care Cancer*, vol. 26, no. 4, Apr, 1019-1028.

Kohli, S, Fisher, SG, Tra, Y, Adams, MJ, Mapstone, ME, Wesnes, KA, Roscoe, JA & Morrow, GR (2009). The effect of modafinil on cognitive function in breast cancer survivors, *Cancer*, vol. 115, no. 12, 2605-2616.

Lange, M, Giffard, B, Noal, S, Rigal, O, Kurtz, JE, Heutte, N, Levy, C, Allouache, D, Rieux, C, Le Fel, J, Daireaux, A, Clarisse, B, Veyret, C, Barthelemy, P, Longato, N, Eustache, F & Joly, F (2014). Baseline cognitive functions among elderly patients with localised breast cancer, *Eur J Cancer*, vol. 50, no. 13, 2181-2189.

Lazic, A, Popovic, J, Paunesku, T, Woloschak, GE & Stevanovic. (M 2020). Insights into platinum-induced peripheral neuropathy-current perspective, *Neural Regen Res*, vol. 15, no. 9, 1623-1630.

Le-Rademacher, J, Kanwar, R, Seisler, D, Pachman, DR, Qin, R, Abyzov, A, Ruddy, KJ, Banck, MS, Lavoie Smith, EM, Dorsey, SG, Aaronson, NK, Sloan, J, Loprinzi, CL & Beutler, AS (2017). Patient-reported (EORTC QLQ-CIPN20) versus physician-reported (CTCAE) quantification of oxaliplatin- and paclitaxel/carboplatin-induced peripheral neuropathy in NCCTG/Alliance clinical trials, *Support Care Cancer*, vol. 25, no. 11, 3537-3544.

Leung, L & Cahill, CM (2010). TNF-alpha and neuropathic pain--a review, *J Neuroinflammation*, vol. 7, 27.

Li, Y, Zhang, H, Kosturakis, AK, Cassidy, RM, Zhang, H, Kennamer-Chapman, RM, Jawad, AB, Colomand, CM, Harrison, DS & Dougherty, PM (2015). MAPK signaling downstream to TLR4 contributes to paclitaxel-induced peripheral neuropathy, *Brain Behav Immun*, vol. 49, 255-266.

Li, Y, Zhang, H, Zhang, H, Kosturakis, AK, Jawad, AB & Dougherty, PM (2014). Toll-like receptor 4 signaling contributes to Paclitaxel-induced peripheral neuropathy, *J Pain*, vol. 15, no. 7, 712-725.

Lindner, OC, Phillips, B, McCabe, MG, Mayes, A, Wearden, A, Varese, F & Talmi, D (2014). A meta-analysis of cognitive impairment following adult cancer chemotherapy, *Neuropsychology*, vol. 28, no. 5, 726-740.

Lomeli, N, Di, K, Czerniawski, J, Guzowski, JF & Bota, DA (2017). Cisplatin-induced mitochondrial dysfunction is associated with impaired cognitive function in rats, *Free Radic Biol Med*, vol. 102, 274-286.

Loprinzi, C, Le-Rademacher, JG, Majithia, N, McMurray, RP, ONeill, CR, Bendel, MA, Beutler, A, Lachance, DH, Cheville, A, Strick, DM, Black, DF, Tilburt, JC & Smith, TJ (2020). Scrambler therapy for chemotherapy neuropathy: a randomized phase II pilot trial, *Support Care Cancer*, vol. 28, no. 3, 1183-1197.

Loprinzi, CL, Lacchetti, C, Bleeker, J, Cavaletti, G, Chauhan, C, Hertz, DL, Kelley, MR, Lavino, A, Lustberg, MB, Paice, JA, Schneider, BP, Lavoie Smith, EM, Smith, ML, Smith, TJ, Wagner-Johnston, N & Hershman, DL (2020). Prevention and Management of Chemotherapy-Induced Peripheral Neuropathy in Survivors of Adult Cancers: ASCO Guideline Update, *J Clin Oncol*, vol. 38, no. 28, 3325-3348.

Loprinzi, CL, Reeves, BN, Dakhil, SR, Sloan, JA, Wolf, SL, Burger, KN, Kamal, A, Le-Lindqwister, NA, Soori, GS, Jaslowski, AJ, Novotny, PJ & Lachance, DH (2011). Natural history of paclitaxel-associated acute pain syndrome: prospective cohort study NCCTG N08C1, *J Clin Oncol*, vol. 29, no. 11, 1472-1478.

Lu, W, Giobbie-Hurder, A, Freedman, RA, Shin, IH, Lin, NU, Partridge, AH, Rosenthal, DS & Ligibel, JA (2020). Acupuncture for Chemotherapy-Induced Peripheral Neuropathy in Breast Cancer Survivors: A Randomized Controlled Pilot Trial, *Oncologist*, vol. 25, no. 4, 310-318.

Lynch, ME, Cesar-Rittenberg, P & Hohmann, AG (2014). A double-blind, placebo-controlled, crossover pilot trial with extension using an oral mucosal cannabinoid extract for treatment of chemotherapy-induced neuropathic pain, *J Pain Symptom Manage*, vol. 47, no. 1, 166-173.

Mancuso, A, Migliorino, M, De Santis, S, Saponiero, A & De Marinis, F (2006). Correlation between anemia and functional/cognitive capacity in elderly lung cancer patients treated with chemotherapy, *Annals of Oncology*, vol. 17, no. 1, 146-150.

Manohar, S, Jamesdaniel, S & Salvi, R (2014). Cisplatin inhibits hippocampal cell proliferation and alters the expression of apoptotic genes, *Neurotox Res*, vol. 25, no. 4, 369-380.

Masocha, W (2016). Gene expression profile of sodium channel subunits in the anterior cingulate cortex during experimental paclitaxel-induced neuropathic pain in mice, *PeerJ*, vol. 4, e2702.

Mayo, SJ, Lustberg, M, H, MD, Nakamura, ZM, Allen, DH, Von Ah, D, M, CJ, Chan, A, Olson, K, Tan, CJ, Toh, YL, Oh, J, Grech, L, Cheung, YT, Subbiah, IM, Petranovic, D, DOlimpio, J, Gobbo, M, Koeppen, S, Loprinzi, CL, Pang, L, Shinde, S, Ntukidem, O & Peters, KB (2021). Cancer-related cognitive impairment in patients with non-central nervous system malignancies: an overview for oncology providers from the MASCC Neurological Complications Study Group, *Support Care Cancer*, vol. 29, no. 6, 2821-2840.

Menning, S, de Ruiter, MB, Veltman, DJ, Boogerd, W, Oldenburg, HS, Reneman, L & Schagen, SB (2017). Changes in brain activation in breast cancer patients depend on cognitive domain and treatment type, *PLoS One*, vol. 12, no. 3, e0171724.

Milbury, K, Chaoul, A, Biegler, K, Wangyal, T, Spelman, A, Meyers, CA, Arun, B, Palmer, JL, Taylor, J & Cohen, L (2013). Tibetan sound meditation for cognitive dysfunction: results of a randomized controlled pilot trial, *Psychooncology*, vol. 22, no. 10, 2354-2363.

Miller, AB, Hoogstraten, B, Staquet, M & Winkler, A (1981). Reporting results of cancer treatment, *Cancer*, vol. 47, no. 1, 207-214.

Miltenburg, NC & Boogerd, W (2014). Chemotherapy-induced neuropathy: A comprehensive survey, *Cancer Treat Rev*, vol. 40, no. 7, 872-882.

Molassiotis, A, Cheng, HL, Leung, KT, Li, YC, Wong, KH, Au, JSK, Sundar, R, Chan, A, Ng, TR, Suen, LKP, Chan, CW, Yorke, J & Lopez, V (2019). Risk factors for chemotherapy-induced peripheral neuropathy in patients receiving taxane- and platinum-based chemotherapy, *Brain Behav*, vol. 9, no. 6, e01312.

Molassiotis, A, Suen, LKP, Cheng, HL, Mok, TSK, Lee, SCY, Wang, CH, Lee, P, Leung, H, Chan, V, Lau, TKH & Yeo, W (2019). A Randomized Assessor-Blinded Wait-List-Controlled Trial to Assess the Effectiveness of Acupuncture in the Management of Chemotherapy-Induced Peripheral Neuropathy, *Integr Cancer Ther*, vol. 18, 1534735419836501.

Murono, K, Nagata, H, Ishimaru, K, Emoto, S, Kaneko, M, Hiyoshi, M, Sasaki, K, Otani, K, Shuno, Y, Nishikawa, T, Tanaka, T, Hata, K, Kawai, K, Nozawa, H, Muro, K & Ishihara, S (2019). Safety of intraperitoneal paclitaxel combined with conventional chemotherapy for colorectal cancer with peritoneal carcinomatosis: a phase I trial, *Cancer Chemother Pharmacol*, vol. 83, no. 1, 145-150.

Nelson, WL & Suls, J (2013). New approaches to understand cognitive changes associated with chemotherapy for non-central nervous system tumors, *J Pain Symptom Manage*, vol. 46, no. 5, 707-721.

Network. NCC (2021). *NCCN Clinical Practice Guidelines in Oncology: Survivorship* National Comprehensive Cancer Network, Plymouth Meeting.

Nudelman, KN, McDonald, BC, Wang, Y, Smith, DJ, West, JD, ONeill, DP, Zanville, NR, Champion, VL, Schneider, BP & Saykin, AJ (2016). Cerebral Perfusion and Gray Matter Changes Associated With Chemotherapy-Induced Peripheral Neuropathy, *J Clin Oncol*, vol. 34, no. 7, 677-683.

Oken, MM, Creech, RH, Tormey, DC, Horton, J, Davis, TE, McFadden, ET & Carbone, PP (1982). Toxicity and response criteria of the Eastern Cooperative Oncology Group, *Am J Clin Oncol*, vol. 5, no. 6, 649-655.

Omran, M, Belcher, EK, Mohile, NA, Kesler, SR, Janelsins, MC, Hohmann, AG & Kleckner, IR 2021, Review of the Role of the Brain in Chemotherapy-Induced Peripheral Neuropathy, *Front Mol Biosci*, vol. 8, p. 693133.

Ownby, KK (2019). Use of the distress thermometer in clinical practice, *J Adv Pract Oncol*, vol. 10, no. 2, 175-179.

Pabla, N, Huang, S, Mi, QS, Daniel, R & Dong, Z (2008). ATR-Chk2 signaling in p53 activation and DNA damage response during cisplatin-induced apoptosis, *J Biol Chem*, vol. 283, no. 10, 6572-6583.

Pachman, DR, Qin, R, Seisler, DK, Smith, EM, Beutler, AS, Ta, LE, Lafky, JM, Wagner-Johnston, ND, Ruddy, KJ, Dakhil, S, Staff, NP, Grothey, A & Loprinzi, CL (2015). Clinical Course of Oxaliplatin-Induced Neuropathy: Results From the Randomized Phase III Trial N08CB (Alliance), *J Clin Oncol*, vol. 33, no. 30, 3416-3422.

Paniagua, N, Sanchez-Robles, EM, Bagues, A, Martin-Fontelles, MI, Goicoechea, C & Giron, R (2021). Behavior and electrophysiology studies of the peripheral neuropathy induced by individual and co-administration of paclitaxel and oxaliplatin in rat, *Life Sci*, vol. 277, 119397.

Park, SB, Goldstein, D, Krishnan, AV, Lin, CS, Friedlander, ML, Cassidy, J, Koltzenburg, M & Kiernan, MC (2013). Chemotherapy-induced peripheral neurotoxicity: a critical analysis, *CA Cancer J Clin*, vol. 63, no. 6, 419-437.

Parsons, MW & Dietrich, J (2019). Assessment and management of cognitive changes in patients with cancer, *Cancer*, vol. 125, no. 12, 1958-1962.

Pasetto, LM, DAndrea, MR, Rossi, E & Monfardini, S (2006). Oxaliplatin-related neurotoxicity: how and why?, *Crit Rev Oncol Hematol*, vol. 59, no. 2, 159-168.

Patel, SK, Meier, AM, Fernandez, N, Lo, TTY, Moore, C & Delgado, N (2017). Convergent and criterion validity of the CogState computerized brief battery cognitive assessment in women with and without breast cancer, *Clin Neuropsychol*, vol. 31, no. 8, 1375-1386.

Pendergrass, JC, Targum, SD & Harrison, JE (2018). Cognitive impairment associated with cancer: A brief review, *Innovations in clinical neuroscience*, vol. 15, no. 1-2, 36-44.

Pike, CT, Birnbaum, HG, Muehlenbein, CE, Pohl, GM & Natale, RB (2012). Healthcare costs and workloss burden of patients with chemotherapy-associated peripheral neuropathy in breast, ovarian, head and neck, and nonsmall cell lung cancer, *Chemother Res Pract*, vol. 2012, 913848.

Prinsloo, S, Novy, D, Driver, L, Lyle, R, Ramondetta, L, Eng, C, McQuade, J, Lopez, G & Cohen, L (2017). Randomized controlled trial of neurofeedback on chemotherapy-induced peripheral neuropathy: A pilot study, *Cancer*, vol. 123, no. 11, 1989-1997.

Raffard, S, Lebrun, C, Bayard, S, Macgregor, A & Capdevielle, D (2020). Self-awareness deficits of cognitive impairment in individuals with schizophrenia. Really?, *Frontiers in Psychiatry*, vol. 11, no. 731.

Reeves, BN, Dakhil, SR, Sloan, JA, Wolf, SL, Burger, KN, Kamal, A, Le-Lindqwister, NA, Soori, GS, Jaslowski, AJ, Kelaghan, J, Novotny, PJ, Lachance, DH & Loprinzi, CL (2012). Further data supporting that paclitaxel-associated acute pain syndrome is associated with development of peripheral neuropathy: North Central Cancer Treatment Group trial N08C1, *Cancer*, vol. 118, no. 20, 5171-5178.

Reid-Arndt, SA & Cox, CR (2012). Stress, coping and cognitive deficits in women after surgery for breast cancer, *J Clin Psychol Med Settings*, vol. 19, no. 2, 127-137.

Riis, CL, Stie, M, Bechmann, T, Jensen, PT, Coulter, A, Moller, S & Steffensen, KD 2021, ePRO-based individual follow-up care for women treated for early breast cancer: impact on service use and workflows, *J Cancer Surviv*, vol. 15, no. 4, Aug, 485-496.

Rostock, M, Jaroslawski, K, Guethlin, C, Ludtke, R, Schroder, S & Bartsch, HH (2013). Chemotherapy-induced peripheral neuropathy in cancer patients: a four-arm randomized trial on the effectiveness of electroacupuncture, *Evid Based Complement Alternat Med*, vol. 2013, 349653.

Salgado, TM, Quinn, CS, Krumbach, EK, Wenceslao, I, Gonzalez, M, Reed, HL, Syverson, JG, Etz, RS, Vangipuram, K, Barker, MR, Henry, NL, Farris, KB & Hertz, DL (2020). Reporting of paclitaxel-induced peripheral neuropathy symptoms to clinicians among women with breast cancer: a qualitative study, *Support Care Cancer*, vol. 28, no. 9, 4163-4172.

Sands, S, Ladas, EJ, Kelly, KM, Weiner, M, Lin, M, Ndao, DH, Dave, A, Vahdat, LT & Bender, JG (2017). Glutamine for the treatment of vincristine-induced neuropathy in children and adolescents with cancer, *Support Care Cancer*, vol. 25, no. 3, 701-708.

Schagen, SB, Muller, MJ, Boogerd, W, Mellenbergh, GJ & van Dam. FSAM (2006). Change in cognitive function after chemotherapy: a prospective longitudinal study in breast cancer patients, *JNCI: Journal of the National Cancer Institute*, vol. 98, no. 23, 1742-1745.

Schmidt, JE, Beckjord, E, Bovbjerg, DH, Low, CA, Posluszny, DM, Lowery, AE, Dew, MA, Nutt, S, Arvey, SR & Rechis, R (2016). Prevalence of perceived cognitive dysfunction in survivors of a wide range of cancers: results from the 2010 LIVESTRONG survey, *Journal of Cancer Survivorship*, vol. 10, no. 2, 302-311.

Shen, H, Perez, RE, Davaadelger, B & Maki, CG (2013). Two 4N cell-cycle arrests contribute to cisplatin-resistance, *PLoS One*, vol. 8, no. 4, e59848.

Smith, EM, Pang, H, Cirrincione, C, Fleishman, S, Paskett, ED, Ahles, T, Bressler, LR, Fadul, CE, Knox, C, Le-Lindqwister, N, Gilman, PB, Shapiro, CL & Alliance for Clinical Trials in, O (2013). Effect of duloxetine on pain, function, and quality of life among patients with chemotherapy-induced painful peripheral neuropathy: a randomized clinical trial, *JAMA*, vol. 309, no. 13, 1359-1367.

Smith, T & Nicholson, RA (2007). Review of duloxetine in the management of diabetic peripheral neuropathic pain, *Vasc Health Risk Manag*, vol. 3, no. 6, 833-844.

Smith, TJ, Razzak, AR, Blackford, AL, Ensminger, J, Saiki, C, Longo-Schoberlein, D & Loprinzi, CL (2020). A Pilot Randomized Sham-Controlled Trial of MC5-A Scrambler Therapy in the Treatment of Chronic Chemotherapy-Induced Peripheral Neuropathy (CIPN), *J Palliat Care*, vol. 35, no. 1, 53-58.

Spaich, S, Kinder, J, Hetjens, S, Fuxius, S, Gerhardt, A & Sutterlin, M (2018). Patient Preferences Regarding Chemotherapy in Metastatic Breast Cancer-A Conjoint Analysis for Common Taxanes, *Front Oncol*, vol. 8, 535.

Staff, NP, Grisold, A, Grisold, W & Windebank, AJ (2017). Chemotherapy-induced peripheral neuropathy: A current review, *Ann Neurol*, vol. 81, no. 6, 772-781.

Su, Y, Huang, J, Wang, S, Unger, JM, Arias-Fuenzalida, J, Shi, Y, Li, J, Gao, Y, Shi, W, Wang, X, Peng, R, Xu, F, An, X, Xue, C, Xia, W, Hong, R, Zhong, Y, Lin, Y, Huang, H, Zhang, A, Zhang, L, Cai, L, Zhang, J & Yuan, Z (2020). The Effects of Ganglioside-Monosialic Acid in Taxane-Induced Peripheral Neurotoxicity in Patients with Breast Cancer: A Randomized Trial, *J Natl Cancer Inst*, vol. 112, no. 1, 55-62.

Subramaniam, CB, Bowen, JM, Gladman, MA, Lustberg, MB, Mayo, SJ & Wardill, HR (2020). The microbiota-gut-brain axis: An emerging therapeutic target in chemotherapy-induced cognitive impairment, *Neurosci Biobehav Rev*, vol. 116, 470-479.

Tang, W, Zhu, H, Feng, Y, Guo, R & Wan, D (2020). The Impact of Gut Microbiota Disorders on the Blood-Brain Barrier, *Infect Drug Resist*, vol. 13, 3351-3363.

Tanguturi, SK & Alexander, BM (2018). Neurologic Complications of Radiation Therapy, *Neurol Clin*, vol. 36, no. 3, 599-625.

Tchounwou, PB, Dasari, S, Noubissi, FK, Ray, P & Kumar, S (2021). Advances in Our Understanding of the Molecular Mechanisms of Action of Cisplatin in Cancer Therapy, *J Exp Pharmacol*, vol. 13, 303-328.

Thibault, K, Calvino, B, Dubacq, S, Roualle-de-Rouville, M, Sordoillet, V, Rivals, I & Pezet, S (2012). Cortical effect of oxaliplatin associated with sustained neuropathic pain: exacerbation of cortical activity and down-regulation of potassium channel expression in somatosensory cortex, *Pain*, vol. 153, no. 8, 1636-1647.

Timmins, HC, Mizrahi, D, Li, T, Kiernan, MC, Goldstein, D & Park, SB (2021). Metabolic and lifestyle risk factors for chemotherapy-induced peripheral neuropathy in taxane and platinum-treated patients: a systematic review, *J Cancer Surviv*.

Trotti, A, Colevas, AD, Setser, A, Rusch, V, Jaques, D, Budach, V, Langer, C, Murphy, B, Cumberlin, R, Coleman, CN & Rubin, P (2003). CTCAE v3.0: development of a comprehensive grading system for the adverse effects of cancer treatment, *Semin Radiat Oncol*, vol. 13, no. 3, 176-181.

Tsuyuki, S, Senda, N, Kanng, Y, Yamaguchi, A, Yoshibayashi, H, Kikawa, Y, Katakami, N, Kato, H, Hashimoto, T, Okuno, T, Yamauchi, A & Inamoto, T (2016). Evaluation of the effect of compression therapy using surgical gloves on nanoparticle albumin-bound paclitaxel-induced peripheral neuropathy: a phase II multicenter study by the Kamigata Breast Cancer Study Group, *Breast Cancer Res Treat*, vol. 160, no. 1, 61-67.

Umfress, A, Speed, HE, Tan, C, Ramezani, S, Birnbaum, S, Brekken, RA, Sun, X, Plattner, F, Powell, CM & Bibb, JA (2021). Neuropathological Effects of Chemotherapeutic Drugs, *ACS Chem Neurosci*, vol. 12, no. 16, 3038-3048.

van Dam, FS, Schagen, SB, Muller, MJ, Boogerd, W, vd Wall, E, Droogleever Fortuyn, ME & Rodenhuis, S (1998). Impairment of cognitive function in women receiving adjuvant treatment for high-risk breast cancer: high-dose versus standard-dose chemotherapy, *J Natl Cancer Inst*, vol. 90, no. 3, 210-218.

van der Hiele, K, Spliethoff-Kamminga, NGA, Ruimschotel, RP, Middelkoop, HAM & Visser, LH (2012). The relationship between self-reported executive performance and psychological characteristics in multiple sclerosis, *European Journal of Neurology*, vol. 19, 562-569.

van Dyk, K, Crespi, CM, Petersen, L & Ganz, PA (2020). Identifying cancer-related cognitive impairment using the FACT-Cog perceived cognitive impairment, *JNCI Cancer Spectrum*, vol. 4, no. 1.

van Heugten, CM (2017). Evidence-Based Treatment, in *Neuropsychological Rehabilitation: The International Handbook*, Taylor and Francis Group, London.

Vannorsdall, TD (2017). Cognitive Changes Related to Cancer Therapy, *Med Clin North Am*, vol. 101, no. 6, 1115-1134.

Vermorken, JB, ten Bokkel Huinink, WW, Eisenhauer, EA, Favalli, G, Belpomme, D, Conte, PF & Kaye, SB (1993). Advanced ovarian cancer. Carboplatin versus cisplatin, *Ann Oncol*, vol. 4 Suppl 4, 41-48.

Wagner, LI, Sweet, J, Butt, Z, Lai, JS & Cella, D (2009). Measuring patient self-reported cognitive function: Development of the Functional Assessment of Cancer Therapy–Cognitive Function Instrument, *Journal of Supportive Oncology*, vol. 7, W32-W39.

Waissengrin, B, Mirelman, D, Pelles, S, Bukstein, F, Blumenthal, DT, Wolf, I & Geva, R (2021). Effect of cannabis on oxaliplatin-induced peripheral neuropathy among oncology patients: a retrospective analysis, *Ther Adv Med Oncol*, vol. 13, 1758835921990203.

Walbert, T & Gilbert, MR (2009). The role of chemotherapy in the treatment of patients with brain metastases from solid tumors, *Int J Clin Oncol*, vol. 14, no. 4, 299-306.

Wardill, HR, Mander, KA, Van Sebille, YZ, Gibson, RJ, Logan, RM, Bowen, JM & Sonis, ST (2016). Cytokine-mediated blood brain barrier disruption as a conduit for cancer/chemotherapy-associated neurotoxicity and cognitive dysfunction, *Int J Cancer*, vol. 139, no. 12, 2635-2645.

Wefel, JS, Lenzi, R, Theriault, RL, Davis, RN & Meyers, CA (2004). The cognitive sequelae of standard-dose adjuvant chemotherapy in women with breast carcinoma: Results of a prospective, randomized, longitudinal trial, *Cancer*, vol. 100, no. 11, 2292-2299.

Wefel, JSP, Vardy, JMD, Ahles, TP & Schagen. SBD (2011). International Cognition and Cancer Task Force recommendations to harmonise studies of cognitive function in patients with cancer, *Lancet Oncol*, vol. 12, no. 7, 703-708.

Weng, HR, Cordella, JV & Dougherty, PM (2003). Changes in sensory processing in the spinal dorsal horn accompany vincristine-induced hyperalgesia and allodynia, *Pain*, vol. 103, no. 1-2, 131-138.

Wilson, BA (2007). *Neuropsychological Rehabilitation: Theory, Models, Therapy and Outcome*, Cambridge University Press, Leiden.

Wilson, BA, Winegardner, J, Heugten, CMv & Ownsworth, T (2017). *Neuropsycho-logical rehabilitation: the international handbook*, Taylor and Francis, London.

Wolf, S, Barton, D, Kottschade, L, Grothey, A & Loprinzi, C (2008). Chemotherapy-induced peripheral neuropathy: prevention and treatment strategies, *Eur J Cancer*, vol. 44, no. 11, Jul, 1507-1515.

Yap, NY, Toh, YL, Tan, CJ, Acharya, MM & Chan A (2021). Relationship between cytokines and brain-derived neurotrophic factor (BDNF) in trajectories of cancer-related cognitive impairment, *Cytokine*, vol. 144, 155556.

Zajaczkowska, R, Kocot-Kepska, M, Leppert, W, Wrzosek, A, Mika, J & Wordliczek, J (2019). Mechanisms of Chemotherapy-Induced Peripheral Neuropathy, *Int J Mol Sci*, vol. 20, no. 6.

Zamble, DB, Mikata, Y, Eng, CH, Sandman, KE & Lippard, SJ 2002, Testis-specific HMG-domain protein alters the responses of cells to cisplatin, *J Inorg Biochem*, vol. 91, no. 3, 451-462.

Zheng, Y, Luo, J, Bao, P, Cai, H, Hong, Z, Ding, D, Jackson, JC, Shu, XO & Dai, Q (2014). Long-term cognitive function change among breast cancer survivors, *Breast Cancer Res Treat*, vol. 146, no. 3, 599-609.

Zimmer, P, Trebing, S, Timmers-Trebing, U, Schenk, A, Paust, R, Bloch, W, Rudolph, R, Streckmann, F & Baumann, FT (2018). Eight-week, multimodal exercise counteracts a progress of chemotherapy-induced peripheral neuropathy and improves balance and strength in metastasized colorectal cancer patients: a randomized controlled trial, *Support Care Cancer*, vol. 26, no. 2, 615-624.

Chapter 5

Ototoxicity Induced by Platinum-Based Chemotherapy

Ignacio A. Cortés-Fuentes[1,2,*], **Mauricio A. Retamal**[3,4,5] **and Juan G. Gormaz**[6]

[1]Hospital Barros Luco-Trudeau, San Miguel, Santiago, Chile
[2]Departamento de Otorrinolaringología, Facultad de Medicina, Universidad de Chile, Chile
[3]Universidad del Desarrollo, Programa de Comunicación Celular en Cáncer. Clínica Alemana Facultad de Medicina. Santiago, Chile
[4]Universidad del Desarrollo, Centro de Fisiología Celular e Integrativa. Clínica Alemana Facultad de Medicina. Santiago, Chile
[5]Department of Cell Physiology and Molecular Biophysics, and Center for Membrane Protein Research, School of Medicine, Texas Tech University Health Sciences Center, Lubbock, TX, United States
[6]Facultad de Medicina, Universidad de Chile, Chile

Abstract

Platinum-based treatments can trigger ototoxicity during cancer treatment. Patients commonly develop bilateral, irreversible sensorineural hearing loss, which is especially critical in the pediatric population, requiring long-term follow-up due to potential detrimental hearing-loss effects on language and social development. The prevalence of ototoxicity following platinum-based chemotherapy in this group is not well established, but incidences as high as 90% have been reported. Among the adult population, it has been reported that up to 80% of patients may develop ototoxicity. Thus, this condition may be an

*Corresponding Author's Email: ignaciocortes@med.uchile.cl.

In: Platinum-Based Chemotherapy
Editors: Kulmira Nurgali and Raquel Abalo
ISBN: 978-1-68507-972-7
© 2022 Nova Science Publishers, Inc.

important cause of decreasing quality of life in cancer survivors. From a clinical point of view, ototoxicity induced by platinum-based chemotherapy exhibits auditory manifestations as well as vestibular symptoms and tinnitus. Ototoxicity can clinically manifest within hours to days following the first chemotherapy cycle or even years after treatment. High-frequency hearing loss typically occurs first, and it can evolve to involve middle frequencies in a dose-dependent manner. Mechanistically, platinum-based chemotherapy induced ototoxicity is mainly caused from the production of pathological levels of reactive oxygen species (ROS) rather than DNA-adduct formation, which has led to test strategies based on direct ROS scavengers to ameliorate hearing loss. Clinically controversial data have been obtained from several trials and thus have increased interest in the development of strategies to protect patients from ototoxicity without altering the anticancer effects of platinum-based treatments.

Keywords: cisplatin, hearing loss, ototoxicity, platinum-based chemotherapy, tinnitus

Introduction

Auditory and vestibular symptoms often occur following platinum-based treatments. They are the clinical expression of ototoxicity or inner ear injury caused by cisplatin and related drugs. Thus, ototoxicity can impair cancer-survivor quality of life, which is especially important in children as hearing loss may hamper language development, but also in adults as hearing deterioration worsens social interaction. Ototoxicity represents an unsolved clinical problem because there are no optimal preventive or restorative treatments. Furthermore, current auditory aids for established hearing loss have technical and access limitations as well as suboptimal adherence.

Epidemiology and Impact

Hearing loss, tinnitus and chronic equilibrium disorders derived from cancer treatments have a major impact on quality of life of survivors (Pearson et al., 2019). As ototoxicity generated by oncological therapies represents one of the most important potentially preventable causes of hearing loss (Laurell, 2019), intensive research has been generated as to possible strategies to delay their apparition or even to restore auditory and vestibular function (Yu et al., 2020). However, to date there are no current treatments or prevention strategies approved to reduce its occurrence (Ramkumar et al., 2021; Sheth et al., 2017). In this context, early recognition, treatment, or avoidance of potentially preventable causes of chemotherapy-induced hearing loss continue to be major objectives for reducing both short- and long-term hearing disability of cancer survivors (Elena et al., 2013).

Ototoxicity incidence reported during platinum-based treatments is variable. In adults, it has been reported that up to 80% develop some degree of ototoxicity (Frisina et al., 2016). It can manifest early during treatment, in days or weeks, or may appear after years during the follow-up (Breglio et al. 2017; Clemens et al. 2017). This is relevant because the prevalence of hearing loss increases throughout the lifespan (Haile et al., 2021), with at least 25% of people older than 60 demonstrating significant hearing deterioration (Lin et al., 2011). Furthermore, by 2050 2.45 billion people are expected to have hearing loss (Haile et al., 2021). In people who received ototoxic treatments it may be difficult or even impossible to know the exact contribution of ototoxicity to their hearing loss; thus, close follow-up is required on termination of platinum-based treatments (Freyer et al., 2020). It has been reported that quality of life is reduced among cancer survivors following platinum-based treatments and this is further worsened when permanent hearing loss, tinnitus or balance problems appear (Pearson et al., 2019; Prayuenyong et al., 2018).

In children, ototoxic treatments may contribute to significant hearing loss (van As et al., 2016). In fact, hearing loss has a major effect on child development, especially when it occurs prior to language acquisition (Knight et al., 2005). It has been reported that up to 90.1% of children experience ototoxicity following platinum-based treatments (van As et al., 2016). This is further increased when it is combined with radiation schemes (Freyer et al., 2020).

Current treatment modalities for ototoxicity such as hearing aids are frequently not accepted by patients, arguing that hearing aids do not provide the expected benefit, are uncomfortable or esthetically unsatisfactory (McCormack & Fortnum, 2013). Furthermore, auditory treatments represent an important cost for health systems (McDaid et al., 2021) and in some non-developed countries, there remain significant drawbacks to access hearing-related health care (Harris & Dodson, 2017; Kamenov et al., 2021).

Vestibular symptoms following platinum-based treatments are not well understood, and their etiology is also obscure (Prayuenyong et al., 2018).

Vestibular dysfunction following platinum-based treatments is not well reported and may be underrated, although the fact that vestibular damage can have a major impact on quality of life is generally accepted (Sun et al., 2014). Drug-induced vestibulotoxicity frequently affects both ears gradually and symmetrically, causing progressive disequilibrium, which can be overlooked during clinical evaluation. Regrettably, cancer patients have a higher risk than the general population for balance problems such as falls and mobility impairment (Wildes et al., 2015), which is associated with increased mortality in the elderly (Bergen et al., 2016).

Ototoxicity Caused by Platinum-Based Treatment in the Clinical Practice

Ototoxicity refers to the damage and functional impairment caused by different insults to the inner ear, thus resulting mainly in sensorineural hearing loss and tinnitus (L. Rybak et al., 2019).

Hearing loss resulting from ototoxic treatments usually starts with bilateral, sensorineural, progressive, and usually permanent hearing loss associated with tinnitus and vestibular symptoms (Freyer et al., 2020). These side effects caused by ototoxic therapies may significantly impact the quality of life of cancer survivors (Brooks & Knight, 2018), especially in young children, whose hearing loss may lead to deterioration in language and social development (Knight et al., 2005).

Usually, hearing loss starts in the high frequencies and progresses, dose-dependently, to involve middle and low frequencies (Rybak et al. 2009). Auditory deterioration severity depends on several factors and most reports are of mild to moderate hearing loss. This is influenced by, among other factors: age, prior hearing loss, concomitant use of aminoglycosides and loop diuretics, renal impairment and concomitant head and neck radiation therapy (Rybak et al. 2009; Theunissen et al. 2015; Clemens et al. 2016).

However, it is a side effect that frequently is not considered or reported in large clinical trials or follow-up during cancer treatments, which has led to underestimation of the real impact. This is especially frequent in the adult population from lower- to middle-income countries, where access to the health system and auditory rehabilitation programs are limited (Kamenov et al., 2021).

To date, different clinical systems have been described to classify and measure ototoxicity, specifically referring to auditory deterioration (King &

Brewer, 2018). These scales have significant variability between them, and efforts have been made to standardize ototoxicity grading (Clemens et al. 2019). This is especially important because an exact classification for hearing loss has implications for accurate auditory rehabilitation options and reporting audiologic outcomes in clinical trials.

Auditory Treatments for Established Hearing Loss

Hearing aids for adults and children represents the mainstay of managing patients who develop clinically significant ototoxicity (Landier, 2016). Their use is associated with a significant improvement in different auditory outcomes (Ferguson et al., 2017), including perception and intelligibility of sounds, social performance, quality of life and others (Cunningham & Tucci, 2017; Kim & Barrs, 2006; Lieu et al., 2020). This is especially obtained when their use is associated with auditory programs of rehabilitation and technical guidance (Cardemil et al., 2014).

Hearing aids basically receive sounds, process and filter them based on certain technical features, and finally amplify them to the inner ear, thus providing further stimulation for the remaining auditory cells instead of restoring auditory function to normal levels (Kim & Barrs, 2006; Landier, 2016). This is relevant because ototoxicity triggers a sensorineural hearing loss caused by damage to cochlear cells and even in neural cells, which in turn determine that patients may have lower auditory outcomes using hearing aids compared to patients with hearing loss due to other etiologies (Einarsson et al., 2011).

Nevertheless, patients with hearing aids also experience several problems, especially cancer patients with chemo-radiation schemes for head and neck malignancies (Nader & Gidley, 2019). They frequently refer to chirps and annoying coupling sounds and complain about difficulties to detect sound and recognize speech in noisy environments, worsening their adherence to the daily use of hearing aids (Lerner, 2019; McCormack & Fortnum, 2013). Therefore, it is reported that hearing aids have a higher rate of misuse or no-use (Cunningham & Tucci, 2017; Kim & Barrs, 2006; McCormack & Fortnum, 2013). In children, the adaptation to hearing aids may be difficult as they do not understand or perceive the importance and gain of their use or children are uncomfortable using behind-the-ear models (Lieu et al., 2020; Muñoz et al., 2016).

Cochlear implantation represents an auditory treatment when severe to profound hearing loss develops. They are surgically placed in the temporal bone and transform acoustic signals to electric impulses by direct cochlear nerve stimulation. However, in the context of cancer patients there is limited data related to their use (Nader & Gidley, 2019).

Mechanisms behind Ototoxicity

Effects of Platinum-Based Chemotherapy on Auditory System

The classic antineoplastic effect of platinum-based drugs is the generation of nuclear DNA adducts leading to apoptosis (Wang & Lippard, 2005). However, this mechanism does not completely explain the effect of cisplatin on auditory cells and several other mechanisms have been involved in the pathogenesis of auditory cell death triggered by platinums, such as oxidative stress and autophagy induction (Gentilin et al., 2019). For a more comprehensive analysis regarding the biologic effects of platinum-based drugs see the related chapter in this book.

Normally, there is limited entry of platinum-based drugs to the inner ear due to the presence of the blood-labyrinth barrier (Zou et al., 2016). However, it has been reported that platinum-based drugs can enter auditory cells through passive diffusion or mediated by transporters (Rybak, Mukherjea, and Ramkumar 2019). There has been increasing interest in some copper transporters, organic cation transporters and others, that have been involved in differing degrees in the ototoxic effects of cisplatin (Ramkumar et al., 2021; Sheth et al., 2017).

Auditory cells have a special susceptibility to platinum-based chemotherapy ototoxic effects, triggering apoptosis of different cells, including supporting cells, stria vascularis, spiral ganglia cells and preferably outer hair cells (Devarajan et al., 2002; Ding et al., 2020; Liang et al., 2005). Marginal cells, which are involved in $K+$ metabolism in the cochlea, may also be injured, causing $K+$ metabolism disruption, in turn enhancing cell death in the organ of Corti (Laurell et al., 2007).

In combination, DNA/RNA direct damage and increased production of ROS are involved in cisplatin-induced ototoxicity (Tang et al., 2021). Cisplatin has been reported to trigger oxidative-mediated injury by increasing

ROS levels by direct production through stimulating enzymes related to these processes or by decreasing antioxidant defenses (Yu et al., 2020).

The human cochlea has a high metabolic activity in certain areas such as stria vascularis and spiral ligament, which lead to leakage of electrons from the mitochondrial respiratory chain with subsequent ROS (Sheth et al., 2017). Therefore, cochlear cells have antioxidant defense systems, including ROS scavengers such as vitamins C and E and glutathione (Yu et al. 2020; Rybak et al. 2009). Glutathione is largely produced in basal and intermediate cells of stria vascularis as well as in spiral ligament cells (Sheth et al., 2017). Antioxidant enzymes also expressed in the cochlea play a key role preventing oxidative-derived injury, including catalase and the glutathione peroxidase-reductase system contributing to glutathione (Rybak et al. 2009). Two isoforms of superoxide dismutase with a Cu-Zn isoform have reportedly been located in the cytosol and the Mn- isoform located in the mitochondria; this isoform is highly expressed in stria vascularis, spiral ligament and the organ of Corti (Sheth et al. 2017; Rybak et al. 2009). Therefore, cisplatin may increase ROS production by impairing antioxidant defenses through direct antioxidant inactivation caused by increased ROS and peroxides production, as occurs with the thioredoxin enzyme system (Dammeyer et al., 2014), or through decreasing redox scavengers (Yu et al., 2020).

Several sources of ROS have been observed in ototoxicity triggered by platinum-based drugs. There is ROS production caused by the activation of the isoform NOX3 of the enzyme NADPH (nicotinamide adenine dinucleotide phosphate-oxidase) triggered by cisplatin, which in turn leads to Ca^{+2} overload and caspase-induced outer hair cell apoptosis (Rybak et al. 2012). Direct mitochondrial damage in the electron transport chain is caused by cisplatin and may also account for toxic effects on auditory cells, increasing ROS production, independently of nuclear DNA damage (Rybak et al. 2012). Similarly, cisplatin may lead to increased mitochondrial-ROS production triggering autophagy, a caspase-independent mechanism of cell death (Rybak et al. 2012).

Furthermore, reactive nitrogen species have also been reported to be produced by cisplatin. The ROS produced may react with nitric oxide, thus forming peroxynitrite, which can alter proteins by S-nitrosylation processes, involved in controlling cell survival, enhancing caspases- and p53-mediated apoptosis in cochlear cells (Rybak et al. 2012).

There are several mechanisms which have also been described to be involved in ototoxic effects caused by cisplatin, including the expression of several pro-inflammatory mediators such as interleukins, tumor necrosis factor-α, nuclear factor κ-B and others, which in turn may enhance apoptotic effects and interact with other mechanisms discussed above (Clemens et al., 2016; Tang et al., 2021).

Current Molecular and Cellular Findings which Account for Auditory Damage

The latest advances in the study of platinum-analogue mechanisms associated with auditory cell damage are in tune with prior findings, giving oxidative stress a key role in ototoxicity (Ramkumar et al., 2021).

Although the evidence has yet to prove the potential importance in ototoxicity of possible hearing damage mechanisms associated with platinum operating independently of oxidative stress, recent molecular studies point to ROS overproduction as being involved at least in part in nearly all pathways.

For example, it was recently reported that in certain apoptotic responses derived to platinum-analogues historically associated with direct DNA damage, early generation of ROS would, at least in part, be involved in the damage (Tang et al., 2021). Specifically, it was demonstrated that in A549 cell lines (adenocarcinomic human alveolar basal epithelial cells) a synthetic platinum complex induced apoptosis trough generation of endoplasmic reticulum stress, as a direct consequence of early ROS generation.

A recent review regarding this field mentions that as the cochlea is relatively isolated in comparison with other tissues, hair cells cannot excrete the platinum-analogues fast enough to compensate their entry, resulting in an accumulation that, among other effects, reduces antioxidant enzyme synthesis (Oun et al., 2018). This is important because it suggests that platinum-analogues damage is not only interceded by enhancing production of oxidative mediators, but also by reducing enzymatic antioxidant capacity.

Main Attempts to Prevent or Reduce Ototoxicity

The use of systemic strategies to ameliorate hearing loss triggered by platinum-based treatments have resulted in mixed results and have raised concerns about decreasing antitumor therapy efficacy. Thus, different agents have been tested to reduce ototoxicity by directly intervening in the inner ear through trans-tympanic injections. However, this has had variable results and there are several practical drawbacks.

Strategies Based on Direct Interventions to the Ear

The use of systemic treatments to diminish or prevent ototoxicity are potentially feasible. However, there are several drawbacks representing critical points in the development of otoprotection strategies. Thus, considering that cisplatin exerts its anticancer effects through mechanisms which are also involved in their side effects, the use of systemic otoprotective agents must be carefully designed due to the possibility of interfering with the anticancer effects of platinum-based drugs (Yu et al., 2020).

The use of direct interventions to deliver drugs such as trans-tympanic drug injections to the inner ear is widely used in ear-nose-and throat clinics to treat several diseases (Rybak et al. 2019). It minimizes or avoids the undesired effects of systemic drug usage, especially the possible interaction (Laurell, 2019) of otoprotective substance with cisplatin which may decrease oncologic effectiveness. The trans-tympanic injections allow direct application of drugs through the tympanic membrane (Laurell, 2019). Trans-tympanic N-acetylcysteine usage has been documented in pilot trials at 2% and 10% concentrations, with 11 (Yoo et al., 2014) and 20 patients (Riga et al., 2013), respectively. No clinically significant otoprotection was reported in the treated ears compared to untreated ones. In a study with 60 patients trans-tympanic N-acetylcysteine provided no significant effect and dexamethasone had some benefit at 8,000 Hz (Sarafraz et al., 2018). Similarly, the use of dexamethasone has produced a limited benefit at 6,000 Hz in some studies (Marshak et al., 2014; Nasr et al., 2018). Trans-tympanic sodium-thiosulfate (STS) gel was recently tried in 12 patients and reported to be feasible and safe, with no decreased oncologic effectiveness (Duinkerken et al., 2021). Another trial tested trans-tympanic STS in 13 patients prior to cisplatin delivery, reporting no significant effects, but the trial was stopped early due to poor accrual (Rolland et al., 2019).

Furthermore, there is increasing research of adjuvant substances that potentially enhance the diffusion of drugs to the inner ear such as nanoparticles, hydrogels, and others (Duinkerken et al., 2021) that probably will provide some benefit in certain cases.

Despite the potential benefits of local drug delivery, significant drawbacks remain, including anatomic middle ear variations that hamper drug diffusion, drug leakage through the Eustachian tube, ear pain caused by the injection, the possibility of causing a permanent tympanic perforation, and the need of an ear-nose-and throat physician to inject the drug, thus limiting its clinical use (Laurell, 2019; Nader & Gidley, 2019; L. P. Rybak et al., 2019).

Strategies Based on Systemic Drug Delivery for Ear Protection

The most used systemic compound for ear protection are thiol compounds. A limited pilot trial with 36 adults with brain tumors reported that the co-administration of STS with carboplatin reduced ototoxicity in the intervention group (Doolittle et al., 2001). The control group showed auditory damage of 84% and the intervention group only 29% ($p < 0.0018$). No side effects were reported.

In pediatrics results were less encouraging. The most relevant results were reported by a multicenter, randomized, controlled, open-label, phase 3 trial published in 2017 (n = 104) (Freyer et al., 2017). In said study STS was administered intravenously six hours after the end of cisplatin chemotherapy. As in adults, in this protocol the STS effectively reduces the risk of ototoxicity in the group exposed to this thiol compound, (OR 0.31; 95% CI 0.13–0.73; $p = 0.0036$). However, the STS intervention reduced the cisplatin antineoplastic effect, and the patients with disseminated disease showed an inferior 3-year event-free survival rate (42%; 95% CI 0.21–0.61) compared to the control group (61%, 95% CI 0.39–0.77) (p value by log-rank test <0.05) as well as lesser overall survival (45%, 95% CI 0.23–0.65) versus the control children (84%, 95% CI 0.62–0.94) (p value by log-rank test <0.05). These results complicate the establishment of otoprotective strategies based on STS in pediatric patients treated with cisplatin, thus necessitating pre-clinical evaluation to establish whether other platinum-based compounds would cause similar effects.

More recently, another randomized multicenter pediatric trial (n = 109) was performed on children with standard-risk hepatoblastoma (Brock et al., 2018). The intervention group received intravenous STS administered six hours after cisplatin chemotherapy. Children exposed to STS showed a minor incidence of grade ≥1 hearing loss (≥40 dB at frequencies ≥8,000 Hz) (RR: 0.52; 95% CI 0.33-0.81; $p = 0.002$) without reporting STS-related effects on the 3-year follow-up of event-free survival and overall survivor. Despite the similarities of this study with the previously mentioned protocol, the trials are not comparable because the former only included patients with hepatoblastoma. In any case, evidence accumulated to date regarding systemic interventions with STS is scarce and too inconsistent to establish any recommendation. Additionally, any future similar studies will need to be performed with great caution.

Another thiol compound tested systemically to prevent ototoxicity derived from platinum-based chemotherapy in pediatric patients is amifostine, with studies showing no consistent results regarding the efficacy of this substance. A summary of these protocols can be reviewed in a meta-analysis which concluded that current evidence does not support the use of amifostine to prevent platinum-analogue induced ototoxicity (Brock et al., 2018).

Non-thiol compounds have also been tested, including antioxidant compounds as well as synthetic drugs. Among the former, a small pilot double-blind trial (n = 15) reported that the group which received a Ginko biloba extract (natural polypenol extract) concomitant with cisplatin therapy showed higher distortion product otoacoustic emissions mean amplitudes and smaller signal-to-noise ratio than the placebo group (Choi et al., 2013). However, due to the small sample size the results cannot be extrapolated to a clinical population. Regarding standard drugs, the most interesting approach was performed with aspirin and (Crabb et al., 2017) pantoprazole (Fox et al., 2018). Despite aspirin demonstrating decreased gentamicin-induced hearing loss without compromising anti-bacterial treatment (Sha et al., 2006), it fails to prevent cisplatin-induced ototoxicity in adults (Crabb et al., 2017). On the other hand, it has been postulated that the pharmacological effect of pantoprazole is through the inhibition of the organic cation transporter 2 which would mediate cisplatin uptake into cochlear hair cells and renal tubular cells. Unfortunately, the small randomized cross-over protocol (n = 12) performed in children and adolescents with newly diagnosed osteosarcoma to evaluate that hypothesis reported that the co-administration of cisplatin with pantoprazole did not ameliorate cisplatin-related ototoxicity or nephrotoxicity (Fox et al., 2018).

Finally, it is important to mention that before trying a new compound as a candidate to prevent ototoxicity, it is necessary to analyze possible biochemical interactions, especially those related to potential interactions with platinum analogues, thus decreasing oncologic effectiveness. The previously mentioned survival reduction reported in pediatric multicenter study could be due to well-known chemical interactions between cisplatin and thiol compounds (Ekborn et al., 2002; Viale et al., 1999), which have been reported to reduce cisplatin anti-neoplastic activity (Aamdal et al., 1987; Inoue et al., 1991).

Conclusion

Ototoxicity often occurs following platinum-based treatments and it mainly manifests as auditory symptoms. It can impair quality of life of cancer survivors; thus, its early recognition, treatment, or avoidance arises as a major objective for reducing hearing disability during lifespan. However, there are no current treatments or prevention strategies approved to reduce its occurrence so far. Auditory treatments such as hearing aids for adults and children represents the mainstay of management of patients who already developed clinically significant ototoxicity, however, it still has several drawbacks and access limitations in some places.

Cochlear cells have a special susceptibility to platinum-based chemotherapy ototoxic effects, triggering apoptosis of different cells, outer hair cells, stria vascularis and others. Increased production of ROS and subsequent oxidative-derived injury is a key event involved in cisplatin-induced ototoxicity. It has been reported that cisplatin triggers oxidative-mediated injury by increasing ROS levels by direct production through stimulating enzymes related to these processes or by decreasing antioxidant defenses.

The use of systemic treatments to diminish or prevent ototoxicity are potentially feasible to perform and have shown some promising results but they also have raised concerns about decreasing oncologic effectiveness of platinum drugs. Thus, considering that cisplatin exerts its anticancer effects through mechanisms which are also involved in their side effects, the use of systemic otoprotective agents must be carefully designed because of the possibility of interfering with anticancer effects.

The use of direct interventions to deliver drugs to the inner ear such as the transtympanic drug injections are frequently used in ear-nose-and throat clinics. It minimizes or avoids the undesired effects of systemic drug usage, especially the interaction with cisplatin that may decrease oncologic effectiveness. Despite the potential benefits of local drug delivery, there still are significant limitations including anatomic variations of middle ear, difficult drug diffusion, drug leakage through the Eustachian tube, ear pain, among others.

References

Aamdal, S., Fodstad, O., & Pihl, A. (1987). Some procedures to reduce cis-platinum toxicity reduce antitumour activity. *Cancer Treatment Reviews*, *14*(3–4), 389–395.

Bergen, G., Stevens, M. R., & Burns, E. R. (2016). Falls and Fall Injuries Among Adults Aged ≥65 Years — United States, 2014. *MMWR. Morbidity and Mortality Weekly Report*, *65*(37), 993–998.

Breglio, A. M., Rusheen, A. E., Shide, E. D., Fernandez, K. A., Spielbauer, K. K., McLachlin, K. M., Hall, M. D., Amable, L., & Cunningham, L. L. (2017). Cisplatin is retained in the cochlea indefinitely following chemotherapy. *Nature Communications*, *8*(1), 1654.

Brock, P. R., Maibach, R., Childs, M., Rajput, K., Roebuck, D., Sullivan, M. J., Laithier, V., Ronghe, M., Dall'Igna, P., Hiyama, E., Brichard, B., Skeen, J., Mateos, M. E., Capra, M., Rangaswami, A. A., Ansari, M., Rechnitzer, C., Veal, G. J., Covezzoli, A., Neuwelt, E. A. (2018). Sodium Thiosulfate for Protection from Cisplatin-Induced Hearing Loss. *New England Journal of Medicine*, *378*(25), 2376–2385.

Brooks, B., & Knight, K. (2018). Ototoxicity monitoring in children treated with platinum chemotherapy. *International Journal of Audiology*, *57*(sup4), S62–S68.

Cardemil, F., Aguayo, L., & Fuente, A. (2014). Programas de rehabilitación auditiva en adultos mayores, ¿qué sabemos de su efectividad? In *Acta Otorrinolaringologica Espanola*, (Vol. 65, Issue 4, pp. 249–257). Elsevier Doyma.

Choi, S. J., Kim, S. W., Lee, J. B., Lim, H. J., Kim, Y. J., Tian, C., So, H. S., Park, R., & Choung, Y.-. H. (2013). Gingko biloba extracts protect auditory hair cells from cisplatin-induced ototoxicity by inhibiting perturbation of gap junctional intercellular communication. *Neuroscience*, *244*, 49–61.

Clemens, E., Brooks, B., de Vries, A. C. H., van Grotel, M., van den Heuvel-Eibrink, M. M., & Carleton, B. (2019). A comparison of the Muenster, SIOP Boston, Brock, Chang and CTCAEv4.03 ototoxicity grading scales applied to 3,799 audiograms of childhood cancer patients treated with platinum-based chemotherapy. *PLOS ONE*, *14*(2), e0210646.

Clemens, E., de Vries, A. C., am Zehnhoff-Dinnesen, A., Tissing, W. J., Loonen, J. J., Pluijm, S. F., van Dulmen-den Broeder, E., Bresters, D., Versluys, B., Kremer, L. C., van der Pal, H. J., Neggers, S. J., van Grotel, M., & M van den Heuvel-Eibrink, M. (2017). Hearing loss after platinum treatment is irreversible in noncranial irradiated childhood cancer survivors. *Pediatric Hematology and Oncology*, *34*(2), 120–129.

Clemens, E., de Vries, A. C., Pluijm, S. F., am Zehnhoff-Dinnesen, A., Tissing, W. J., Loonen, J. J., van Dulmen-den Broeder, E., Bresters, D., Versluys, B., Kremer, L. C., van der Pal, H. J., van Grotel, M., & van den Heuvel-Eibrink, M. M. (2016). Determinants of ototoxicity in 451 platinum-treated Dutch survivors of childhood cancer: A DCOG late-effects study. *European Journal of Cancer*, *69*, 77–85.

Crabb, S. J., Martin, K., Abab, J., Ratcliffe, I., Thornton, R., Lineton, B., Ellis, M., Moody, R., Stanton, L., Galanopoulou, A., Maishman, T., Geldart, T., Bayne, M., Davies, J., Lamb, C., Popat, S., Joffe, J. K., Nutting, C., Chester, J., … King, E. (2017). COAST (Cisplatin ototoxicity attenuated by aspirin trial): A phase II double-blind, randomised controlled trial to establish if aspirin reduces cisplatin induced hearing-loss. *European Journal of Cancer*, *87*, 75–83.

Cunningham, L. L., & Tucci, D. L. (2017). Hearing Loss in Adults. *New England Journal of Medicine*, *377*(25), 2465–2473.

Dammeyer, P., Hellberg, V., Wallin, I., Laurell, G., Shoshan, M., Ehrsson, H., Arnér, E. S. J., & Kirkegaard, M. (2014). Cisplatin and oxaliplatin are toxic to cochlear outer hair cells and both target thioredoxin reductase in organ of Corti cultures. *Acta Oto-Laryngologica*, *134*(5), 448–454.

Devarajan, P., Savoca, M., Castaneda, M. P., Park, M. S., Esteban-Cruciani, N., Kalinec, G., & Kalinec, F. (2002). Cisplatin-induced apoptosis in auditory cells: Role of death receptor and mitochondrial pathways. *Hearing Research*, *174*(1–2), 45–54.

Ding, D., Zhang, J., Jiang, H., Xuan, W., Qi, W., & Salvi, R. (2020). Some Ototoxic Drugs Destroy Cochlear Support Cells Before Damaging Sensory Hair Cells. *Neurotoxicity Research*, *37*(3), 743–752.

Doolittle, N. D., Muldoon, L. L., Brummett, R. E., Tyson, R. M., Lacy, C., Bubalo, J. S., Kraemer, D. F., Heinrich, M. C., Henry, J. A., & Neuwelt, E. A. (2001). Delayed sodium thiosulfate as an otoprotectant against carboplatin-induced hearing loss in patients with malignant brain tumors. *Clinical Cancer Research: An Official Journal of the American Association for Cancer Research*, *7*(3), 493–500.

Duinkerken, C. W., de Weger, V. A., Dreschler, W. A., van der Molen, L., Pluim, D., Rosing, H., Nuijen, B., Hauptmann, M., Beijnen, J. H., Balm, A. J. M., de Boer, J. P., Burgers, J. A., Marchetti, S., Schellens, J. H. M., & Zuur, C. L. (2021). Transtympanic Sodium Thiosulfate for Prevention of Cisplatin-Induced Ototoxicity. *Otology & Neurotology*, Publish Ah.

Einarsson, E.-J., Petersen, H., Wiebe, T., Fransson, P.-A., Magnusson, M., & Moëll, C. (2011). Severe difficulties with word recognition in noise after platinum chemotherapy in childhood, and improvements with open-fitting hearing-aids. *International Journal of Audiology*, *50*(10), 642–651.

Ekborn, A., Laurell, G., Johnström, P., Wallin, I., Eksborg, S., & Ehrsson, H. (2002). D-Methionine and cisplatin ototoxicity in the guinea pig: D-methionine influences cisplatin pharmacokinetics. *Hearing Research*, *165*(1–2), 53–61.

Elena, J. W., Travis, L. B., Simonds, N. I., Ambrosone, C. B., Ballard-Barbash, R., Bhatia, S., Cerhan, J. R., Hartge, P., Heist, R. S., Kushi, L. H., Lash, T. L., Morton, L. M., Onel, K., Pierce, J. P., Robison, L. L., Rowland, J. H., Schrag, D., Sellers, T. A., Seminara, D., … Freedman, A. N. (2013). Leveraging Epidemiology and Clinical Studies of Cancer Outcomes: Recommendations and Opportunities for Translational Research. *JNCI: Journal of the National Cancer Institute*, *105*(2), 85–94.

Ferguson, M. A., Kitterick, P. T., Chong, L. Y., Edmondson-Jones, M., Barker, F., & Hoare, D. J. (2017). Hearing aids for mild to moderate hearing loss in adults. In *Cochrane Database of Systematic Reviews*, (Vol. 2017, Issue 9). John Wiley and Sons Ltd.

Fox, E., Levin, K., Zhu, Y., Segers, B., Balamuth, N., Womer, R., Bagatell, R., & Balis, F. (2018). Pantoprazole, an Inhibitor of the Organic Cation Transporter 2, Does Not Ameliorate Cisplatin-Related Ototoxicity or Nephrotoxicity in Children and Adolescents with Newly Diagnosed Osteosarcoma Treated with Methotrexate, Doxorubicin, and Cisplatin. *The Oncologist*, *23*(7), 762.

Freyer, D. R., Brock, P. R., Chang, K. W., Dupuis, L. L., Epelman, S., Knight, K., Mills, D., Phillips, R., Potter, E., Risby, D., Simpkin, P., Sullivan, M., Cabral, S., Robinson, P. D., & Sung, L. (2020). Prevention of cisplatin-induced ototoxicity in children and adolescents with cancer: a clinical practice guideline. *The Lancet Child & Adolescent Health*, *4*(2), 141–150.

Freyer, D. R., Chen, L., Krailo, M. D., Knight, K., Villaluna, D., Bliss, B., Pollock, B. H., Ramdas, J., Lange, B., Van Hoff, D., VanSoelen, M. L., Wiernikowski, J., Neuwelt, E. A., & Sung, L. (2017). Effects of sodium thiosulfate versus observation on development of cisplatin-induced hearing loss in children with cancer (ACCL0431): a multicentre, randomised, controlled, open-label, phase 3 trial. *The Lancet Oncology*, *18*(1), 63–74.

Frisina, R. D., Wheeler, H. E., Fossa, S. D., Kerns, S. L., Fung, C., Sesso, H. D., Monahan, P. O., Feldman, D. R., Hamilton, R., Vaughn, D. J., Beard, C. J., Budnick, A., Johnson, E. M., Ardeshir-Rouhani-Fard, S., Einhorn, L. H., Lipshultz, S. E., Dolan, M. E., & Travis, L. B. (2016). Comprehensive Audiometric Analysis of Hearing Impairment and Tinnitus After Cisplatin-Based Chemotherapy in Survivors of Adult-Onset Cancer. *Journal of Clinical Oncology*, *34*(23), 2712–2720.

Gentilin, E., Simoni, E., Candito, M., Cazzador, D., & Astolfi, L. (2019). Cisplatin-Induced Ototoxicity: Updates on Molecular Targets. *Trends in Molecular Medicine*, *25*(12), 1123–1132.

Haile, L. M., Kamenov, K., Briant, P. S., Orji, A. U., Steinmetz, J. D., Abdoli, A., Abdollahi, M., Abu-Gharbieh, E., Afshin, A., Ahmed, H., Rashid, T. A., Akalu, Y., Alahdab, F., Alanezi, F. M., Alanzi, T. M., Al Hamad, H., Ali, L., Alipour, V., Al-Raddadi, R. M., … Chadha, S. (2021). Hearing loss prevalence and years lived with disability, 1990-2019: Findings from the Global Burden of Disease Study 2019. *The Lancet*, *397*(10278), 996–1009.

Harris, M. S., & Dodson, E. E. (2017). Hearing health access in developing countries. In *Current Opinion in Otolaryngology and Head and Neck Surgery*, (Vol. 25, Issue 5, pp. 353–358). Lippincott Williams and Wilkins.

Inoue, M., Shimizu, C., Shimizu, H., & Tanizawa, O. (1991). Neutralizing effect of sodium thiosulfate on antitumor efficacy of cisplatin for human carcinoma xenografts in nude mice. *Gynecologic Oncology*, *40*(1), 34–37.

Kamenov, K., Martinez, R., Kunjumen, T., & Chadha, S. (2021). Ear and Hearing Care Workforce: Current Status and its Implications. *Ear and Hearing*, 249–257.

Kim, H. H., & Barrs, D. M. (2006). Hearing Aids: A Review of What's New. *Otolaryngology–Head and Neck Surgery*, *134*(6), 1043–1050.

King, K. A., & Brewer, C. C. (2018). Clinical trials, ototoxicity grading scales and the audiologist's role in therapeutic decision making. *International Journal of Audiology*, *57*(sup4), S19–S28.

Knight, K. R. G., Kraemer, D. F., & Neuwelt, E. A. (2005). Ototoxicity in Children Receiving Platinum Chemotherapy: Underestimating a Commonly Occurring Toxicity That May Influence Academic and Social Development. *Journal of Clinical Oncology*, *23*(34), 8588–8596.

Landier, W. (2016). Ototoxicity and cancer therapy. *Cancer*, *122*(11), 1647–1658.

Laurell, G. (2019). Pharmacological intervention in the field of ototoxicity. *HNO*, *67*(6), 434–439.

Laurell, G., Ekborn, A., Viberg, A., & Canlon, B. (2007). Effects of a Single High Dose of Cisplatin on the Melanocytes of the Stria Vascularis in the Guinea Pig. *Audiology and Neurotology*, *12*(3), 170–178.

Lerner, S. (2019). Limitations of Conventional Hearing Aids: Examining Common Complaints and Issues that Can and Cannot Be Remedied. In *Otolaryngologic Clinics of North America*, (Vol. 52, Issue 2, pp. 211–220). W.B. Saunders.

Liang, F., Schulte, B. A., Qu, C., Hu, W., & Shen, Z. (2005). Inhibition of the calcium- and voltage-dependent big conductance potassium channel ameliorates cisplatin-induced apoptosis in spiral ligament fibrocytes of the cochlea. *Neuroscience*, *135*(1), 263–271.

Lieu, J. E. C., Kenna, M., Anne, S., & Davidson, L. (2020). Hearing Loss in Children. *JAMA*, *324*(21), 2195.

Lin, F. R., Niparko, J. K., & Ferrucci, L. (2011). Hearing loss prevalence in the United States. *Archives of Internal Medicine*, *171*(20), 1851–1852.

Marshak, T., Steiner, M., Kaminer, M., Levy, L., & Shupak, A. (2014). Prevention of cisplatin-induced hearing loss by intratympanic dexamethasone: A randomized controlled study. *Otolaryngology - Head and Neck Surgery (United States)*, *150*(6), 983–990.

McCormack, A., & Fortnum, H. (2013). Why do people fitted with hearing aids not wear them? *International Journal of Audiology*, *52*(5), 360–368.

McDaid, D., Park, A. La, & Chadha, S. (2021). Estimating the global costs of hearing loss. *International Journal of Audiology*, *60*(3), 162–170.

Muñoz, K., Rusk, S. E. P., Nelson, L., Preston, E., White, K. R., Barrett, T. S., & Twohig, M. P. (2016). Pediatric Hearing Aid Management: Parent-Reported Needs for Learning Support. *Ear & Hearing*, *37*(6), 703–709.

Nader, M.-E., & Gidley, P. (2019). Challenges of Hearing Rehabilitation after Radiation and Chemotherapy. *Journal of Neurological Surgery Part B: Skull Base*, *80*(02), 214–224.

Nasr, W., Abdelhady, M., Abd Elbary, M., & Nada, E. (2018). Treatment of cisplatin-induced ototoxicity by intra-tympanic corticosteroid injection. *Indian Journal of Otology*, *24*(1), 33–37.

Oun, R., Moussa, Y. E., & Wheate, N. J. (2018). The side effects of platinum-based chemotherapy drugs: a review for chemists. *Dalton Transactions*, *47*(19), 6645–6653.

Pearson, S. E., Taylor, J., Patel, P., & Baguley, D. M. (2019). Cancer survivors treated with platinum-based chemotherapy affected by ototoxicity and the impact on quality of life: a narrative synthesis systematic review. *International Journal of Audiology*, *58*(11), 685–695.

Prayuenyong, P., Taylor, J. A., Pearson, S. E., Gomez, R., Patel, P. M., Hall, D. A., Kasbekar, A. V, & Baguley, D. M. (2018). Vestibulotoxicity Associated with Platinum-Based Chemotherapy in Survivors of Cancer: A Scoping Review. *Frontiers in Oncology*, *8*, 363.

Ramkumar, V., Mukherjea, D., Dhukhwa, A., & Rybak, L. P. (2021). Oxidative Stress and Inflammation Caused by Cisplatin Ototoxicity. *Antioxidants*, *10*(12), 1919.

Riga, M. G., Chelis, L., Kakolyris, S., Papadopoulos, S., Stathakidou, S., Chamalidou, E., Xenidis, N., Amarantidis, K., Dimopoulos, P., & Danielides, V. (2013). Transtympanic injections of N-acetylcysteine for the prevention of cisplatin-induced ototoxicity: A feasible method with promising efficacy. *American Journal of Clinical Oncology: Cancer Clinical Trials*, *36*(1), 1–6.

Rolland, V., Meyer, F., Guitton, M. J., Bussières, R., Philippon, D., Bairati, I., Leclerc, M., & Côté, M. (2019). A randomized controlled trial to test the efficacy of trans-tympanic injections of a sodium thiosulfate gel to prevent cisplatin-induced ototoxicity in patients with head and neck cancer. *Journal of Otolaryngology - Head & Neck Surgery*, *48*(1), 4.

Rybak, L., Mukherjea, D., & Ramkumar, V. (2019). Mechanisms of Cisplatin-Induced Ototoxicity and Prevention. *Seminars in Hearing*, *40*(02), 197–204.

Rybak, L. P., Dhukhwa, A., Mukherjea, D., & Ramkumar, V. (2019). Local Drug Delivery for Prevention of Hearing Loss. *Frontiers in Cellular Neuroscience*, *13*.

Rybak, L. P., Mukherjea, D., Jajoo, S., Kaur, T., & Ramkumar, V. (2012). siRNA-mediated knock-down of NOX3: therapy for hearing loss? *Cellular and Molecular Life Sciences*, *69*(14), 2429–2434.

Rybak, L. P., Mukherjea, D., Jajoo, S., & Ramkumar, V. (2009). Cisplatin Ototoxicity and Protection: Clinical and Experimental Studies. *The Tohoku Journal of Experimental Medicine*, *219*(3), 177–186.

Sarafraz, Z., Ahmadi, A., & Daneshi, A. (2018). Transtympanic Injections of N-acetylcysteine and Dexamethasone for Prevention of Cisplatin-Induced Ototoxicity: Double Blind Randomized Clinical Trial. *The International Tinnitus Journal*, *22*(1).

Sha, S.-H., Qiu, J.-H., & Schacht, J. (2006). Aspirin to Prevent Gentamicin-Induced Hearing Loss. *New England Journal of Medicine*, *354*(17), 1856–1857.

Sheth, S., Mukherjea, D., Rybak, L. P., & Ramkumar, V. (2017). Mechanisms of Cisplatin-Induced Ototoxicity and Otoprotection. *Frontiers in Cellular Neuroscience*, *11*.

Sun, D. Q., Ward, B. K., Semenov, Y. R., Carey, J. P., & Della Santina, C. C. (2014). Bilateral Vestibular Deficiency. *JAMA Otolaryngology–Head & Neck Surgery*, *140*(6), 527.

Tang, Q., Wang, X., Jin, H., Mi, Y., Liu, L., Dong, M., Chen, Y., & Zou, Z. (2021). Cisplatin-induced ototoxicity: Updates on molecular mechanisms and otoprotective strategies. *European Journal of Pharmaceutics and Biopharmaceutics*, *163*, 60–71.

Theunissen, E. A. R., Bosma, S. C. J., Zuur, C. L., Spijker, R., van der Baan, S., Dreschler, W. A., de Boer, J. P., Balm, A. J. M., & Rasch, C. R. N. (2015). Sensorineural hearing loss in patients with head and neck cancer after chemoradiotherapy and radiotherapy: A systematic review of the literature. *Head & Neck*, *37*(2), 281–292.

van As, J. W., van den Berg, H., & van Dalen, E. C. (2016). Platinum-induced hearing loss after treatment for childhood cancer. *Cochrane Database of Systematic Reviews*, *2019*(4).

Viale, M., Zhang, J. G., Pastrone, I., Mariggiò, M. A., Esposito, M., & Lindup, W. E. (1999). Cisplatin combined with tiopronin or sodium thiosulfate: cytotoxicity *in vitro* and antitumor activity *in vivo*. *Anti-Cancer Drugs*, *10*(4), 419–428.

Wang, D., & Lippard, S. J. (2005). Cellular processing of platinum anticancer drugs. *Nature Reviews. Drug Discovery*, *4*(4), 307–320. https://doi.org/10.1038/nrd1691.

Wildes, T. M., Dua, P., Fowler, S. A., Miller, J. P., Carpenter, C. R., Avidan, M. S., & Stark, S. (2015). Systematic review of falls in older adults with cancer. In *Journal of Geriatric Oncology*, (Vol. 6, Issue 1, pp. 70–83). Elsevier Ltd.

Yoo, J., Hamilton, S. J., Angel, D., Fung, K., Franklin, J., Parnes, L. S., Lewis, D., Venkatesan, V., & Winquist, E. (2014). Cisplatin otoprotection using transtympanic L-N-acetylcysteine: A pilot randomized study in head and neck cancer patients. *Laryngoscope*, *124*(3), E87–E94.

Yu, D., Gu, J., Chen, Y., Kang, W., Wang, X., & Wu, H. (2020). Current Strategies to Combat Cisplatin-Induced Ototoxicity. *Frontiers in Pharmacology*, *11*.

Zou, J., Pyykkö, I., & Hyttinen, J. (2016). Inner ear barriers to nanomedicine-augmented drug delivery and imaging. *Journal of Otology*, *11*(4), 165–177.

Chapter 6

Cardiovascular Side Effects of Platinum-Based Chemotherapy

Kristen Renee McSweeney*, Laura Kate Gadanec and Anthony Zulli†
Institute for Health and Sport, Victoria University, Melbourne, Victoria, Australia

Abstract

Platinum-based drugs are a potent class of antineoplastic drugs used to treat a broad spectrum of solid cancers. Despite their efficacy, the use of these agents is often accompanied by toxicities, including ototoxicity, nephrotoxicity, myelosuppression, neurotoxicity, and cardiotoxicity. Several clinical cases of heart complications following treatment with platinum-based chemotherapies have been reported. The most concerning cardiac conditions associated with platinum treatment include vascular toxicity, thrombosis, hypertension, hypotension, atherosclerosis, and dysrhythmia. Most large-scale clinical studies of cardiotoxicity are retrospective, and as such provide some information but lack key details. In this regard, specifically designed prospective studies are required to better establish causes and potential therapies for these complications. Pre-clinical studies refer to cardiotoxicity as an umbrella term with most studies investigating the prevention of cardiotoxicity with the use of antioxidant and anti-inflammatory pharmacotherapies. Pre-clinical studies to date do not fully mimic the specificity of conditions associated with platinum-based treatment. Establishing superior animal models of cardiotoxicity to identify and

*Corresponding Author's Email: kristen.mcsweeney@live.vu.edu.au.
†Corresponding Author's Email: anthony.zulli@vu.edu.au.

In: Platinum-Based Chemotherapy
Editors: Kulmira Nurgali and Raquel Abalo
ISBN: 978-1-68507-972-7
© 2022 Nova Science Publishers, Inc.

treat specific cardiac complications may benefit clinical prevention of cardiac conditions following platinum-based chemotherapeutic treatment. There are many clinical and pre-clinical studies investigating cardiotoxicity associated with the treatment of cancer patients with platinum-based chemotherapies. Many retrospective clinical studies lack long term follow up periods whilst animal studies lack clinical relevancy in investigating some of the most frequent cardiac conditions. More specific studies in both pre-clinic and clinical settings are needed to provide valuable data to identify causes and preventative strategies to better patient outcomes following platinum-based treatment.

Keywords: cardiotoxicity, cisplatin, hypertension, platinum-based chemotherapy, thrombosis

Introduction

Platinum-based chemotherapies are widely used as a first-line cancer therapy. Despite their efficacy they have been associated with multiple toxicities, such as ototoxicity, nephrotoxicity, myelosuppression, neurotoxicity, and cardiotoxicity (Dasari et al. 2014, Oun et al. 2018). First class and analogues of platinum-based chemotherapies are used to treat a broad range of cancers, including cisplatin (CDDP) (Ghosh 2019), carboplatin (Ming et al. 2017), oxaliplatin (Goldberg 2000), nedaplatin, heptaplatin (Choi et al. 2004), lobaplatin (McKeage 2001), satraplatin (Bhargava et al. 2009), triplatin tetranitrate (Oberoi et al. 2013), picoplatin (Tang et al. 2011), iproplatin (Kreisman et al. 1987), and ormaplatin (Rischin et al. 1996). Cisplatin is the most potent and prescribed platinum-containing anti-neoplastic drug and despite efforts to create novel analogues (e.g., carboplatin and oxaliplatin) that have reduced toxicity profiles, a decrease in toxicity has been positively correlated with reduced cytotoxicity against cancer (Oun et al. 2018). In addition to reducing toxicity, development and clinical trials of these analogues aim to override cancer cell resistance, which frequently develops with cis-diamminedichloroplatinum (CDDP) usage (Dasari et al. 2014). The dose limiting side effects of these platinum-based drugs are well documented. Cardiotoxicity, although a concerning side effect, is not a focus except in extreme circumstances when cases arise during treatment. Often patient discomfort or symptomology facilitate cardiac investigations irrespective of the frequency of cardiac complications. There are multiple cardio-related conditions associated with treatment with various platinum containing agents.

Often some conditions are more prevalent with certain chemotherapies, such as the development of CDDP-induced venous thromboembolism (VTE). Complications and potentially life-threatening conditions that target the cardiovascular system are shown in Figure 1 and include, vascular toxicity, coronary vasospasm induced myocardial infarction, atherosclerosis, hypertension, endothelial dysfunction, endothelial activation, abnormal lipid profile, hypotension, pre-clinical cardiotoxicity, tachycardia, arrhythmia, bradycardia, and thrombosis. Literature, clinical studies, and patient case studies relating to the cardiovascular side effects associated with platinum chemotherapeutic treatment have been reviewed and analyzed. Results and findings have been further discussed in this book chapter.

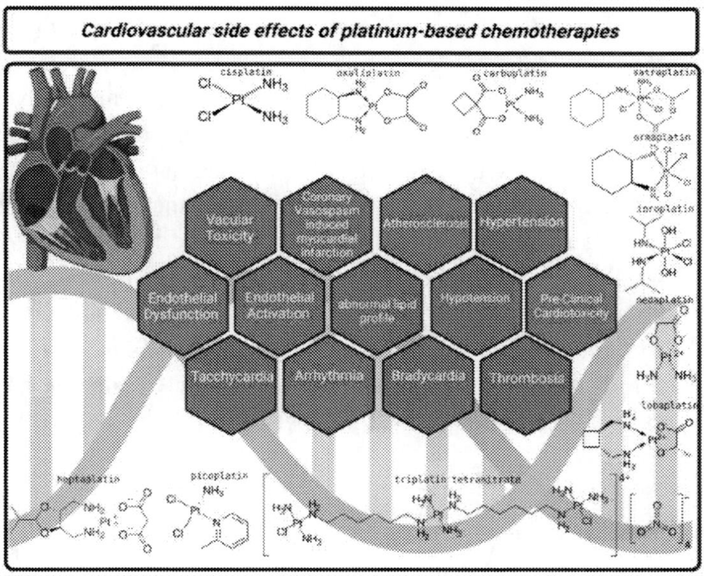

Figure 1. Cardiovascular side effects associated with the use of platinum-based chemotherapies, including vascular toxicity, coronary vasospasm induced myocardial infarction, atherosclerosis, hypertension, endothelial dysfunction, endothelial activation, abnormal lipid profile, hypotension, pre-clinical cardiotoxicity, tachycardia, arrhythmia, bradycardia, and thrombosis.

Vascular Toxicity

Coronary Vasospasm-Induced Acute Myocardial Infarction

Coronary vasospasm (CVS) is a mechanism of myocardial ischemia and is characterised by vasoconstriction, resulting in total or partial occlusion of coronary arteries (Lanza et al. 2011). CVS is attributed to myocardial infarction reported in patients treated with CDDP-based chemotherapy. A case study of a 30-year-old male with testicular seminoma presented with chest pain radiating down the left arm, tachycardia (120 bpm) and hypertension (150/100 mmHg) the day before beginning a fourth cycle of the BOP (bleomycin, vincristine, and CDDP) regimen. Investigations reported hyperlipidaemia, left ventricular dysfunction and a reduction in left ventricular ejection fraction (LVEF) to 35%. Angiography confirmed an absence of thrombosis with the final diagnosis ruled as CVS-induced acute myocardial infarction (Hanchate et al. 2017). Interestingly, the same diagnosis was made in a 55-year-old male patient diagnosed with small cell lung cancer. Following the second cycle of a platinum-based regimen, the patient developed breathlessness, chest pain, tachycardia (180 bpm) and hypotension. Shortly after investigations, symptoms subsided and radiotherapy was continued; however, chemotherapy was not recommenced. The final diagnosis of acute myocardial infarction-induced by vasospastic angina was made (Rao et al. 2015). In addition to the CVS observed following CDDP treatment, it has also been linked to oxaliplatin treatment (Chang et al. 2013).

Endothelial Activation

Endothelial activation refers to transition of endothelial cells from a quiescent state to an activated and pro-inflammatory state, resulting in increased expression of adhesion molecules (i.e., intercellular adhesion molecule 1 (ICAM-1), vascular cell adhesion molecule 1 (VCAM-1), E-selectin and P-selectin) (Page and Liles 2013), cytokines and chemokines (i.e., tumour necrosis factor alpha (TNF-α), interleukin-1 (IL-1), interleukin-4 (IL-4), interferon gamma (IFNγ) and vascular endothelial growth factor A (VEGFA) (Pober et al. 2007). Endothelial activation is associated with platinum-based cardiotoxicity and may provide a comprehensible insight as to the involvement of adhesion molecules and other inflammatory processes in cardiotoxicity manifestation. A study in human umbilical vein endothelial cells (HUVECs) demonstrated upregulation of ICAM-1 expression after CDDP; however, it did not influence mRNA or protein expression levels of other adhesion molecules, including P-selectin and E-selectin. Interestingly, VCAM-1 expression is often measured instead of ICAM-1 or vice versa in models of CDDP cardiotoxicity; however, both are often assessed in models of nephrotoxicity and thus may also be beneficial in models of cardiotoxicity to establish the mechanism of pathogenesis. Additionally, another study showed a dose-dependent increase in E-selectin mRNA expression in Human umbilical vein endothelial cells (HUVECs) incubated with CDDP (Kawase et al. 2009). Serum ICAM-1 is not often investigated in the context of cardiotoxicity clinically; but may be useful as an early biomarker particularly given the link between endothelial activation, endothelial dysfunction, and thrombosis, which is one of the most concerning clinical manifestations of platinum treatment.

Endothelial Dysfunction

Many platinum-based chemotherapies, particularly CDDP, are associated with endothelial dysfunction (ED). Vascular injury is linked to elevations in oxidative stress, resulting in a sequence of metabolic disturbances. CDDP treatment leads to oxidative stress induced by reactive oxygen species (ROS) and impaired function of the antioxidant scavenging system (Holditch et al. 2019). ROS produced excessively include superoxide (O_2^-), hydroxyl radical (HO•), hydrogen peroxide (H_2O_2), peroxynitrite ($ONOO^-$), nitrogen oxide (NO), and hypochlorous acid (HOCl). Increased oxidative stress leads to endothelial damage resulting in impaired endothelial-dependent vascular relaxation. Endothelial-dependent vascular smooth muscle cell (VSMC) relaxation is mediated by NO and alterations in its production or bioavailability disrupt relaxation. Additionally, endothelial nitric oxide synthase (eNOS) function is impaired when ROS production is not regulated (Coats et al. 2017). The production of NO from eNOS is reliant upon L-arginine (Dasari et al. 2014). NO reacts with the NO scavenger O_2^- to produce ROS in the form of $ONOO^-$ (Hussain et al. 2012, Mandic et al. 2003, Pabla et al. 2008, Price et al. 2006), resulting in reduced NO bioavailability and ultimately endothelial dysfunction (Guzik et al. 2002).

A study in HUVECs pre-incubated with the calcium ionophore A23187 to induce NO production demonstrated that incubation with CDDP reduces

NO production, indicative of endothelial dysfunction (Sekijima et al. 2011). In addition to CDDP reducing NO, endothelial dysfunction has been observed in rats following treatment with oxaliplatin, suggesting reduced NO (Kataoka et al. 2021). A clinical study from 2018 to 2020 (NCT04681560) investigated the effects of platinum-based chemotherapies on endothelial function in patients with gastrointestinal, ovarian, bladder and breast cancers. Three methods were used to evaluate vascular system function, including measurement of blood pressure, flow-mediated vasodilation and pulse-wave velocity, and blood sampling to quantify eNOS and Big-endothelin concentrations. The results of this study are yet to be published; however, outcomes will identify and describe an important cardiovascular correlation between platinum induced endothelial dysfunction and long-term cardiovascular complications.

A key clinical concern regarding endothelial dysfunction associated with platinum treatment is the direct link between endothelial dysfunction and atherosclerotic development, which may be due to chronic (years) elevated platinum following cessation of treatment. Chemotherapy-induced endothelial dysfunction has been suggested as a precursor to cardiovascular events and correlates with other cardiovascular risk factors (Soultati et al. 2012), such as venous thromboembolism (Prasad et al. 2016), hypertension (Kannel 1993) and atherosclerosis (Hadi et al. 2005).

Thrombosis

Thrombosis is recognized as blood clot formation in either the arterial or venous vasculature, which can partially or completely obstruct blood flow. Reduced circulation can lead to the development of potentially catastrophic clinical complications, comorbidities and mortality (Ashorobi et al. 2021, Oklu 2017). Thrombosis is a condition known to influence and increase the risk of other cardiovascular conditions including, myocardial infarction, stroke, pulmonary embolism (PE), and limb ischemia. The most widely reported thrombotic condition described following treatment with platinum containing antineoplastic agents is venous thromboembolism (VTE).

Venous Thromboembolism (VTE)

VTE occurs when blood clots develop within veins and is divided into two subcategories: deep vein thrombosis (DVT) and pulmonary embolism (PE). DVT is a largely preventable condition; however, PE is a complication associated with DVT and can increase the risk of mortality (Stone et al. 2017). The incidence of VTE following treatment with platinum-based chemotherapies is an extensively researched side effect, particularly in the clinical setting (Edvardsen, Hansen, et al. 2021, Kim et al. 2017, Lee et al. 2015, Mellema et al. 2014, Mitani et al. 2018). Table 1 describes the broad spectrum of clinical findings of multiple studies investigating the incidence of VTEs at various time points in cancer patients treated with platinum-based chemotherapeutics.

A 2021 study by (Yuk et al. 2021) used information obtained from the Korean Health Insurance Review and Assessment Services Database to determine the incidence of VTE in women diagnosed with ovarian cancer between 2009 and 2018. A total of 23, 863 patients were included in the study, with 7, 553 (28%) treated with platinum-based chemotherapy. VTEs were identified as occurring within either the first 6 months following initiation of the primary treatment or after the total follow up period (mean follow up time of 3.5 years). During the first 6 months post-treatment with platinum-based chemotherapies, 149 individuals presented with VTE and within the total follow up period 240 patients developed VTE. Further investigations were completed to identify the specific type of VTE (DVT/PE) in these patients; however, this was not separated by chemotherapy type. Although this provides insightful data it does not yield a correlation between VTE incidence and platinum-based chemotherapy regimens (Yuk et al. 2021). Compared with other agent's platinum chemotherapy only showed a minor increase in VTE development over the total follow up period. Platinum chemotherapy yielded 3.18% VTE incidence while other agents and surgery alone presented 2.15% and 1.32% respectively. Of these 61%, 45% and 52% occurred within the first 6 months of treatment. There is a 2.4-fold increase in VTE development in those treated with platinum chemotherapy compared with those treated with surgery alone. Thus, suggesting that platinum chemotherapy may have an influence on increased VTE risk. A longer follow up period may prove beneficial to establish the long-term effect of various treatment options on VTE risk.

A recent publication by (Moik et al. 2020) investigated the development of VTE in cancer patients (total: 1, 409) treated with gemcitabine (235), platinum-based agents (501), or a combination (167). This study determined a strong univariable association between VTE risk and platinum-based therapy; however, upon addition of other variables (tumor type and D-dimer) the correlation dampened, and CDDP treatment was suggested to be a limited independent risk factor for cancer-associated VTE rather than a direct cause.

Table 1. Publications indicating clinical incidence of vein thromboembolism (VTE) events in cohort studies of cancer patients treated with platinum based anticancer agents

PARTICIPANT numbers	Treatment	TEE	TEE TYPE	Year
7,553	CDDP/Carboplatin	240	Unspecified	(2021) (Yuk et al. 2021)
501	Unspecified Platinum agent	191	Unspecified	(2020) (Moik et al. 2020)
277	CDDP/Carboplatin	30	PE; n=15 AT; n=7 DVT; n=4 DVT + PE; n=4	(2015) (Lee et al. 2015)
1677	CDDP	110	VTE/PE; n=96 AT; n=14	(2018) (Abdel-Razeq et al. 2018)
300	CDDP + Docetaxel	29	Pre-operatively; n=21 During chemotherapy; n=4 During chemoradiotherapy; n=17 Post-operatively; n=8 (5/8 were PE, 3/5 PEs were fatal)	(2020) (Fehr et al. 2020)
165	CDDP	8	PE; n=3 CI; n=5	(2018) (Joshi et al. 2018)
200	CDDP/non-CDDP-based chemotherapy	CDDP based; n=31 Non-CDDP based; n=11	DVT; n=18 Unspecified; n=13	(2017) (Zahir et al. 2017)

Abbreviations: VTE: venous thromboembolism (including DVT: deep vein thrombosis and PE: pulmonary embolism), CI: cerebral infarction, AT: arterial thrombosis, TEEs: thromboembolic events *Please note TEE event refers to the total number of identified events not patient numbers, some patients may have presented with multiple TEEs*.

CDDP vs Carboplatin Comparative Incidence of VTE

Large clinical studies often group platinum-based chemotherapeutic agents without identifying the specific platinum-based drug used when discussing the risk of VTEs. However, there are differences between the risks associated with the use of each individual platinum agent. The incidence of VTE development in CDDP and carboplatin treated patients provide conflicting data. There is one study showing a higher incidence of VTEs in CDDP treated patients compared to those treated with carboplatin and another study reporting the opposite. Yun-Gyoo Lee and colleagues investigated the risk of VTEs in lung cancer patients. A retrospective study of 277 patients diagnosed with small cell lung carcinoma between 2006 and 2012 identified VTEs through radiographic or nuclear medicine scanning. It was reported that 11% of patients (30/277) involved in the study developed VTE and incidence of VTEs increased over time following the cessation of treatment. Patients were monitored 3-, 6- and 12-months post-treatment with VTE incidence being 5%, 9.1% and 10.2%, respectively. Of the 30 VTEs identified, all presented in patients treated with platinum-based chemotherapies. 20 of those were in patients treated with CDDP, and two during treatment with carboplatin. 90% of CDDP VTEs occurred between the initiation of treatment and four weeks following the last dose (Lee et al. 2015). Two retrospective studies in lung cancer patients showed no significant difference in VTE incidence in patients treated with CDDP compared to carboplatin (Kim et al. 2017, Mellema et al. 2014). Interestingly a large-scale retrospective analysis comparing the incidence of VTEs between CDDP treated lung cancer patients and patients treated with carboplatin and the less commonly used platinum analogue nedaplatin. The study excluded patients who received more than one platinum treatment suggesting that carboplatin and nedaplatin were not given as adjuvant treatments; however, data is presented combining the two as comparative to CDDP. Presenting a comparative of the three may provide a clearer delineation as to the specific influence of nedaplatin on VTE development. Despite this CDDP displayed a higher percentage of DVT development (0.24%) compared to carboplatin/nedaplatin (0.15%); however, PE incidence was uniform (0.08%) amongst the two categories (Mitani et al. 2018). Interestingly despite the higher frequency of VTEs in CDDP treated patients, the duration of hospital stays, and mortality rates were lower compared to carboplatin and nedaplatin. Although patients treated with carboplatin and nedaplatin develop fewer VTEs they correlate with increased hospital stay duration and mortality rates implying worsened severity compared with CDDP. Thus, implying that although VTEs are less common in other platinum-based analogues, they may not be the best treatment for cancer patients as they could potentially present more severe symptoms of other conditions including VTEs in addition to their reduced efficacy as antitumor agents.

Limitations to VTE Identification: Chemotherapy Contribution

Cancer activates a pro-thrombotic state and is postulated to be via tumor induced activation of the coagulation system (Caine et al. 2002). Therefore, a limitation to thrombosis studies following treatment with platinum-based chemotherapy is the thrombotic risk of cancer itself, independent of chemotherapeutic intervention. Interestingly, it has been suggested that chemotherapy induced arterial thrombosis is rarely observed in patients following tumor resection, indicating a more prominent role for tumors in VTEs.

Studies to date provide a link between platinum-based chemotherapy and VTE development. Despite considering other risk factors by using common methods, such as the Khorana risk assessment, identifying the incidence of VTEs induced directly by platinum agents proves inconsistencies. Furthermore, varying assessment time points amongst studies yield inconclusive results. Most studies investigate VTE development within the first 4 weeks following cessation of treatment or shortly thereafter (Abdel-Razeq et al. 2018, Fehr et al. 2020, Joshi et al. 2018, Lee et al. 2015). Most clinical publications are retrospective studies with authors capable of providing data obtained from that time frame and within study criteria. One of the critical flaws of retrospective studies is the validity and accuracy of records (Huang 2021). Additionally, bias is more frequent in retrospective studies compared to prospective studies. Prospective studies may benefit from more extensive and specific data collection and records to better understand platinum-induced cardiotoxicity pathology. However, a staggered and more extensive follow up period may provide invaluable data on VTEs given the known long-term cardiovascular effects of platinum-based chemotherapy treatment and the mortality risk of VTEs.

Upregulation of Von Willebrand Factor (VWF)

Von Willebrand factor (VWF) is a multimeric protein released by damaged endothelial cells and displays pro-thrombotic physiological mechanisms (Edvardsen, Hindberg, et al. 2021). VWF is responsible for binding and transportation of the blood clotting protein Factor VIII. VWF also facilitates platelet adhesion, aggregation, and thrombus growth. A 2021 study by Edvardsen identified a dose-dependent relationship between plasma concentrations of VWF and the risk of VTE development in non-cancer patients, with similar results observed in cancer patients (Obermeier et al. 2019). They also determined that VWF may be a promising VTE risk biomarker (Edvardsen, Hansen, et al. 2021). Initial reports from the 1980s first suggested a role for CDDP in elevating plasma VWF concentration (Dieckmann et al. 2011, Licciardello et al. 1985, Lubberts et al. 2016, Nuver et al. 2005), indicating endothelial activation and damage. It also may be a contributing factor to the prevalence and incidence of thrombosis observed during and following treatment with platinum-based chemotherapies. Strikingly, although thrombosis compared to cisplatin is reduced following treatment with carboplatin and oxaliplatin, the influence of VWF is not widely reported. This might be a key pathological investigation independent of other prothrombotic factors.

Hypertension

Hypertension is defined as a chronic systemic increase in arterial blood pressure (above 120/80 mmHg). (Oparil et al. 2018). Systemic hypertension is one of the most observed vascular toxicities in patients treated with platinum-based chemotherapies and increases the risk of cardiovascular complications, including heart failure, stroke, myocardial infarction, and cardiac arrhythmias (van Dorst et al. 2021). Reports of hypertension in patients receiving platinum-based chemotherapy are less common within the literature compared to other conditions, such as arrhythmia and thrombosis. Endothelial dysfunction is the suggested mechanism associated with CDDP induced hypertension. The disrupted balance between NO and O_2^- caused by elevated ROS resulting in reduced NO bioavailability reducing vasodilation capacity. A 26-year-old treated with doxorubicin, ifosfamide, MESNA and CDDP, and a 61-year-old female treated with docetaxel, CDDP, and 5-

fluorouracil (5-FU) after being diagnosed with carcinosarcoma and metastatic gastric carcinoma, both developed generalized seizures combined with hypertension. Blood pressure readings were 180/110 and 140-180/90-110 mmHg, respectively (Limor et al. 2012). Hypertension following chemotherapy treatment appears a significantly common complication, however hypotension is a significantly rarer side effect.

Hypotension

Hypotension refers to low blood pressure (lower than 90/60 mmHg) and results in inadequate systemic oxygen supply to organs. Low blood pressure may remain undetected or present with physiological symptoms, including light headedness, dizziness, weakness, confusion, nausea, heart palpitations and hypotensive shock (Sharma et al. 2021). Reports of hypotension following adjunct treatment with CDDP, and 5-FU were recorded in the 1980s. Incidence of cardiotoxicity is rare in isolated CDDP and 5-FU treatment and the cardiotoxic effects observed in this paper are hypothesized to be linked to the concomitant administration of CDDP and 5-FU rather than CDDP or 5-FU alone. Three hypotensive cases in patients diagnosed with adenocarcinoma (44-year-old women, a 59-year-old man and a 53-year-old man) were recorded in the 1980s, following its approval in 1978. Case 1 and 2 both tolerated day one to day three well; however, presented with symptoms on day four. Case 3 tolerated day one, with symptoms observed on day two. Symptoms are relatively consistent amongst all three patients. Pre-CDDP blood pressures were 120/70, 140/90 and 130/90 mmHg respectively, which on the day of symptoms dropped to 80/60, 90/60 and systolic 60-70mmHg (no record of diastolic reading) (Jakubowski et al. 1988). These values are all indicators of hypotension. Despite three very clear cases of hypotension suggested to be linked to CDDP-based chemotherapy treatment, it is a side effect that has rarely been reported since the 1980s, possibly explained by pre-hydration therapy increasing blood volume.

Atherosclerosis

Atherosclerosis is characterised by the formation and deposition of plaques (composed of fat, cholesterol, immune cells and debris, and calcium) within the vasculature (Weaver 2013). Atherosclerosis progression is slow and develops over a significant amount of time, resulting in hardening of arteries, lumen narrowing, weakening, and rupturing of plaques (Insull Jr 2009), and in severe cases ischemia and hypoxia (Birnbaum et al. 1997). Acute treatment with CDDP results in ED. ED is hypothesised as the earliest and 'silent' vascular abnormality of atherosclerosis and disrupts the homeostatic balance between vasodilation and vasoconstriction factors, resulting in reduced NO (Davignon et al. 2004). Atherosclerosis is the leading cause of stroke and myocardial infarction (Lusis 2000) and there have been multiple reports of myocardial infarction in cases of patients treated with CDDP-based regimens; however, findings have suggested a non-atherosclerotic cause (Fukunaga et al. 2006, Hanchate et al. 2017, Rao et al. 2015). Despite this, there is the potential for atherosclerotic progression following platinum-based regimen treatment through endothelial dysfunction and hyperlipidaemia (Sekijima et al. 2011). Hyperlipidaemia is a common clinical symptom associated with platinum-based treatments. (Koc et al. 2011, Lander et al. 2020, Sekijima et al. 2011).

Lipid Profiling

Serum lipid levels are considered a key pathology in atherogenesis, as increased total cholesterol (TC), triacylglycerol (TAG) and low-density lipoprotein cholesterol (LDL) and reduced high-density lipoprotein cholesterol (HDL) are hallmarks of atherogenic progression (Linton et al. 2019). There is an interesting variation regarding the LDL and HDL balance following platinum chemotherapy treatment. One study investigated levels of LDL and HDL following treatment with platinum-based chemotherapy carboplatin with a follow up period of one year and another using CDDP with a 4-6 year follow up period. In ovarian and endometrial cancer patients undergone either surgery or surgery with a carboplatin-based chemotherapy regimen showed a trend towards increased LDL levels in patients treated with surgery and chemotherapy compared with surgery alone (Sekijima et al. 2011). This same study investigated changes in HDL content, demonstrating that HDL was reduced in ovarian cancer patients without chemotherapy; but increased in patients with chemotherapy. The opposite trend was observed in patients with endometrial cancer. In testicular cancer patients treated with a CDDP-based regimen it was determined that after 8 years, CDDP had no long-term effect on alterations in blood lipid levels (Willemse et al. 2014). Another study showed that LDL, serum TC and insulin were significantly elevated 3-

months following CDDP treatment; however, returned to baseline 9 months post-treatment (Koc et al. 2011). Previous studies have shown a link between elevated triglycerides and the development and progression of atherosclerosis through the identification of triglyceride-containing remnant lipoproteins in human atherosclerotic plaque (Peng et al. 2017). Triglyceride content was measured following surgery and treatment with a carboplatin-based regimen. There was a statistically significant increase in triglyceride and LDL levels in both ovarian and endometrial cancer patients following chemotherapy treatment compared to without (Sekijima et al. 2011). This suggests that hyperlipidemia, although a risk factor for atherosclerotic development, may not be a contributor to atherosclerotic development following CDDP treatment; but may following other therapies such as carboplatin (Sekijima et al. 2011).

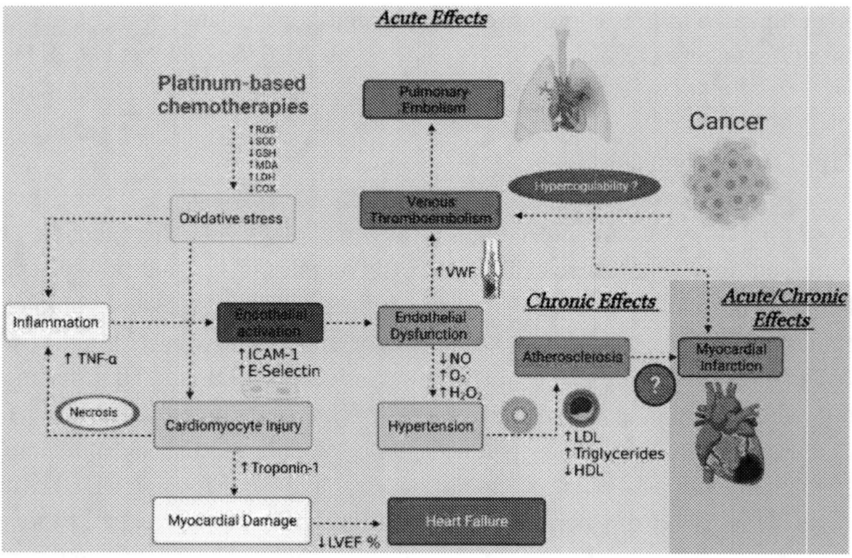

Abbreviations: ROS: reactive oxygen species, SOD: superoxide dismutase, GSH: glutathione, MDA: malondialdehyde, LDH: lactate dehydrogenase, COX: cyclooxygenase 2, ICAM-1: intracellular adhesion molecule 1, LVEF: left ventricular ejection fraction, H_2O_2: hydrogen peroxide, O_2^-: superoxide, NO: nitric oxide, VWF: von Willebrand factor, LDL: low-density lipoprotein, HDL: high-density lipoprotein.

Figure 2. Molecular mechanisms associated with platinum-based chemotherapy induced cardiotoxicity include, inflammation, endothelial activation, endothelial dysfunction, cardiomyocyte injury, hypertension, atherosclerosis, venous thromboembolism, pulmonary embolism, and myocardial infarction.

It is plausible that the follow up period post chemotherapy may not be a long enough period to observe atherosclerotic progression. Despite the acute hyperlipidaemia observed and its normalization over time, the fundamental concern is ED. The time frame from the manifestation of ED progressing to rupture and acute myocardial infarction development can vary from short duration in the case of accelerated atherosclerosis (2-3 months) or over a long duration (many years) (Shah et al. 2015). This indicates that although lipid levels may return to normal following platinum-based treatment the ED may not, increasing the development and progression of atherosclerotic development. This suggests that increased follow up time may identify and further elucidate the role of CDDP and other platinum analogue induced EDs in long term progression of atherosclerosis.

Arrhythmia

Cardiac arrhythmia refers to any physiologically deviation from normal heart rate or rhythm. Two major categories are used to determine the general mechanism associated with cardiac arrhythmias initiated in both the atrium or ventricle: (1) altered impulse formation and (2) conduction disturbances (Antzelevitch et al. 2011). Treatment with platinum-based chemotherapies have been linked to both tachycardic and bradycardic arrhythmias (Bang et al. 2020, Fassio et al. 1986, Ozcan et al. 2011, Raja et al. 2013). Interestingly, despite the incidence and variety of cardiac arrhythmias reported during or following infusions of platinum-based chemotherapies little pre-clinical research has been completed to identify cause.

Tachycardia

Tachycardia describes a heart rate $\geq$ 100 bpm and is clinically important because it can cause or be an indicator of myocardial ischemia, hypotension, low cardiac output, cardiomyopathy, and cardiac arrest (Gopinathannair et al. 2015). Tachycardia following CDDP treatment has been associated with paroxysmal supraventricular tachycardia (PSVT), atrial fibrillation and vasospasm-induced myocardial infarction.

Paroxysmal Supraventricular Tachycardia (PSVT)

Multiple reports of paroxysmal supraventricular tachycardia (PSVT) have been published following treatment with CDDP based regimens (Fassio et al. 1986, Raja et al. 2013). A 55-year-old patient diagnosed with SCLC solely in the right lung was diagnosed with PSVT by electrocardiogram (ECG) during the second cycle of CDDP, as the patient complained of heart palpitations. Pre-treatment ECG and blood pressure was normal, with no evidence of cardiac disease or heart complications observed during the first chemotherapy cycle. At the time of PSVT presentation, patient blood samples were taken and indicated normal electrolyte levels. Chemotherapy was ceased at the time of heart complications; however, a subsequent ECG returned a normal heart rate with no PSVT reported. No further cardiac events occurred during any following cycles following pre-treatment with bisoprolol (Raja et al. 2013). This suggests that pre-treatment with bisoprolol or other beta blockers may be a treatment in high-risk patients to prevent the development of PSVT.

Atrial Fibrillation (AF)

One of the more concerning arrhythmias reported following platinum-based treatment is atrial fibrillation (AF). AF is considered the most common continuous arrhythmia, and its incidence is associated with elevated morbidity and mortality rates (Heijman et al. 2014). AF is usually referred to as a progressive illness with three stages: (1) paroxysmal, which is often seen in short duration and resolves without intervention; (2) persistent, multiple episodes requiring pharmacological therapies to reestablish a normal heart rhythm; and (3) permanent, sinus rhythm that cannot be restored using treatment (Wyndham 2000). There have been multiple reports of AF following treatment with CDDP (Pastorino et al. 2016); however, a lack of combined case statistics is lacking, therefore research into the epidemiology of the condition may provide better insight into the frequency and severity of this condition in patients.

A 2016 publication outlined the occurrence of AF in a patient diagnosed with stage 3 testicular seminoma treated with a bleomycin, etoposide, and cisplatin (PEB) chemotherapy regimen. Pre-chemotherapy investigations determined that the patient had no pre-existing co-morbidities or history of cardiologic disease, negative ECG, and normal cardiac rhythm, physical exam, blood count and electrolyte levels of Na^+, K^+ and Ca^{2+}.However, the patient displayed hypomagnesemia. On the third day of the first cycle, during the CDDP infusion the patient began to experience heart palpitations. A physical examination demonstrated pulse arrhythmia with AF confirmed by an ECG; however, despite the AF a normal (86 BPM) ventricular rate was observed. Based on the normal ventricular rhythm the chemotherapy infusion of CDDP was maintained; however adjunct treatment with the blood thinners, heparin, and enoxaparin was initiated. The evening after AF was diagnosed a tachycardic heart rate (110 BPM) was observed and the patient was given a 12-hour infusion of saline and digoxin, which returned heart rhythm to normal, determined by ECG. In addition to the determination of electrolyte levels within a normal range. Following this, the PEB regimen was continued with no subsequent cardiac events (Pastorino et al. 2016). In addition to treatment with CDDP, AF has been observed following infusion with oxaliplatin (Hancox et al. 2016). Based on the magnitude of research indicating the reduction of magnesium and cardiac events seen in patients treated with CDDP, cardiac arrhythmias are still observed in patients treated with CDDP when baseline electrolyte levels are normal, and it is difficult to determine if the AF was caused by the treatment or by other factors.

Bradycardia

Bradycardia is a frequently observed cardiac arrhythmia and is defined as a heart rate below 50-60 BPM. Symptoms of bradycardia include fatigue, dizziness, confusion, syncope (fainting) and dyspnea (shortness of breath) (Sidhu et al. 2020). There are various subsets of bradycardia. Sinus bradycardia refers to an issue in conductivity of the sinoatrial node (the hearts natural primary pacemaker) resulting in stimulation of less than 60 electrical impulses per minute (Palatnik et al. 2003). Bradycardia has been seen following platinum-based chemotherapy treatment, frequently associated with atrioventricular (AV) block, although it has also been observed in vasospastic myocardial ischemia.

Atrioventricular (AV) Block

There have been multiple reports of AV blockages in cancer patients treated with platinum-based chemotherapy regimens (Bang et al. 2020, Ozcan et al. 2011). AV block is a subtype of bradycardic arrythmias and is characterized by a disruption or interference in the transmission of electrical impulses from the atria to the ventricles (Kashou et al. 2021). AV blocks are categorized as being first degree, second degree or third degree. Second degree AV blocks are further subtyped as being Mobitz type 1 or 2 (Mangi et al. 2020).

A paper published in 2020 gives extensive details into two patients diagnosed with CDDP-induced AV block. A 65-year-old woman with Metastatic Klatskin's tumors and 75-year-old man with esophageal cancer, both with no underlying heart disease, presented with dyspnea without chest pain and bradycardia following CDDP treatment. Both patients demonstrated normal vital signs, electrolyte levels and ECG pre-therapy. Symptoms of AV block occurred following the sixth cycle of a platinum-based regimen for both patients. Heart rates were 38 and 44 BPM, 2D ECG showed normal left ventricular systolic function with ejection fractions of 71 and 73% respectively and neither patient showed any signs of wall motion abnormality. It was determined that both patients had severe, irreversible AV blocks and underwent pacemaker insertions. ECG results of the 65-year-old woman after surgery showed normal ECG functioning and CDDP treatment was resumed, with no evidence of further cardiovascular complications (Bang et al. 2020). Another case of AV block showed a 50-year-old man diagnosed with squamous cell carcinoma develop syncope on the fifth day of a five-day CDDP infusion schedule. The patient underwent routine testing on admission which showed a normal ECG, electrolyte levels and blood count pre-treatment. A second 5-day regimen resulted in syncope on the third day, where the patient become unconscious and hypotensive with a blood pressure reading of 60/40 mmHg. An ECG confirmed AV block, and as seen with other patients, the AV block was irreversible, and a permanent pacemaker was inserted. Normal ventricular ejection fraction was seen in all patients with no further cardiovascular complications observed following the resumption of chemotherapeutic, no further cardiovascular complication arose at the resumption of treatment following pacemaker insertion (Ozcan et al. 2011). Following reports of AV blocks in clinical presentation, pre-clinical evaluations have suggested that oxidative damage induced by CDDP may be causal to disturbances in AV conduction (Rosic et al. 2015), potentiating it as a contributor to the incidence of AV blocks in patients treated with CDDP.

Cardiopulmonary Arrest

One of the most severe cardiac cases seen following treatment with CDDP was observed in a 53-year-old woman with stage IV mesothelioma in the right lung, with pre-existing arterial hypertension. During the second cycle of

CDDP the patient complained of malaise and fatigue. Before the next cycle the patient was administered the pre-medications folic acid and cyanocobalamin (dietary supplements), mannitol (to force urine production), and ondansetron (to prevent nausea). Following this the patient received a CDDP infusion. During this infusion the patient developed cardiopulmonary arrest and became unresponsive. Cardiorespiratory resuscitation was initiated following asystole algorithm and administration of adrenaline. The patient was intubated, and the airway stabilized, with resuscitation continued. 12 minutes following beginning of resuscitation a cardiac sinus rhythm was restored along with spontaneous circulation.

Platinum Chemotherapy Induced Hypomagnesemia

Hypomagnesemia is a common occurrence in cancer patients treated with the three most prescribed platinum-based chemotherapies (i.e., CDDP, carboplatin and oxaliplatin). Hypomagnesemia is present in 40-90% of patients treated with CDDP; however, is only observed in 10% of patients treated with carboplatin or oxaliplatin (Workeneh et al. 2020). Hypomagnesemia is an electrolyte imbalance and is highly linked to dysrhythmia. Interestingly, hypomagnesemia and dysrhythmia are common pathologies presented in platinum treated cancer patients and are often asynchronous. However, many of the clinical studies outlining various dysrhythmia cases are often accompanied by homeostatic electrolyte levels, particularly magnesium (Fassio et al. 1986, Jakubowski et al. 1988, Pastorino et al. 2016). Thus, suggesting that cardiac arrhythmias although linked to hypomagnesemia in other conditions, in most instances of dysrhythmia during/following platinum-based chemotherapy treatment it is not causal. This prompted further investigations into the cause of platinum-based chemotherapy inducing arrhythmias and any specific roles for hypomagnesemia or other mechanisms in its pathogenesis. One of the fundamental considerations regarding arrythmias following CDDP treatment is the unlikelihood that CDDP is prescribed as a stand-alone treatment. CDDP-based chemotherapy suggests CDDP is the principal chemotherapy administered. However, it is often prescribed as a regimen, with other chemotherapies, such as the PEB regimen (CDDP, etoposide and bleomycin) (Christensen et al. 2014). Despite this, cardiac arrythmias are often observed specifically during CDDP infusions; however, it is generally unclear as to the involvement of the other compounds influencing arrhythmic generation.

Hypomagnesemia has also been induced by carboplatin treatment, with patients presenting with mild, moderate, and severe magnesium deficiency and as such further investigations into the clinical relevancy of carboplatin-induced magnesium deficiency is required (Gaughran et al. 2020). Understanding the role of other platinum analogues inducing magnesium deficiency would be beneficial, particularly in understanding cardiac complications associated with treatment.

Pre-Clinical Cardiotoxicity

Multiple pre-clinical studies have investigated pharmacological prevention of CDDP-induced cardiotoxicity. CDDP is considered the most potent of the platinum chemotherapeutic analogues and is often the agent of choice in pre-clinical evaluations. The definition of cardiotoxicity remains an evolving concept with many subdivisions that have continued to change and may continue to be redefined as time progresses. Cardiotoxicity is widely defined as development or worsened ventricular function and increased myocardial damage (Zamorano 2020). Clinically cardiotoxicity is diagnosed by a percentage reduction compared to baseline in left ventricular ejection fraction in addition to key biomarkers, such as troponin and natriuretic peptides indicative of early myocardial damage (Henri et al. 2016, Pistillucci et al. 2015, Zamorano 2020). However, many studies refer to cardiotoxicity as an umbrella term to collectively group all forms of cardiac complication associated with pharmacological treatments. This largely correlates with pre-clinical studies that often do not divide cardiotoxicity into specific subtypes and instead refer to cardiotoxicity as a single entity. The initial step would be to identify a protocol and treatment regimen to establish these conditions, such as thrombosis in animal models, which is a recent avenue within the field (Filonova et al. 2020). Establishing models that target specific conditions may be beneficial. For example, creating a suitable model that uses platinum-based chemotherapy drugs to induce thrombosis in both a healthy and tumor bearing animal model may provide useful insight into the role of cancer progression on thrombosis risk. It may also aid the identification of potential adjuvant treatments to prevent thrombosis formation. Pre-clinical studies have largely linked increased oxidative stress to platinum-based chemotherapy induced cardiotoxicity, through a variety of mechanisms shown in figure 2. Recent publications have found multiple potential treatments to prevent oxidative stress in models of platinum-based chemotherapy-induced cardiotoxicity.

Interestingly, many lack cancer bearing models or studies showing the effects of these treatments on CDDP cytotoxicity; however, inducing cancer in these models may be the progression from commonly used non-cancer models. Key serum and cardiac tissue biomarkers in addition to histopathological changes in cardiac tissue are key methodological evaluations used to identify cardiotoxicity in pre-clinical models. Biochemical analysis of serum lactate dehydrogenase (LDH), creatine phosphokinase (CPK), troponin-1 and cardiac tissue levels of ROS, malondialdehyde (MDA), superoxide dismutase (SOD), TNF-α, NO and catalase (CAT) are primary identifiers used in diagnosis of cardiotoxicity in animal studies, whilst Troponin-1 is one of the common biomarkers used in pre-clinic and clinical evaluations. Table 2 outlines some of the pre-clinical evaluations and therapeutic interventions targeting the umbrella term of cardiotoxicity with a primary focus on antioxidation mechanisms. Interestingly a fundamental challenge in pre-clinical to clinic translation is the variation of cardiovascular complications presented clinically. Namely the key and highly specific complications observed following platinum treatments are not represented in pre-clinical studies, which may highlight a need for animal models with a higher clinical relevancy in representation of clinical conditions.

Conclusion

Cardiac complications arising during and following treatment with platinum-based chemotherapy is an evolving and often overlooked side effect. Pre-clinically these complications are placed under the umbrella term cardiotoxicity and these studies have mostly focused largely on therapeutic targets for oxidative stress to reduce ROS formation and restore the oxidant/antioxidant defense system. Clinically, cardiotoxicity is reported more specifically compared to animal studies and based on the precise diagnosis and clinical conditions rather than the generalized cardiotoxicity classification. Some of the most common cardiovascular complications include vascular toxicity, including coronary vasospasm, endothelial activation, ED, and upregulation of prothrombotic factors. Thrombosis, hypertension, hypotension, and arrhythmia are other key reported clinical complications. Despite the array of clinical reports of cardiac complications, it is interesting that pre-clinical research lacks the same specificity. Future research may benefit from producing more clinically relevant models to reproduce these specific conditions to better understand their pathology.

Table 2. Pre-Clinical evaluations investigate the pathological mechanisms and therapeutic options for CDDP induced cardiotoxicity

Intervention	Mechanism	Species	Type	Key findings	Year
Curcumin Nanoparticles	Antioxidant	Wistar Albino Rats	CDDP 12 mg/kg	↓ MDA ↓ NO ↓ TNF-α ↑ GSH ↓ AchEs ↑ LDH ↓ NA^+/K^+	2020 (Khadrawy et al. 2021)
Acetyl-L-carnitine	Antioxidant	Athymic nude Mice	CDDP 16 mg/kg culled after 7 days	↓ SOD-2 ↑ COX-2	2020 (Bayrak et al. 2020)
All-Trans Retinoic acid	Antioxidant	Wistar Albino Rats	CDDP 7 mg/kg Culled on 7th day	↓ Necrosis ↓Cytoplasmic Vacuolization ↓ Congestion	2021 (Ekmekci et al. 2021)
Tinospora cordifolia	Anti-inflammatory/ Antioxidant	Wistar Rats	CDDP 7.5 mg/kg	↓ LDH ↓ CPK ↓ Troponin Moderate → mild congestion Moderate → mild myocardial degenerative changes Moderate → mild haemorrhages Moderate → mild disruption of cardiac muscle	2021 (Begum et al. 2021)
Vitamin C	Antioxidant	Wistar Rats	CDDP 7.5 mg/kg	↓ LDH ↓ CPK ↓ Troponin very mild evidence of histopathological cardiac tissue injury	2021 (Begum et al. 2021)
Blackberry (bb) loaded Ag@AuNPs	Antioxidant/ Antilipidemic	Albino Rats	Dose of CDDP 20 mg/kg,	↓ MDA ↓ AOPP ↑ TAC ↓ LDH ↓ Troponin-1	2020 (Hussein et al. 2020)

Table 2. (Continued)

Intervention	Mechanism	Species	Type	Key findings	Year
Rosuvastatin and simvastatin	Statins (Anti-inflammatory)	Wistar Rats	CDDP 10 mg/kg	↓ Serum Troponin-1 ↓ Serum LDH ↓ Serum CK-MB ↑ Cardiac SOD ↑ GSH ↑ GRP78 ↑ Calpain-1 ↑ Active Caspase 3	2020 (Saleh et al. 2020)
Trimetazidine and coenzyme Q10 pre-treatment	Anti-ischemic/anti-oxidant	Isolated Rat Cardiomyocytes	CDDP 200 μM	↓ ROS ↓ MDA ↑ SOD ↑ CAT	2019 (Zhao 2019)

Abbreviations: MDA: malondialdehyde, NO: nitric oxide, TNF-α: tumor necrosis factor Alpha, GSH: glutathione, AchEs: acetylcholinesterase, LDH: lactate dehydrogenase, SOD-2: superoxide dismutase 2, COX-2: cyclooxygenase 2, CPK: creatine phosphokinase, AOPP: advanced oxidation protein products, TAC: total antioxidant capacity, CK-MB: creatine kinase MB, GRP78: glucose regulating protein 78, ROS: reactive oxygen species, CAT: Catalase. Key: ↑ = increased; ↓ = decreased.

References

Abdel-Razeq, Hikmat, Asem Mansour, Hazem Abdulelah, Anas Al-Shwayat, Mohammad Makoseh, Mohammad Ibrahim, Mahmoud Abunasser, Dalia Rimawi, Abeer Al-Rabaiah, and Rozan Alfar. 2018. "Thromboembolic events in cancer patients on active treatment with cisplatin-based chemotherapy: another look!" *Thrombosis journal* 16 (1):1-7.

Antzelevitch, Charles, and Alexander Burashnikov. 2011. "Overview of basic mechanisms of cardiac arrhythmia." *Cardiac electrophysiology clinics* 3 (1):23-45.

Ashorobi, Damilola, Muhammad Atif Ameer, and Roberto Fernandez. 2021. "Thrombosis." In *StatPearls [Internet]*. Treasure Island (FL): StatPearls Publishing

Bang, Hyun-Jin, Ho Young Lee, Hyeon-Jong Kim, Namsik Yoon, Ik-Joo Chung, and Woo Kyun Bae. 2020. "Cisplatin-induced Atrioventricular Block Requiring a Pacemaker: Two Case Reports and a Literature Review." *Electrolytes & Blood Pressure: E & BP* 18 (2):49.

Bayrak, Serdar, Safiye Aktaş, Zekiye Altun, Yasemin Çakir, Merve Tütüncü, Selen Kum Özşengezer, Osman Yilmaz, and Nur Olgun. 2020. "Antioxidant effect of acetyl-l-carnitine against cisplatin-induced cardiotoxicity." *Journal of International Medical Research* 48 (8):0300060520951393.

Begum, Nisaath, P Shivakumar, A Gopala Reddy, B Ramya, and B Anil. 2021. "Cardio protective actions of Tinospora cordifolia and vitamin C against experimental toxicity due to Cisplatin."

Bhargava, Ashish, and Ulka N Vaishampayan. 2009. "Satraplatin: leading the new generation of oral platinum agents." *Expert opinion on investigational drugs* 18 (11):1787-1797.

Caine, Graham J, Paul S Stonelake, Gregory YH Lip, and Sean T Kehoe. 2002. "The hypercoagulable state of malignancy: pathogenesis and current debate." *Neoplasia (New York, NY)* 4 (6):465.

Chang, Rei-Yeuh, Ming-Yang Lee, Chung-Ben Kan, Wei-Pang Hsu, and Pei-Ching Hsiao. 2013. "Oxaliplatin-induced acquired long QT syndrome with torsades de pointes and myocardial injury in a patient with dilated cardiomyopathy and rectal cancer." *Journal of the Chinese Medical Association* 76 (8):466-469.

Choi, Cheol-Hee, Yoon-Jung Cha, Chun-San An, Kyung-Jong Kim, Kweon-Cheon Kim, Sung-Pyo Moon, Zang Hee Lee, and Young-Don Min. 2004. "Molecular mechanisms of heptaplatin effective against cisplatin-resistant cancer cell lines: less involvement of metallothionein." *Cancer Cell International* 4 (1):1-12.

Christensen, Jesper Frank, LW Jones, Anders Tolver, LW Jørgensen, JL Andersen, L Adamsen, P Højman, RH Nielsen, Mikkel Rørth, and Gedske Daugaard. 2014. "Safety and efficacy of resistance training in germ cell cancer patients undergoing chemotherapy: a randomized controlled trial." *British journal of cancer* 111 (1):8-16.

Coats, A, and S Jain. 2017. "Protective effects of nebivolol from oxidative stress to prevent hypertension-related target organ damage." *Journal of human hypertension* 31 (6):376-381.

Dasari, Shaloam, and Paul Bernard Tchounwou. 2014. "Cisplatin in cancer therapy: molecular mechanisms of action." *European journal of pharmacology* 740:364-378.

Davignon, Jean, and Peter Ganz. 2004. "Role of endothelial dysfunction in atherosclerosis." *Circulation* 109 (23_suppl_1):III-27-III-32.

Dieckmann, Klaus-Peter, Werner Jan Struss, and Ulrich Budde. 2011. "Evidence for acute vascular toxicity of cisplatin-based chemotherapy in patients with germ cell tumour." *Anticancer research* 31 (12):4501-4505.

Edvardsen, Magnus S, Ellen-Sofie Hansen, Kristian Hindberg, Vânia M Morelli, Thor Ueland, Pål Aukrust, Sigrid K Brækkan, Line H Evensen, and John-Bjarne Hansen. 2021. "Combined effects of plasma von Willebrand factor and platelet measures on the risk of incident venous thromboembolism." *Blood* 138 (22):2269-2277.

Edvardsen, Magnus S, Kristian Hindberg, Ellen-Sofie Hansen, Vânia M Morelli, Thor Ueland, Pål Aukrust, Sigrid K Brækkan, Line H Evensen, and John-Bjarne Hansen. 2021. "Plasma levels of von Willebrand factor and future risk of incident venous thromboembolism." *Blood Advances* 5 (1):224-232.

Ekmekci, Cenk, Sümeyye Ekmekci, Cem Yücel, and Ebru ÇAKIR. 2021. "Cardioprotective effect of all-trans retinoic acid on cisplatin induced cardiotoxicity in rats." *Cukurova Medical Journal* 46 (3):1230-1236.

Fassio, Tiziana, Luciano Canobbio, Giampietro Gasparini, and Fabrizio Villani. 1986. "Paroxysmal supraventricular tachycardia during treatment with cisplatin and etoposide combination." *Oncology* 43 (4):219-220.

Fehr, Martin, Hanne Hawle, Stefanie Hayoz, Peter Thuss-Patience, Sabina Schacher, Jorge Riera Knorrenschild, Donat Dürr, Wolfram T Knoefel, Holger Rumpold, and Michael Bitzer. 2020. "High thromboembolic event rate in patients with locally advanced oesophageal cancer during neoadjuvant therapy. An exploratory analysis of the prospective, randomised intergroup phase III trial SAKK 75/08." *BMC cancer* 20 (1):1-9.

Filonova, MV, EP Fedorova, AA Churin, L Yu Kotlovskaya, MA Solov'ev, and VV Udut. 2020. "Changes in Hemostasis System in Outbred Female Mice with Cisplatin-Induced Procoagulant Status." *Bulletin of Experimental Biology and Medicine* 170 (1):15-18.

Fukunaga, Takashi, Hirofumi Soejima, Koichi Sugamura, Sunao Kojima, Seigo Sugiyama, Tomohiro Sakamoto, Michihiro Yoshimura, Toshihide Tanoue, Toshiro Kageshita, and Tomomichi Ono. 2006. "Acute myocardial infarction induced by cisplatin-based combination chemotherapy for malignant melanoma: a case report." *J Cardiol* 47 (4):191-195.

Gaughran, Gregory, Kiran Qayyum, Lillian Smyth, and Alison Davis. 2020. "Carboplatin and hypomagnesemia: Is it really a problem?" *Asia-Pacific Journal of Clinical Oncology*.

Ghosh, Sumit. 2019. "Cisplatin: The first metal based anticancer drug." *Bioorganic chemistry* 88:102925.

Goldberg, Richard. 2000. "Oxaliplatin in colorectal cancer: current studies." *Oncology (Williston Park, NY)* 14 (12 Suppl 11):42-47.

Gopinathannair, Rakesh, and Brian Olshansky. 2015. "Management of tachycardia." *F1000prime reports* 7.

Guzik, Tomasz J, Nick EJ West, Ravi Pillai, David P Taggart, and Keith M Channon. 2002. "Nitric oxide modulates superoxide release and peroxynitrite formation in human blood vessels." *Hypertension* 39 (6):1088-1094.

Hadi, Hadi AR, Cornelia S Carr, and Jassim Al Suwaidi. 2005. "Endothelial dysfunction: cardiovascular risk factors, therapy, and outcome." *Vascular health and risk management* 1 (3):183.

Hanchate, Lalith Prabhakar, Shimpa Rakesh Sharma, and Sadhana Madyalkar. 2017. "Cisplatin induced acute myocardial infarction and dyslipidemia." *Journal of clinical and diagnostic research: JCDR* 11 (6):OD05.

Hancox, Jules C, Rachel E Caves, Stéphanie CM Choisy, and Andrew F James. 2016. "QT interval prolongation and torsades de pointes with oxaliplatin." *Therapeutic advances in drug safety* 7 (6):261-263.

Heijman, Jordi, Niels Voigt, Stanley Nattel, and Dobromir Dobrev. 2014. "Cellular and molecular electrophysiology of atrial fibrillation initiation, maintenance, and progression." *Circulation research* 114 (9):1483-1499.

Henri, Christine, Therese Heinonen, and Jean-Claude Tardif. 2016. "The role of biomarkers in decreasing risk of cardiac toxicity after cancer therapy: supplementary issue: biomarkers and their essential role in the development of personalised therapies (A)." *Biomarkers in cancer* 8:BIC. S31798.

Holditch, Sara J, Carolyn N Brown, Andrew M Lombardi, Khoa N Nguyen, and Charles L Edelstein. 2019. "Recent Advances in Models, Mechanisms, Biomarkers, and Interventions in Cisplatin-Induced Acute Kidney Injury." *International journal of molecular sciences* 20 (12):3011.

Huang, Peng. 2021. "Retrospective Study." *Pain Physician* 24:E117-E125.

Hussain, SA, DH Palmer, B Lloyd, SI Collins, D Barton, J Ansari, and ND James. 2012. "A study of split-dose cisplatin-based neo-adjuvant chemotherapy in muscle-invasive bladder cancer." *Oncology letters* 3 (4):855-859.

Hussein, Jihan, Mehrez E El-Naggar, Moustafa MG Fouda, Osama M Morsy, Jamaan S Ajarem, Ahmed M Almalki, Ahmed A Allam, and Enas Mahmoud Mekawi. 2020. "The efficiency of blackberry loaded AgNPs, AuNPs and Ag@ AuNPs mediated pectin in the treatment of cisplatin-induced cardiotoxicity in experimental rats." *International Journal of Biological Macromolecules* 159:1084-1093.

Insull Jr, William. 2009. "The pathology of atherosclerosis: plaque development and plaque responses to medical treatment." *The American journal of medicine* 122 (1):S3-S14.

Jakubowski, Ann A, and Nancy Kemeny. 1988. "Hypotension as a manifestation of cardiotoxicity in three patients receiving cisplatin and 5-fluorouracil." *Cancer* 62 (2):266-269.

Joshi, Amit, Shruti Kate, Vanita Noronha, Vijay Patil, Vaishakhi Trivedi, Supriya Goud, Sucheta More, Sandeep Bhairva, and Kumar Prabhash. 2018. "Thromboembolic events in patients with advanced stage non-small cell lung cancer treated with platinum-based chemotherapy: a prospective observational study." *ecancermedicalscience* 12.

Kannel, William B. 1993. "Hypertension as a risk factor for cardiac events--epidemiologic results of long-term studies." *Journal of cardiovascular pharmacology* 21:S27-37.

Kashou, Anthony H, Amandeep Goyal, Tran Nguyen, Lovely Chhabra, and Laura G Kukuc. 2021. "Atrioventricular Block (Nursing)." In *StatPearls [Internet]*. Treasure Island (FL): StatPearls Publishing.

Kataoka, Tomoya, Taiki Mori, Jun Suzuki, Yuto Kawaki, Yohei Kito, Yuji Hotta, Yoshihiro Kawade, Yasuhiro Maeda, and Kazunori Kimura. 2021. "Oxaliplatin, an Anticancer Agent, Causes Erectile Dysfunction in Rats due to Endothelial Dysfunction." *The Journal of Sexual Medicine* 18 (8):1337-1345.

Kawase, Jin, Soji Ozawa, Kenichi Kobayashi, Yoshihiro Imaeda, Shunji Umemoto, Sumio Matsumoto, and Masakazu Ueda. 2009. "Increase in E-selectin expression in umbilical vein endothelial cells by anticancer drugs and inhibition by cimetidine." *Oncology reports* 22 (6):1293-1297.

Khadrawy, Yasser A, Eman N Hosny, Mayada M El-Gizawy, Hussein G Sawie, and Heba S Aboul Ezz. 2021. "The Effect of Curcumin Nanoparticles on Cisplatin-Induced Cardiotoxicity in Male Wistar Albino Rats." *Cardiovascular Toxicology* 21 (6):433-443.

Kim, Eric S, Andrea M Baran, Esther L Mondo, Thomas D Rodgers, Gradon C Nielsen, David W Dougherty, Kishan J Pandya, David Q Rich, and Edwin van Wijngaarden. 2017. "Risk of thromboembolism in cisplatin versus carboplatin-treated patients with lung cancer." *PloS one* 12 (12):e0189410.

Koc, Gokhan, Taner Rauf Divrik, Nuri Unlu, Volkan Bulut, and Ferruh Zorlu. 2011. "Does cisplatin-based chemotherapy effect on blood lipid levels of patients with germ cell testicular tumor in long-term follow-up?" *International urology and nephrology* 43 (4):1095-1100.

Kreisman, Harvey, Sandra Ginsberg, Kathleen J Propert, Frederick Richards, Stephen Graziano, and Mark Green. 1987. "Carboplatin or iproplatin in advanced non-small cell lung cancer: a Cancer and Leukemia Group B Study." *Cancer Treat. Rep.* 71 (11):1049-1052.

Lander, Megan, Yasmin Abedin, Sofia Gabrilovich, and Jenna Z Marcus. 2020. "Severe hypertriglyceridemia during treatment with intraperitoneal cisplatin and paclitaxel for advanced stage fallopian tube carcinoma." *Gynecologic oncology reports* 32:100552.

Lanza, Gaetano Antonio, Giulia Careri, and Filippo Crea. 2011. "Mechanisms of coronary artery spasm." *Circulation* 124 (16):1774-1782.

Lee, Yun-Gyoo, Eunyoung Lee, Inho Kim, Keun-Wook Lee, Tae Min Kim, Se-Hoon Lee, Dong-Wan Kim, and Dae Seog Heo. 2015. "Cisplatin-based chemotherapy is a strong risk factor for thromboembolic events in small-cell lung cancer." *Cancer research and treatment: official journal of Korean Cancer Association* 47 (4):670.

Licciardello, Jere TW, Joel L Moake, Christine K Rudy, Daniel D Karp, and Waun Ki Hong. 1985. "Elevated plasma von Willebrand factor levels and arterial occlusive complications associated with cisplatin-based chemotherapy." *Oncology* 42 (5):296-300.

Limor, Amit, Ben-Aharon Irit, Tichler Thomas, Inbar Edna, Sulkes Aaron, and Stemmer Salomon M. 2012. "Cisplatin-induced posterior reversible encephalopathy syndrome—brief report and review of the literature." *Journal of Behavioral and Brain Science* 2012.

Linton, MacRae F, Patricia G Yancey, Sean S Davies, W Gray Jerome, Edward F Linton, Wenliang L Song, Amanda C Doran, and Kasey C Vickers. 2019. "The role of lipids and lipoproteins in atherosclerosis." *Endotext [Internet].*

Lubberts, S, H Boer, R Altena, C Meijer, AM Van Roon, N Zwart, SF Oosting, PW Kamphuisen, J Nuver, and AJ Smit. 2016. "Vascular fingerprint and vascular damage markers associated with vascular events in testicular cancer patients during and after chemotherapy." *European Journal of Cancer* 63:180-188.

Lusis, A. 2000. "Atherosclenrosis." *Nature* 407:233-241.

Mandic, Aleksandra, Johan Hansson, Stig Linder, and Maria C Shoshan. 2003. "Cisplatin induces endoplasmic reticulum stress and nucleus-independent apoptotic signaling." *Journal of Biological Chemistry* 278 (11):9100-9106.

Mangi, Muhammad Asif, Wesley M Jones, Mohamed K Mansour, and Laura Napier. 2020. "Atrioventricular Block Second-Degree." In *StatPearls [Internet]*. Treasure Island (FL): StatPearls Publishing.

McKeage, Mark J. 2001. "Lobaplatin: a new antitumour platinum drug." *Expert opinion on investigational drugs* 10 (1):119-128.

Mellema, Wouter W, Dorien van der Hoek, Pieter E Postmus, and Egbert F Smit. 2014. "Retrospective evaluation of thromboembolic events in patients with non-small cell lung cancer treated with platinum-based chemotherapy." *Lung cancer* 86 (1):73-77.

Ming, Ming, Zhao-long Ma, Yong-tao Xu, Feng-Yin Sun, and Xin-hai Cui. 2017. "Carboplatin-based Nanomedicine to Enhance the Anticancer Effect in SK-NEP-1 Wilms'Tumor Cells." *Iranian journal of pharmaceutical research: IJPR* 16 (4):1305.

Mitani, Akihisa, Taisuke Jo, Hideo Yasunaga, Yukiyo Sakamoto, Wakae Hasegawa, Hirokazu Urushiyama, Yasuhiro Yamauchi, Hiroki Matsui, Kiyohide Fushimi, and Takahide Nagase. 2018. "Venous thromboembolic events in patients with lung cancer treated with cisplatin-based versus carboplatin/nedaplatin-based chemotherapy." *Anti-cancer drugs* 29 (6):560-564.

Moik, Florian, Nick van Es, Florian Posch, Marcello Di Nisio, Thorsten Fuereder, Matthias Preusser, Ingrid Pabinger, and Cihan Ay. 2020. "Gemcitabine and platinum-based agents for the prediction of cancer-associated venous thromboembolism: results from the Vienna Cancer and Thrombosis Study." *Cancers* 12 (9):2493.

Nuver, Janine, Andries J Smit, Jan van der Meer, Maarten P van den Berg, Winette TA van der Graaf, Martin T Meinardi, Dirk Th Sleijfer, Harald J Hoekstra, Anne I van Gessel, and Arie M van Roon. 2005. "Acute chemotherapy-induced cardiovascular changes in patients with testicular cancer." *Journal of clinical oncology* 23 (36):9130-9137.

Obermeier, Hanna L, Julia Riedl, Cihan Ay, Silvia Koder, Peter Quehenberger, Rupert Bartsch, Alexandra Kaider, Christoph C Zielinski, and Ingrid Pabinger. 2019. "The role of ADAMTS-13 and von Willebrand factor in cancer patients: Results from the Vienna Cancer and Thrombosis Study." *Research and practice in thrombosis and haemostasis* 3 (3):503-514.

Oberoi, Hardeep S, Natalia V Nukolova, Alexander V Kabanov, and Tatiana K Bronich. 2013. "Nanocarriers for delivery of platinum anticancer drugs." *Advanced drug delivery reviews* 65 (13-14):1667-1685.

Oklu, Rahmi. 2017. "Thrombosis." *Cardiovascular diagnosis and therapy* 7 (Suppl 3):S131.

Oparil, Suzanne, Maria Czarina Acelajado, George L. Bakris, Dan R. Berlowitz, Renata Cífková, Anna F. Dominiczak, Guido Grassi, Jens Jordan, Neil R. Poulter, Anthony Rodgers, and Paul K. Whelton. 2018. "Hypertension." *Nature reviews. Disease primers* 4:18014-18014. doi: 10.1038/nrdp.2018.14.

Oun, Rabbab, Yvonne E Moussa, and Nial J Wheate. 2018. "The side effects of platinum-based chemotherapy drugs: a review for chemists." *Dalton transactions* 47 (19):6645-6653.

Ozcan, T, A Cirit, and A Kiykim. 2011. "Recurrent complete atrioventricular block during cisplatin infusion: a case report." *J Clin Exp Cardiol* 2:151.

Pabla, N, and Zheng Dong. 2008. "Cisplatin nephrotoxicity: mechanisms and renoprotective strategies." *Kidney international* 73 (9):994-1007.

Palatnik, AnneMarie, and Rosemary Kates. 2003. "Bradycardia and medications: identify the dangerous pace." *Nursing management* 34 (6):56A.

Pastorino, Alessandro, G Bregni, A Damiani, M Grassi, A Puccini, and G Fornarini. 2016. "Cisplatin-related atrial fibrillation during PEB chemotherapy for testicular seminoma: a case report." *Journal of Health & Medical Informatics* 7 (3).

Peng, Jia, Fei Luo, Guiyun Ruan, Ran Peng, and Xiangping Li. 2017. "Hypertriglyceridemia and atherosclerosis." *Lipids in health and disease* 16 (1):1-12.

Pistillucci, G, AA Ciorra, V Sciacca, M Raponi, R Rossi, and E Veltri. 2015. "Troponin I and B-type Natriuretic Peptide (BNP) as biomarkers for the prediction of cardiotoxicity in patients with breast cancer treated with adjuvant anthracyclines and trastuzumab." *La Clinica Terapeutica* 166 (1):e67-71.

Pober, Jordan S, and William C Sessa. 2007. "Evolving functions of endothelial cells in inflammation." *Nature Reviews Immunology* 7 (10):803-815.

Prasad, Megha, Robert McBane, Martin Reriani, Lilach O Lerman, and Amir Lerman. 2016. "Coronary endothelial dysfunction is associated with increased risk of venous thromboembolism." *Thrombosis research* 139:17-21.

Price, Peter M, Fang Yu, Philipp Kaldis, Eiman Aleem, Grażyna Nowak, Robert L Safirstein, and Judit Megyesi. 2006. "Dependence of cisplatin-induced cell death in vitro and in vivo on cyclin-dependent kinase 2." *Journal of the American Society of Nephrology* 17 (9):2434-2442.

Raja, Waseem, M Hussain Mir, Imtiyaz Dar, Muzamil Ahmad Banday, and Irfan Ahmad. 2013. "Cisplatin induced paroxysmal supraventricular tachycardia." *Indian journal of medical and paediatric oncology: official journal of Indian Society of Medical & Paediatric Oncology* 34 (4):330.

Rao, Arpitha S, Rishabh Kumar, and Geeta S Narayanan. 2015. "A rare case of cisplatin-induced acute myocardial infarction in a patient receiving chemoradiation for lung cancer." *Journal of cancer research and therapeutics* 11 (4):983.

Rischin, D, and V Ling. 1996. "Ormaplatin resistance is associated with decreased accumulation of its platinum (II) analogue, dichloro (D, L-trans) 1, 2-diaminocyclohexaneplatinum (II)." *British journal of cancer* 74 (4):590-596.

Rosic, Gvozden, Ivan Srejovic, Vladimir Zivkovic, Dragica Selakovic, Jovana Joksimovic, and Vladimir Jakovljevic. 2015. "The effects of N-acetylcysteine on cisplatin-induced cardiotoxicity on isolated rat hearts after short-term global ischemia." *Toxicology reports* 2:996-1006.

Saleh, Dalia O, Dina F Mansour, and Rasha E Mostafa. 2020. "Rosuvastatin and simvastatin attenuate cisplatin-induced cardiotoxicity via disruption of endoplasmic reticulum stress-mediated apoptotic death in rats: targeting ER-Chaperone GRP78 and Calpain-1 pathways." *Toxicology Reports* 7:1178-1186.

Sekijima, T, A Tanabe, R Maruoka, N Fujishiro, S Yu, S Fujiwara, H Yuguchi, Y Yamashita, Y Terai, and M Ohmichi. 2011. "Impact of platinum-based chemotherapy on the progression of atherosclerosis." *Climacteric* 14 (1):31-40.

Shah, Priyank, Sharad Bajaj, Hartaj Virk, Mahesh Bikkina, and Fayez Shamoon. 2015. "Rapid progression of coronary atherosclerosis: A review." *Thrombosis* 2015.

Sharma, Sandeep, Muhammad F Hashmi, and Priyanka T Bhattacharya. 2021. "Hypotension." In *StatPearls [Internet]*. Treasure Island (FL): StatPearls Publishing.

Sidhu, Sunjeet, and Joseph E Marine. 2020. "Evaluating and managing bradycardia." *Trends in cardiovascular medicine* 30 (5):265-272.

Soultati, Aspasia, Giannis Mountzios, Chrysoula Avgerinou, George Papaxoinis, Dimitrios Pectasides, Meletios-Athanassios Dimopoulos, and Christos Papadimitriou. 2012. "Endothelial vascular toxicity from chemotherapeutic agents: preclinical evidence and clinical implications." *Cancer treatment reviews* 38 (5):473-483.

Stone, Jonathan, Patrick Hangge, Hassan Albadawi, Alex Wallace, Fadi Shamoun, M Grace Knuttien, Sailendra Naidu, and Rahmi Oklu. 2017. "Deep vein thrombosis: pathogenesis, diagnosis, and medical management." *Cardiovascular diagnosis and therapy* 7 (Suppl 3):S276.

Tang, Chi-Hui, Christi Parham, Ellyn Shocron, Gerald McMahon, and Neela Patel. 2011. "Picoplatin overcomes resistance to cell toxicity in small-cell lung cancer cells previously treated with cisplatin and carboplatin." *Cancer chemotherapy and pharmacology* 67 (6):1389-1400.

van Dorst, Daan CH, Stephen JH Dobbin, Karla B Neves, Joerg Herrmann, Sandra M Herrmann, Jorie Versmissen, Ron HJ Mathijssen, AH Jan Danser, and Ninian N Lang. 2021. "Hypertension and Prohypertensive Antineoplastic Therapies in Cancer Patients." *Circulation Research* 128 (7):1040-1061.

Weaver, Janelle. 2013. "Insights into how calcium forms plaques in arteries pave the way for new treatments for heart disease." *PLoS biology* 11 (4):e1001533.

Willemse, Peter-Paul M, Rutger W van der Meer, Jacobus Burggraaf, Saskia GC van Elderen, Marieke L de Kam, Albert de Roos, Hildo J Lamb, and Susanne Osanto. 2014. "Abdominal visceral and subcutaneous fat increase, insulin resistance and hyperlipidemia in testicular cancer patients treated with cisplatin-based chemotherapy." *Acta Oncologica* 53 (3):351-360.

Workeneh, Biruh T, Nupur N Uppal, Kenar D Jhaveri, and Helbert Rondon-Berrios. 2020. "Hypomagnesemia in the cancer patient." *Kidney360*.

Wyndham, Christopher RC. 2000. "Atrial fibrillation: the most common arrhythmia." *Texas Heart Institute Journal* 27 (3):257.

Yuk, Jin-Sung, Banghyun Lee, Kidong Kim, Myoung Hwan Kim, Yong-Soo Seo, Sung Ook Hwang, Sang-Hee Yoon, and Yong Beom Kim. 2021. "Incidence and risk of venous thromboembolism according to primary treatment in women with ovarian cancer: A retrospective cohort study." *Plos one* 16 (4):e0250723.

Zahir, Muhammad Nauman, Quratulain Shaikh, Munira Shabbir-Moosajee, and Adnan Abdul Jabbar. 2017. "Incidence of Venous Thromboembolism in cancer patients treated with Cisplatin based chemotherapy—a cohort study." *BMC cancer* 17 (1):1-8.

Zamorano, JL. 2020. "'Cardiotoxicity': time to define new targets?" *European Heart Journal*.

Zhao, Li. 2019. "Protective effects of trimetazidine and coenzyme Q10 on cisplatin-induced cardiotoxicity by alleviating oxidative stress and mitochondrial dysfunction." *Anatolian journal of cardiology* 22 (5):232.

Chapter 7

Gastrointestinal Side Effects of Platinum-Based and Other Chemotherapeutic Drugs

Petra Semenye[1], Rachel McQuade[2,3], Raquel Abalo[4,5,6,7,*] and Kulmira Nurgali[1,2,8,†]

[1]Institute for Health and Sport, Victoria University, Melbourne, Australia
[2]Department of Medicine Western Health, The University of Melbourne, Melbourne, Australia
[3]Florey Institute of Neuroscience and Mental Health, Melbourne, Australia
[4]Area of Pharmacology and Nutrition, Department of Basic Health Sciences, Faculty of Health Sciences, Universidad Rey Juan Carlos, Alcorcón, Madrid, Spain
[5]High Performance Research Group in Physiopathology and Pharmacology of the Digestive System (NeuGut-URJC), Universidad Rey Juan Carlos, Alcorcón, Madrid, Spain
[6]Associated Unit to Institute of Medicinal Chemistry (Unidad Asociada I+D+i del Instituto de Química Médica, IQM), Spanish National Research Council (CSIC), Madrid, Spain
[7]Working Group of Basic Sciences in Pain and Analgesia of the Spanish Pain Society, Madrid, Spain
[8]Regenerative Medicine and Stem Cells Program, Australian Institute of Musculoskeletal Science (AIMSS), Melbourne, Australia

---

*Corresponding Author's Email: raquel.abalo@urjc.es.
†Corresponding Author's Email: kulmira.nurgali@vu.edu.au.

In: Platinum-Based Chemotherapy
Editors: Kulmira Nurgali and Raquel Abalo
ISBN: 978-1-68507-972-7
© 2022 Nova Science Publishers, Inc.

Abstract

Chemotherapy is the first-line treatment for many cancers. Despite effectively improving survival rates by 5 to 10 years, beneficial treatment outcomes are impeded by undesirable side effects. Chemotherapy-induced toxicities commonly present in the gastrointestinal tract, are a major contributing factor to dose reductions, delays, and cessation of treatment, resulting in sub-optimum treatment outcomes. Gastrointestinal side effects such as oral and gastrointestinal mucositis, nausea, vomiting, constipation, and diarrhea may persist many years after termination of treatment, significantly reducing the patient's quality of life. Although some chemotherapy-induced gastrointestinal symptoms can be managed through lifestyle modifications, many of the currently recommended drugs induce adverse effects themselves. Thus, new approaches are pertinent to address this problem. A better understanding of the mechanisms underlying gastrointestinal dysfunction associated with chemotherapeutic drugs may serve to expose potential therapeutic targets to alleviate and prevent chemotherapy-induced toxicity. This review will discuss the etiology, incidence, and treatment of gastrointestinal toxicities associated with platinum-based and other chemotherapeutic drugs.

Keywords: cisplatin, constipation, diarrhea, gastrointestinal mucositis, nausea and vomiting

Introduction

The gastrointestinal (GI) tract, including the oral cavity, is home to 70-80% of the body's immune cells, 100 000 extrinsic nerve endings, and a vast and complex network of neurons – over 100 million neurons (Furness et al., 2014, Yoo and Mazmanian, 2017, Grundy and Brookes, 2011). Functionally, the GI tract transports, absorbs and digests food, whilst aiding the excretion of waste and potentially ingested pathogens and toxins (Goldstein et al., 2013). This orchestrated symphony is coordinated by the enteric nervous system (ENS), often referred to as the 'second brain', corresponding to its primarily independent, complex, and autonomous function (Goldstein et al., 2013, Furness et al., 2014). The GI tract is a sophisticated system that is able to sense and respond to external cues, through diverse cellular interactions amenable to change. As such, the interaction between luminal constituents and interdependent cellular pathways in the gut and periphery may underlie GI dysfunction comorbid to non-intestinal conditions and treatments, such as chemotherapy (Peery et al., 2012, Yoo and Mazmanian, 2017).

Over the past 70 years, chemotherapeutics had been implemented as a mainstream adjuvant therapy, either before or subsequent to surgery or in combination with radiotherapy (Escalante et al., 2017, Sak, 2012). Chemotherapeutic drugs are classified based on their chemical nature and function. Of particular interest are platinum-based drugs and their combinations with other chemotherapeutics, which have widened the prospects of more effective cancer treatment.

Current platinum-based chemotherapeutics used in clinical practice include cisplatin, carboplatin, and oxaliplatin. Cisplatin is a first-generation platinum-based anti-cancer chemotherapeutic drug (Mlcouskova et al., 2012, Stojanovska et al., 2015). Despite being effective, cancer cells show a primary and acquired resistance to cisplatin, as a result of the reduced formation of cytotoxic platinum DNA adducts due to decreased drug accumulation or increased inactivation; increased repair or tolerance to platinum DNA damage; and increased replicative bypass (Raymond et al., 1998, El-Akawi et al., 1996, Hanigan et al., 1994). The use of cisplatin is strongly correlated with unfavourable side effects, including severe GI complications. Thus, efforts to develop cisplatin analogues with equivalent or higher anti-tumour activity and diminished toxicity have been made (Choi et al., 2004). Among them, carboplatin – a second-generation platinum analogue, displayed reduced renal and GI side effects, with equivalent therapeutic efficacy, and potent anti-cancer activity in cisplatin-resistant cells (Fram, 1992, Temple et al., 2002). Unlike cisplatin and carboplatin, oxaliplatin has been shown to be effective in some cisplatin-resistant cell lines (Wiseman et al., 1999). Advancements in medicine over the last 20 years have widened prospects of anti-cancer agents with diminished side effects that would otherwise compromise beneficial immune responses against tumours. Recently, new platinum drugs with a greater potent anti-tumour activity and efficacy against resistant cells have been investigated (Choi et al., 2004). Nedaplatin and heptaplatin have exhibited decreased renal and GI toxicities, greater anti-tumour activity against a number of human cancer cell lines and moderate emetic risk in clinical practice, compared to the high risk of emesis associated with cisplatin (Shimada et al., 2013, Niioka et al., 2007, Choi et al., 2004, Kim et al., 1994, Ahn et al., 2002). More recently, multiple studies demonstrated that lobaplatin and miriplatin have promising anti-cancer efficacy, and reduced GI side effects, such as nausea and appetite loss, indicating safety in patients with a decreased hepatic reserve and other organ complications (Zhou et al., 2020,

Shan et al., 2018, Yin et al., 2014, Xie et al., 2012, Chen et al., 2018, Okabe et al., 2011). Although structurally different, all aforementioned platinum-based agents exert their positive anti-tumour effects via the formation of DNA platinum monoadducts or intra- or interstrand cross-links in DNA, which ultimately cause DNA strand breaks, cell cycle arrest, and the activation of apoptotic pathways (Alcindor and Beauger, 2011, Stojanovska et al., 2015). In so doing, these platinum analogues essentially reduce tumour cell replication.

Although proven to be individually effective, multi-agent regimens given in combination are the most promising approaches to curative and non-curative cancer management (McQuade et al., 2017). Current platinum-based chemotherapeutic agents given alone or in combination with irinotecan, 5-fluorouracil (5-FU), vincristine, lomustine, doxorubicin, cyclophosphamide, etoposide, paclitaxel or capecitabine, show great therapeutic potential by enhancing antitumor efficacy. However, the combination of these cytotoxic therapies promotes more severe and undesirable side effects, including central and peripheral neurotoxicity, nephrotoxicity, cardiotoxicity, ototoxicity and hematopoietic depression (McQuade et al., 2014, McQuade et al., 2017, Stojanovska et al., 2015). Of particular interest are GI side effects such as nausea, vomiting, esophagopharyngitis, abdominal pain, oral and gastrointestinal mucositis, bloating, constipation and diarrhoea, which are initiated by singular cytotoxic agents and perpetuated by their novel combinations (McQuade et al., 2014, McQuade et al., 2017, Stojanovska et al., 2015, Escalante et al., 2017, Abalo et al., 2017). Prominent changes to the ENS such as neuronal loss and nerve fibre damage, morphological changes to the GI mucosa, such as crypt hypoplasia, villus atrophy, upregulation of pro-inflammatory cytokines, and changes in intestinal and faecal microbiota, have been revealed to contribute to underlying pathophysiological processes behind the aforementioned GI side effects (McQuade et al., 2017, Andrea et al., 2009, Stringer et al., 2009b, Stringer et al., 2009a, Rivera et al., 2011, Bowen et al., 2019, Al-Qadami et al., 2022, Bowen and Wardill, 2022). Recent statistics highlight that the incidence of GI side effects increases from 40% in patients receiving standard-dose chemotherapy, to 100% in patients receiving high dose chemotherapy (McQuade et al., 2014). Furthermore, these GI side effects can persist for many years after treatment cessation due to the presence of reactive platinum compounds retained within the body for as long as 20 years post-treatment (Stojanovska et al., 2015, De Gramont et al., 2000, Gelevert et al., 2001). Fundamentally, the frequent plethora of chronic GI complications often contribute to dose reductions, dose delays, and, in severe circumstances, cessation of the anti-cancer treatment, significantly impacting the clinical efficacy and outcome of the treatment (Escalante et al., 2017, McQuade et al., 2014, Stojanovska et al., 2015). Often the patient's quality of life is greatly compromised, contributing to longer hospitalisations thus, placing a greater burden on health care systems.

This review will focus on the mechanisms underlying the debilitating GI side effects that hinder the success of platinum-based and other anti-cancer drugs, and current methods and new strategies that ameliorate chemotherapy-induced GI toxicity.

Gastrointestinal Side Effects of Platinum-Based Therapies and Their Combinations

Although effective, GI side effects concomitant with the use of platinum-based chemotherapeutics hinder the administration of anticancer agents, limiting their therapeutic potential (McQuade et al., 2017). Most pivotal studies suggest that diarrhoea, constipation, nausea and vomiting are attributable to mucosal damage, presenting as severe inflammation and ulceration, also known as mucositis (McQuade et al., 2014, Sharma et al., 2005a, Kuebler et al., 2007). The aforementioned side effects, discussed below in more detail, are poorly controlled and lead to impaired functioning, decreased patient quality of life (QoL), potential treatment postponement and/or dose reduction of anticancer agent, compromising optimal chemotherapeutic effect (Stojanovska et al., 2015, McQuade et al., 2014, Sharma et al., 2005a).

Chemotherapy-Induced Nausea and Vomiting

Chemotherapy-induced nausea and vomiting (CINV), is the most feared and anticipated toxicity of antineoplastic chemotherapy, including platinum-based drugs (Adel, 2017). About 70-80% of patients receiving standard dose platinum-based chemotherapy exhibit CINV, and if left untreated may lead to malnutrition, dehydration, rapid weight loss (cachexia) and poor QoL, ultimately hindering beneficial treatment outcomes (Adel, 2017, Stojanovska et al., 2015, Mitchell, 2006, Hawkins and Grunberg, 2009, Sommariva et al., 2016, Jordan et al., 2007b, Hesketh et al., 2018).

Although often grouped together in CINV, nausea and vomiting may present independently (Table 1) (Adel, 2017). Nausea is defined as the wave-like feeling at the back of the throat which may or may not culminate in vomiting, whilst vomiting, a reflex, is the forceful elimination of the stomach's content through the mouth, by the sustained action of abdominal muscles and the opening of the gastric cardia (Shelke et al., 2004). Although nausea and vomiting can be elicited by stimuli such as autonomic dysfunction, pain, taste, smell, motion and exposure to toxins, the incidence and severity of CINV are dependent upon dose, type of chemotherapy administered (individual platinum analogues or their novel combinations), treatment schedule and individual patient characteristics (Shelke et al., 2004). For example, in the absence of antiemetic prophylaxis, cisplatin has the highest emetogenic potential (>90%), followed by oxaliplatin and carboplatin with moderate emetogenic risk (30-90%) and 5-FU with low emetogenic potential (10-30%) (Table 2) (Feeney et al., 2007). As such, efficacious antiemetic prophylaxis to control CINV is paramount (Shelke et al., 2004, Hesketh et al., 2018) (Tables 1. and 2.).

Table 1. Grading of vomiting and nausea according to the National Cancer Institute Common Criteria for Adverse Events version 4.0 (Bayo et al., 2012)

Grade	1	2	3	4	5
Nausea	Loss of appetite. No change in eating habits	Oral intake decreased. No significant weight loss, dehydration or malnutrition	Inadequate oral caloric or fluid intake. Tube feeding, total parenteral nutrition (TPN) or hospitalization		
Vomiting	1-2 episodes (separated by 5 mins) in 24 hours	3-5 episodes (separated by 5 mins) in 24 hours	≥ 6 episodes (separated by 5 mins) in 24 hours; tube feeding, total parenteral nutrition (TPN) or hospitalization	Life threatening. Urgent intervention needed	Death

CINV can be divided into five major categories – acute, delayed, anticipatory, breakthrough and refractory – depending on the timing of the symptoms relative to the administration of chemotherapeutic agents (Feeney et al., 2007, Adel, 2017, Jordan et al., 2007a). Acute CINV occurs within few minutes to several hours after chemotherapeutic treatment, with peak intensity occurring after 5-6 hours, but resolves within 24 hours (Bayo et al., 2012, Adel, 2017, Feeney et al., 2007). Frequently reported with cisplatin, carboplatin and doxorubicin, delayed CINV encompasses episodes occurring 24 hours post-treatment and may last up to 5 days, with the maximal effect being felt 48–72 hours after platinum drug administration (Bayo et al., 2012, Rapoport, 2017). Repeated exposure to platinum chemotherapy can often result in a conditioned response known as anticipatory emesis, where a patient will experience CINV prior to subsequent administration of a chemotherapeutic regimen (Adel, 2017). While acute CINV is well managed, delayed CINV is not completely understood, thus there is still a paucity of data regarding antiemetic regimes for patients experiencing delayed emesis (Rapoport, 2017, Ranganath et al., 2015). Persistent CINV, despite the use of recommended antiemetic protocols (breakthrough CINV < 5 days; refractory CINV), remains a challenge in achieving complete control of CINV (Rapoport, 2017).

Table 2. Emetogenic potential of chemotherapeutic drugs (Feeney et al., 2007)

Emetogenic risk of chemotherapeutic agents without antiemetics	Examples
High (>90%)	Cisplatin, dacarbazine, lomustine, doxorubicin or epirubicin combined with cyclophosphamide
Moderate (30-90%)	Irinotecan, oxaliplatin, doxorubicin, carboplatin, temozolomide
Low (10-30%)	Capecitabine, cetuximab, gemcitabine, fluorouracil, etoposide, pemetrexed
Minimal (<10%)	Bevacizumab, bleomycin, vinorelbine, vincristine, trastuzumab, gefitinib

Mechanisms of Chemotherapy-Induced Nausea and Vomiting

The pathophysiology of CINV involves pathways from the central and peripheral nervous systems (Rapoport, 2017). It has been suggested that chemotherapy-induced release of neurotransmitters, 5-hydroxytryptamine (5-HT)$_3$ (serotonin) and substance P, and their interaction with their respective receptors (5-HT$_3$ receptors and neurokinin-1 (NK-1) receptors, respectively) propagates the transmission of an emetic signal to the brain, resulting in CINV (Ranganath et al., 2015, Rapoport, 2017, Adel, 2017, Bayo et al., 2012). The stimulated receptors are abundant on the terminals of afferent nerves in the GI tract, vestibular region and area postrema (also known as the chemoreceptor trigger zone), all of which project to the nucleus tractus solitarius (NTS)

(Rapoport, 2017, Costa et al., 2015, Babic and Browning, 2014, Navari and Aapro, 2016). The accumulation of free radicals generated by platinum-based cytotoxic agents, induces damage to the GI tract, triggering the calcium-dependent exocytic release of serotonin from enterochromaffin cells situated in the intestinal mucosa (Navari and Aapro, 2016, Hornby, 2001, Janelsins et al., 2013, Rapoport, 2017). Thereafter, serotonin interacts with 5-HT_3 receptors on vagal afferent nerves in the intestinal wall, that project into the area postrema and NTS, which coordinates the autonomic process involved in vomiting such as respiration, swallowing, salivation and synergistic contraction and relaxation of abdominal and intestinal muscles (Babic and Browning, 2014, Aapro, 2005, Hesketh et al., 2003). More specifically, damage to the GI tract culminating in gastric distension, delayed emptying and retrograde contractions all contribute to the development of emesis. The acute phase of CINV is largely mediated by the 5-HT_3 receptor signalling cascade, however, 5-HT_3 receptor antagonists although effective in diminishing symptoms of acute CINV, have little impact on delayed CINV suggesting that a different pathophysiological mechanism is involved (Janelsins et al., 2013, Aapro, 2005). As such, delayed CINV is suggested to be driven by the neurotransmitter/neuromodulator substance P (Garcia-Recio and Gascón, 2015). Chemotherapeutic drugs, including platinum-based agents and other drugs, stimulate the neuronal release of substance P, which then binds to NK-1 receptors widely located in the GI tract, NTS and area postrema, mediating the induction of vomiting (Adel, 2017, Garcia-Recio and Gascón, 2015, Rapoport, 2017). The principal role of substance P in delayed CINV stems from the effectiveness of NK-1 receptor antagonists in preventing delayed emesis (Navari and Aapro, 2016). This rationale is supported by preclinical animal studies that highlight the potency of NK-1 receptor antagonists in diminishing cisplatin-induced delayed CINV (Sanger, 2004, Ranganath et al., 2015). Interestingly, dopamine antagonists have also been found to be effective in treating delayed CINV, owing to the profusion of dopamine receptors in the area postrema.

Risk Factors Associated with Chemotherapy-Induced Nausea and Vomiting

Although predictable, the likelihood of CINV is perpetuated by a variety of patient and treatment-associated risk factors. Recent retrospective pooled analyses of two randomised phase III trials have elucidated a strong positive correlation between patients aged < 60 years, female and have a history of motion sickness and/or pregnancy-related nausea and vomiting, with a heightened risk of developing CINV (Adel, 2017, Tageja and Groninger, 2014, Hesketh et al., 2010, Molassiotis et al., 2014). These results are characteristics of highly emetogenic anti-cancer drugs such as platinum-based chemotherapeutic agents (Rapoport, 2014). For instance, an analysis conducted by Takemoto et al. (2017) deemed gender as the most influential patient characteristic of CINV, as they found that the rate of CINV was significantly higher in women than in men in colorectal cancer patients treated with oxaliplatin (Takemoto et al., 2017). Additionally, the habitual consumption of alcohol (> 5 drinks/week) desensitises the area postrema, lowering the risk of CINV (Tageja and Groninger, 2014).

Current Treatments for Chemotherapy-Induced Nausea and Vomiting

Several existing treatments are available to prevent acute and chronic CINV independently. Given that multiple biological pathways contribute to the occurrence of emesis, the search for potent compounds and novel antiemetic combinations that interact with both 5-HT_3 and NK-1 receptors, and that target both categories of CINV is paramount. Even though well-structured guidelines have been put in place to guide the management of CINV, avenues for treatment are limited due to their hazardous side effects that may worsen the diagnosed symptoms. This section will discuss both existing and emerging pharmaceutical treatments for CINV.

5-HT_3 Receptor Antagonists

The interaction between serotonin and 5-HT_3 receptors triggers the emetic centre in the brain stem inducing emesis. 5-HT_3 antagonists work by blocking serotonin released from enterochromaffin cells from interacting with the 5-HT_3 receptor peripherally on vagal nerve terminals and/or centrally in the chemoreceptor trigger zone (CTZ); thereby inhibiting the stimulation of vagal afferents and the subsequent signalling to the nucleus tractus solitarius (NTS) (Grunberg et al., 2013). The most commonly used 5-HT_3 receptor antagonists include ondansetron, granisetron, dolasetron, and tropisetron (Feeney et al., 2007, Grunberg et al., 2013). These first-generation antagonists are highly effective antiemetics for acute CINV in patients receiving cisplatin-based regimens (Rao and Faso, 2012). They are administered before and after highly or moderately emetogenic chemotherapeutic regimes (Feeney et al., 2007). Up until 2003, palonosetron, a second-generation 5-HT_3 receptor antagonist, was approved by US Food and Drug Administration (FDA) (Rao and Faso, 2012). Palonosetron exhibits a higher binding affinity, a longer plasma half-life (40 hours), and greater potency – 30 and 100-fold more potent than granisetron and ondansetron, respectively (Eisenberg et al., 2003, Gralla et al., 2003, Saito et al., 2009). The unique pharmacology of palonosetron offers prevention against both acute and delayed CINV. The tricyclic ring system structure attached to a quinuclidine moiety increases the affinity of palonosetron to the 5-HT_3 receptors, downregulates and internalizes the 5-HT_3 receptor into the cell, providing a long-term antagonistic effect (Rojas et al., 2008, Rojas et al., 2010, Grunberg et al., 2013). Interestingly, an animal study revealed that palonosetron indirectly blocks the NK-1 signalling pathway (Thomas et al., 2014). 5-HT_3 receptor antagonists are prevalent in the clinical setting due to their advantageous effectiveness and tolerable side-effect profile, headache, and constipation (Feeney et al., 2007, Rao and Faso, 2012). A randomised double-blind controlled trial conducted by Tsuji et al. (2019), published that palonosetron-treated patients with at least one risk factor had significantly higher rates of complete response (CR - defined as no vomiting and no use of rescue antiemetics) 120 hours after cisplatin administration than granisetron-treated patients (Tsuji et al., 2019).

NK_1 Receptor Antagonists

NK_1 receptor antagonists work to prevent both acute and delayed emesis, by inhibiting substance P in peripheral and central emetic pathways (Grunberg et al., 2013, Rao and Faso, 2012). Aprepitant and fosaprepitant (water-soluble prodrug of aprepitant) are the only drugs in this class currently approved by the FDA in 2003 and 2008, respectively (Feeney et al., 2007, Rao and Faso, 2012). Among patients receiving carboplatin and pemetrexed (including or excluding bevacizumab), the aprepitant group demonstrated a better CR rate in the acute phase and delayed phase of CINV (Ito et al., 2014). This stands true for other platinum-based chemotherapy drugs, with two recent studies denoting a significantly better acute and delayed CR in groups treated with aprepitant compared to those treated with corticosteroid dexamethasone (He et al., 2021). Nonetheless, second-generation NK_1 receptor antagonists, netupitant and rolapitant, are in the late stages of clinical development (Grunberg et al., 2013). These potent antiemetics are reserved for highly emetogenic chemotherapy regimens or when breakthrough CINV is observed (Phillips et al., 2016). NK_1 receptor antagonists are mediated centrally in higher cortical centres and the dorsal vagal complex in the brain stem (Grunberg et al., 2013). Aprepitant is used for 3 consecutive days with high-risk emetogenic regimes. The approved oral doses are – day 1: 125mg; day 2: 80mg; day 3: 80mg (Feeney et al., 2007). As aprepitant is primarily metabolised by cytochrome (CY)P-450 3A4, it interacts with other orally administered drugs. For example, co-administration of aprepitant with dexamethasone requires a 50% dose reduction in dexamethasone, and when combined with warfarin, a decrease in the internal normalised ratio is recommended (Depré et al., 2005, Sanchez et al., 2004, Rao and Faso, 2012, Warr et al., 2005). Contrastingly, fosaprepitant is administered intravenously as a one-time dose of 150mg on day 1. This one-time dose is non-inferior when compared to the 3-day recommended aprepitant dose (Grunberg et al., 2011, Rao and Faso, 2012). Although both drugs are generally well-tolerated, some adverse effects commonly noted include fatigue, headache, anorexia, diarrhea, hiccups, and increased transaminases (Rao and Faso, 2012). Infusion site adverse events (ISAE) are appreciably higher using fosaprepitant than aprepitant in the first cycle of cisplatin-based chemotherapy (2.7 vs. 0.3%, respectively) (Herrstedt et al., 2022). In corroboration with this study, Saito et al. (2013) showed significantly higher rates of adverse effects including pain, erythema, swelling, and phlebitis in patients receiving both cisplatin and fosaprepitant (Saito et al., 2013). However, it is important to note that this venous toxicity is associated with the peripheral administration of the drug as opposed to central venous access administration (Hegerova et al., 2015).

Corticosteroids

Dexamethasone is the most commonly used corticosteroid in clinical practice. Although not approved by the FDA, dexamethasone is considered a mainstay of antiemetic regimens for the prevention of acute and delayed CINV in patients receiving low emetogenic chemotherapy (Feeney et al., 2007, Rao and Faso, 2012, Basch et al., 2011). The mechanisms of action for corticosteroids have not been elucidated. Hypotheses suggest that through multiple mechanisms, corticosteroids increase low cortisol levels, antagonize serotonin receptors, inhibit the release of prostaglandins and endorphins, thus having an anti-inflammatory effect, and/or compensating for acute adrenal hypofunction induced by platinum-based chemotherapy, ultimately relieving symptoms of nausea and vomiting (Ho et al., 2004, Tanihata et al., 2004, Rao and Faso, 2012, Janelsins et al., 2013, Basch et al., 2011, Fram, 1992, Janowitz et al., 2021). While dexamethasone is the most potent antiemetic, its efficacy is additive when combined with 5-HT_3 receptor antagonists in patients receiving chemotherapeutic drugs with moderate and high emetogenic potential (Rao and Faso, 2012, Grunberg et al., 2013, Janelsins et al., 2013). This is consistent with evidence suggesting that CINV is mediated by stimulated abdominal vagal afferent neurons in the area postrema (Janowitz et al., 2021, Hesketh, 2008). The National Comprehensive Cancer Network and the American Society of Clinical Oncology (ASCO) recommend the daily use of dexamethasone at doses of 8–12 mg on days 1–4 of each cycle of highly emetogenic chemotherapy (Hesketh et al., 2020, Berger et al., 2017, Janowitz et al., 2021). In support of this, a randomized controlled trial in cisplatin-treated patients observed that the combination of 5 mg olanzapine once daily on days 1–4 and a standard dose of dexamethasone as prophylaxis substantially increased the proportion of patients without vomiting from 66% to 79% (Hashimoto et al., 2020). Despite the potent antiemetic properties of corticosteroids, their tolerability is challenged by their adverse effects such as insomnia, epigastric discomfort, agitation, weight gain, and hyperglycaemia, further validating their synergistic use with other antiemetic agents (Vardy et al., 2006). As such, the lowest effective dose should be prescribed until more is understood about their negative side effects.

Dopamine Receptor Antagonists

With the current approval and availability of potent antiemetics, dopamine receptor antagonists are mostly reserved for low-risk regimes or used as rescue antiemetics, in the management of breakthrough and refractory emesis (Feeney et al., 2007, Rao and Faso, 2012, Herrstedt and Dombernowsky, 2007, Herrstedt, 2008, Ryan, 2010). Dopamine antagonists are classified as phenothiazines (e.g., prochlorperazine), butyrophenones (e.g., haloperidol, droperidol), and substituted benzamides (e.g., metoclopramide) – with metoclopramide being the most commonly used. These agents antagonise dopamine (D2) receptors in the periphery, CTZ and emetic centre (Grunberg et al., 2011, Rao and Faso, 2012). At high doses, metoclopramide has been shown to antagonize 5-HT_3 receptors, which may account for its use over its analogues. Of chemotherapy naïve patients treated with cisplatin ($\geq$50 mg/m^2) and metoclopramide as the antiemetic drug (10 mg orally, three times per day until 5 days after chemotherapy) 60% did not experience nausea and/or vomiting (Perwitasari et al., 2011). Contrastingly, Kenward et al. (2017), concluded that metoclopramide did not exhibit any antiemetic or anti-nausea efficacy and nausea-like behaviours in a novel low dose beagle dog cisplatin model (Kenward et al., 2017). Dose-limiting extrapyramidal symptoms of dopamine antagonists include dystonia and drowsiness (Rao and Faso, 2012).

Nonetheless, due to the paucity of data and adverse effects, the clinical use of dopamine antagonists is restricted in part (Ranganath et al., 2015).

Olanzapine

Olanzapine is an antipsychotic agent approved by the FDA. This atypical antipsychotic agent has been shown to antagonise dopamine receptors (D_1 - D_4); serotonin receptors (5-HT_{2a}, 5-HT_{2c}, 5-HT_3, and 5-HT_6); adrenergic receptors (α_1); muscarinic receptors; and histamine receptors (H_1) in the CNS (Navari et al., 2016, Navari, 2014, Hocking and Kichenadasse, 2014). Institution phase III trials have demonstrated the safety and efficacy of olanzapine in mitigating acute, delayed and refractory CINV, with augmented antiemetic properties observed when combined with palonosetron and dexamethasone (Tan et al., 2009, Ryan, 2010). Olanzapine's use in patients receiving moderate and high emetogenic chemotherapy is limited as it may promote sedation, weight gain, orthostatic hypotension, diabetes mellitus and hyperglycaemia (Navari et al., 2016, Passik et al., 2004, Rao and Faso, 2012, Tan et al., 2009). For instance, a randomized, controlled, assessor-blinded study on 100 chemotherapy-naïve patients treated with cisplatin, carboplatin or oxaliplatin, observed better control of delayed emesis, a decline in the incidence and severity of nausea, and improved QoL among patients receiving olanzapine (10 mg/day from day 1 for five consecutive days). Despite no dose-limiting side effects, sedation was pronounced in this group (Mukhopadhyay et al., 2017).

Benzodiazepines

Anxiolytics such as benzodiazepines are effective in reducing anxiety in patients receiving cytotoxic chemotherapy (Feeney et al., 2007). Despite little efficacy as single agents, they are used as adjuvant therapies and administered synergistically with other antiemetic drugs (Howard et al., 2014). Lorazepam and alprazolam are the primary agents used in this class, with sedation and amnesia being the most common aftereffect. Oral lorazepam (2 mg) given the night before and morning of antineoplastic treatment (containing cisplatin) for 5 consecutive days in adult cancer patients provided complete control of anticipatory CINV compared to the control group (52% vs. 32%; $p < 0.05$). However, 76% of those treated with lorazepam experienced mild sedation (Dupuis et al., 2014). The ability of benzodiazepines to induce anterograde amnesia has been favourable in alleviating and attenuating anticipatory CINV linked to repeated exposure to chemotherapy (Patel et al., 2017, Rao and Faso, 2012).

Cannabinoids

Cannabinoids, specific isolates of medical cannabis, have been shown to reduce nausea, vomiting, and diarrhoea during chemotherapy (Mortimer et al., 2019, Abalo et al., 2017). In particular, the FDA has approved the use of dronabinol and nabilone in oncological patients unresponsive to conventional antiemetics (Rao and Faso, 2012). They inhibit the vomiting reflex by suppressing the release of serotonin from enterochromaffin cells in the small intestine and by agonising cannabinoid receptors, CB_1 and possibly CB_2 (Mortimer et al., 2019, Martin and Wiley, 2004). More specifically, *Cannabis sativa* hexane fraction (*CS*-HexFr; 10 mg/kg) has been shown to attenuate cisplatin-induced emesis by 65.85%; decrease the concentration of serotonin in the area postrema, brain stem and intestine; and attenuate the upsurge of serotonin in the brain stem and intestine and dopamine in the area postrema in healthy pigeons (Ullah et al., 2018). One study elucidated that a combination of ondansetron, dexamethasone and dronabinol was equally effective as ondansetron, dexamethasone, and placebo (Meiri et al., 2007). The lack of added potency, and severe adverse effects such as vertigo, euphoria, and somnolence associated with cannabinoids, have restricted its use in the clinical milieu (Herrstedt and Dombernowsky, 2007, Rao and Faso, 2012, Ryan, 2010, Grimison et al., 2020).

Combination of Antiemetic Regimes

Often, the aforementioned treatments for CINV are used synergistically, to achieve better treatment outcomes. For example, some empirical evidence highlighted that an antiemetic regimen consisting of ondansetron, dexamethasone, and aprepitant was able to protect 66-78% of patients from emesis and 50% from nausea during the first cycle of cisplatin-based chemotherapy (Herrstedt, 2008, Ryan, 2010). Additionally, the combination of antiemetic medications decreased the use of rescue medications in patients treated with highly emetogenic chemotherapy (Schmoll et al., 2006). However, the use of multiple oral agents can further perpetuate feelings of nausea and vomiting. Thus, the search for new potent antiemetic drugs with little or no side effects is essential.

Chemotherapy-Induced Mucositis

Anti-cancer therapies have long been associated with a high risk of mucosal damage (Parkhill, 2013). Mucositis is a term used to encompass mucosal damage in areas of the GI tract; for example, mucositis can present in the oral cavity, oesophagus, intestines and rectum, ultimately leading to region-specific symptoms such as gastric dysmotility that culminates in diarrhoea or constipation and other comorbid complications (compromised nutrition and speech, prolong hospital stays, and bloodstream infections) (Treister and Sonis, 2007, Lalla and Peterson, 2005, Lalla et al., 2008, Peterson et al., 2016). Historically, mucositis was viewed as the direct consequence of antineoplastic therapies on rapidly proliferating basal epithelial cells resulting in tolerogenic cell death, tissue atrophy and ulceration. However, more recently, the complex aetiology of mucositis has been appreciated to include aberrant immune signalling, oxidative stress and microbial dysbiosis (Bowen et al., 2019, Al-Qadami et al., 2022, Bowen and Wardill, 2022).

Oral mucositis (OM) describes a major nonhematologic complication of cytotoxic chemotherapy and radiotherapy (Naidu et al., 2004). Annually, there are more than 400 000 cases of anti-cancer treatment-induced damage to the oral mucosa (Naidu et al., 2004). OM is particularly encountered in platinum-based chemotherapeutics, namely combination chemotherapeutic agents, 5-FU/leucovorin with oxaliplatin (FOLFOX); 5-FU/leucovorin with oxaliplatin and irinotecan (FOLFOXIRI) (Naidu et al., 2004). With symptoms ranging from erythema to ulcerative lesions of the oral mucosa, OM inhibits the ability of a patient to tolerate the consumption of foods and fluids (Lalla et al., 2008, Naidu et al., 2004). As such, nutrition and oral hygiene are compromised, heightening the susceptibility of opportunistic local and systemic infectious complications in neutropenic patients (Lalla et al., 2008, Al-Ansari et al., 2015, Bowen et al., 2019). Viral infections such as recrudescent herpes simplex virus (HSV) and fungal infections like candidiasis can be superimposed in OM, complicating its diagnosis and management (Lalla et al., 2008).

Whilst the prevalence and severity of chemotherapy-induced OM varies greatly from patient to patient, OM is categorised and treated using a grade scale (Parkhill, 2013, Naidu et al., 2004). Several grading scales exist for OM, including World Health Organization (WHO) Oral Toxicity scale, Radiation Therapy Oncology Group (RTOG) scale, and the common terminology criteria for adverse events (CTCAE) (Villa et al., 2021). The most widely used in routine clinical practice and trials is the WHO Oral Toxicity Scale (Naidu et al., 2004). OM is graded from 0 to 5; 0 accentuating no signs and symptoms, and 1 to 5 demonstrating increments in the severity of OM (Table 3).

Table 3. World Health Organization (WHO) Oral Toxicity Scale (Bensinger et al., 2008, Parkhill, 2013, Atay et al., 2015)

Grade	Symptoms
Grade 0	No signs and symptoms
Grade 1	Swelling, oral soreness and painless erythema
Grade 2	Painful erythema, oedema and ulcers but able to eat and swallow
Grade 3	Painful erythema, oedema and ulcers that prevent the oral consumption of food. Can only consume liquids
Grade 4	Severe ulceration. Oral alimentation is impossible. Patient requires parenteral or enteral support
Grade 5	Death from toxic effects

Mechanisms of Chemotherapy-Induced Mucositis

Recent animal studies have identified the involvement of connective tissue coupled with epithelial tissue, in the complicated pathobiology of mucositis (Al-Ansari et al., 2015, Sonis, 2004). Based on the above consideration, the pathophysiological concept of oral and GI mucositis follows a five discrete phase process that includes: 1. Initiation, 2. Upregulation, 3. Signal amplification, 4. Ulceration, and 5. Healing (Bowen et al., 2019).

The initiation phase is delineated by chemotherapy-induced cellular damage, resulting in the injury of basal epithelial, submucosal, and endothelial cells (Al-Ansari et al., 2015, Lalla et al., 2008). In response to this damage, injured cells release endogenous damage-associated molecular patterns (DAMPs), forming an enzyme-substrate complex that initiates inflammation and toxicity (Sonis, 2004). Subsequently, lipid peroxidation and the formation of reactive oxygen species (ROS) within injured cells (oxidative stress), stimulates macrophages and other inflammatory mediators (Parkhill, 2013, Sonis, 2009, Yeoh et al., 2005). The activation of transcription factors including nuclear factor (NF)-κB precedes peaks of inflammatory cytokines namely tumour necrosis factor (TNF)-α, interleukin (IL)-6 (Bajic et al., 2018, Sonis, 2004), and IL-1β, and upregulates cyclooxygenase-2 (COX-2) in submucosal fibroblasts and endothelial cells (Al-Dasooqi et al., 2010, Logan et al., 2007). The upregulation of proinflammatory mediators amplifies mucosal injury, due to activated positive feedback mechanisms. For example,

TNF-α may prompt a positive feedback loop on NF-κB to amplify its response, initiating mitogen-activated protein kinase (MAPK) signalling, leading to activation of c-Jun N-terminal kinase (JNK) signalling, all of which prolong tissue injury, apoptosis and vascular permeability (signal amplification) (Al-Ansari et al., 2015, Parkhill, 2013, Sonis, 2007). Exudation and loss of epithelia induce the opportunistic colonisation of gram-negative bacteria and yeast that signal infiltrating macrophages to produce additional pro-inflammatory cytokines, perpetuating mucosal damage and formation of pseudomembranes and ulcers (ulceration) (Al-Ansari et al., 2015, Lalla et al., 2008, Naidu et al., 2004, Sonis, 2007). Inflammation and concurrent barrier disruption induced by platinum-based and other chemotherapeutic drugs cause morphological alterations and increase in the proportion of neuronal nitric oxide synthase (nNOS)-immunoreactive (IR) neurons, all of which are correlated with impaired colonic motility (Wafai et al., 2013; Stojanovska et al., 2015; McQuade et al., 2016a); this will be discussed later in this chapter. Healing of ulcerations is dependent upon epithelial migration, proliferation and differentiation, hematopoietic recovery, reestablishment of the local microbial flora and absence of mechanical irritation (Blijlevens and Sonis, 2007, Yeoh et al., 2005, Al-Qadami et al., 2022). Ulcerations usually resolve 2-4 weeks post-treatment.

According to the five-phase model outlined above, the intestinal microbiota plays a minimal role in the pathophysiology of mucositis. However, several studies have demonstrated that bacterial dysbiosis may lead to the formation of active toxic metabolites, augment intestinal permeability, corrupt the composition of the mucus layer and epithelial repair mechanisms, all of which impact the progression of intestinal mucositis (Van Vliet et al., 2010, Sougiannis et al., 2021, Al-Qadami et al., 2022). 16S rRNA sequencing has been broadly adopted to detect gut microbiota changes and analyse the microbial community information in multiple samples (Wei et al., 2021). It was found that the number of *Lactobacillus* is significantly reduced in patients receiving cisplatin, 5-FU, and docetaxel combined chemotherapy (Motoori et al., 2017). This occurrence has been shown to interfere with the expression of mucin genes, ultimately prompting inflammation in the ulcerative phase of the mucositis, by altering the composition of the mucus layer and increasing the risk of bacterial translocation (Van Vliet et al., 2010, Kim et al., 2008). Additionally, the number of *Bifidobacterium* decreased significantly following irinotecan administration in rats, leading to an increase in NFκB activation, endotoxin levels and plasma IL-6 levels, which has been proposed to augment intestinal inflammation and thus intestinal mucositis (Lin et al.,

2012, Chen et al., 2007, Matsumoto and Benno, 2007, Wei et al., 2021). In male Kunming mice treated with oxaliplatin (5 mg/kg, i.p.) for four consecutive days, an increase in *Proteobacteria* was observed (Xia et al., 2019). A similar increase in *Proteobacteria* was evidenced in C57BL/6 mice induced with colon cancer, receiving three cycles of 5-FU (35 mg/kg) (Sougiannis et al., 2019). A positive correlation was found between *Proteobacteria* and colonic expression of TNFα, monocyte chemoattractant protein-1 (MCP1), IL-6, interferon-gamma (IFNγ), IL-1β, IL-10, forkhead box P3 (FOXP3), and NOS2, all of which heighten the progression of chemotherapy-induced mucositis (Sougiannis et al., 2019, Sougiannis et al., 2021). Although available evidence suggests a link between mucositis and gut microbes, inconsistencies stemming from variable dosages and chemotherapy regimens make it hard to identify the exact bacterial species driving these unwanted side effects (Sougiannis et al., 2019). Future research into the mechanisms and treatment of intestinal mucositis should consider the impact of dysbiosis (Sougiannis et al., 2021).

Risk Factors Associated with Mucositis

The incidence of mucositis is often underreported, as relatively few clinical trials have focused on this debilitating side effect as a specific outcome, and due to sporadic clinical monitoring between treatment cycles (Parkhill, 2013, Trotti et al., 2003). Further to this, the incidence of mucositis is highly variable depending on treatment-related and patient-related risk factors (Wardill et al., 2020).

Treatment-related risk factors include the type of chemotherapy, cumulative dose, schedule, and the route of administration as well as concomitant use of radiotherapy with platinum-based and other chemotherapeutic drugs as well as non-chemotherapeutic drugs (Raber-Durlacher et al., 2010, Sonis et al., 2010, Parkhill, 2013, Wardill et al., 2020, Nishii et al., 2020). A direct correlation between cumulative dose, a combination of chemotherapy with radiotherapy, and severity of mucositis has been identified. The severity of mucositis is positively associated with the number of chemotherapy cycles, due to increased exposure accruing damage to the oral mucosa (Parkhill, 2013, Epstein et al., 2012). In addition, several anti-cancer drugs affecting DNA synthesis, in particular platinum-based drugs, cisplatin, and carboplatin, and other chemotherapeutics such as doxorubicin and 5-FU exhibit more pronounced stomatotoxic effects

(Bensinger et al., 2008, Parkhill, 2013, Watters et al., 2011, Boers-Doets et al., 2012, Martins et al., 2013). As such, platinum-based novel combination therapies and chemoradiation regimens (combined with cisplatin and carboplatin), exhibit a strong positive correlation with reported incidences of mucositis (approximately 75-80%) (Vera-Llonch et al., 2007, Al-Ansari et al., 2015, Ang et al., 2014). In addition, polypharmacy (common in cancer patients) viz. antidepressants, opiates, phenothiazines, antihypertensives, antihistamines and sedatives, have anticholinergic activities, which contribute to xerostomia (dry mouth) and gastrointestinal disturbances leading to oral and GI mucositis (Goh et al., 2018).

Genetic variants in drug-metabolizing pathways, immune signalling, and cell injury/repair mechanisms, have also been associated with mucositis risk (Wardill et al., 2020). Mutations in drug-metabolizing pathways influence the risk of mucositis. More specifically, dihydropyrimidine dehydrogenase and thymidylate synthase polymorphisms are significantly associated with an increased risk of GI mucositis induced by fluoropyrimidines and platinum-based therapies (Campbell et al., 2016). Polymorphism of several other genes and their pathways involved in the metabolism of various chemotherapeutic drugs has been described (Reyes-Gibby et al., 2017; Wardill et al., 2020).

Chemotherapeutic agents secreted in saliva (methotrexate and etoposide) and genetic polymorphisms associated with the expression of inflammatory mediators such as TNF-α have been implicated in mucositis risk (Bogunia-Kubik et al., 2006, Al-Ansari et al., 2015, Naidu et al., 2004). Genetic variability of toll-like receptor (TLR)2, IL-1β and TNF-α are candidate predictors for 5-FU-induced severe mucositis (Coller et al., 2015, Korver et al., 2019).

The type of cancer might be associated with the development and severity of mucositis. A high incidence of severe oral mucositis has been reported for oral, oropharyngeal and other head and neck cancers (Van den Broek et al., 2006, Elad and Zadik 2016, Nishii et al., 2020). Mucositis has been reported in 51% of patients receiving chemotherapy for lymphomas (Elting et al., 2003, Lalla et al., 2008). Overall, the correlation between various types of solid tumours and the severity of mucositis is not well documented and varies significantly among published studies. Most studies follow patients only during their first chemotherapy cycle but not subsequent cycles when the incidence of mucositis may significantly increase due to the cumulative effect of the chemotherapeutic drugs (Al-Ansari et al., 2015).

Patient-associated risk factors are also poorly defined due to dissimilarity in patients, and limited, inconsistent and unpowered research data (Wardill et al., 2020). Patients' gender, age, type of cancer, comorbidities, nutritional and smoking status are variably linked to mucositis outcomes (Raber-Durlacher et al., 2010). A clinical trial conducted by Krishna et al. (2011) revealed a positive correlation between increased risk of GI mucositis and decreased body surface area (BSA), renal function and blood albumin levels. Reports suggest that the rapid epithelial mitotic rate and presence of epidermal growth factor observed in younger patients predisposes them to mucositis (Sonis, 2009). Similarly, poor mucosal regeneration has been observed in immunosuppressed and malnourished patients, contributing to the development of severe (grade 3 or 4) mucositis (Naidu et al., 2004). Poor oral hygiene and health contribute to the severity of OM (Raber-Durlacher et al., 2010, Wuketich et al., 2012). Sex and smoking status showed some association with the risk of chemotherapy-induced mucositis (Raber-Durlacher et al., 2010, Wardill et al., 2020). Some adult studies have concluded that women endured more extensive 5-FU-induced GI mucositis compared to their counterparts (Schwab et al., 2008, Kuiken et al., 2015). Unfortunately, for the majority of patients, no effective interventions are currently available, and those that are marginally effective are primarily palliative (Parkhill, 2013).

Current Treatments for Chemotherapy-Induced Mucositis

The psychosocial implications of OM may manifest as diminished self-esteem and disrupted speech and communication, further compromising the patient's response to treatment and/or palliative care (Miranzadeh et al., 2014, Jemal et al., 2011, Brunner, 2010). In cases of severe oral lesions, patients may be prescribed dose reductions between 25% to 100% in their platinum-based anticancer regimen, due to associated pain, odynophagia, dysgeusia, and subsequent indigestion, dehydration and malnutrition (Oun et al., 2018, Naidu et al., 2004). At times, treatment is discontinued to allow for resolution of oral lesions and enhancement of patient survivorship, drastically affecting cancer treatment outcomes (Miranzadeh et al., 2014, Pavesi et al., 2011, Naidu et al., 2004). These clinical consequences are associated with an increased burden on healthcare resources including, gastrostomy, inflation in the use of antifungals and opioid analgesics and extended periods of hospitalisations (Al-Ansari et al., 2015, Parkhill, 2013). Gastrointestinal mucositis currently faces an unmet need for effective interventions. Although treatments for OM are relatively effective, the morphological and microbial differences characteristic of the distal regions of the GI tract render the diagnosis, inspection, and treatment of GI mucositis more clinically challenging (Ranna et al., 2019). To date, clinical management has focused on the supportive care of the symptoms. For example, mucositis-induced mild abdominal pain can often be treated with paracetamol or ibuprofen, however, their use is contraindicated in those at high risk of thrombocytopenia. In addition, morphine is recommended for mild abdominal pain. Nonetheless, its prolonged use in consecutive episodes of GI mucositis has been shown to insufficiently manage pain, and, therefore, adding ketamine therapy is often required (WHO, 2012, White et al., 2011, Kuiken et al., 2015). It is therefore paramount to identify strategies to prevent or reduce mucositis. At present, no standard therapy exists however, clinical trials have assessed many strategies for the management of chemotherapy-induced mucositis (Sharma et al., 2005b). Several of these strategies will be discussed briefly below in the context of the Mucositis Study Group of the Multinational Association for Supportive Care in Cancer and the International Society of Oral Oncology (MASCC/ISOO) guidelines (Elad et al., 2020).

Basic Oral Health

Reducing oral bacterial load and mucosal trauma caused by ill-fitting dental prostheses and offending teeth, combined with effective oral hygiene, has been demonstrated to lower the incidence and severity of OM (Soga et al., 2009, Da Silva Santos et al., 2011, Kashiwazaki et al., 2012, Wuketich et al., 2012). The MASCC/ISOO guidelines recommend implementing multi-agent combination oral care protocols for the prevention of OM during radiotherapy, chemotherapy, and hematopoietic stem cell transplantation in patients with head and neck cancer (Hong et al., 2019; Elad et al., 2020). No guidelines were developed for professional oral care, patient education, and the use of saline and sodium bicarbonate; these require further studies to provide sufficient evidence for the development of specific guidelines.

Cryotherapy

Cryotherapy or the topical application of ice to the oral mucosa has been shown to reduce the severity of OM in patients receiving bolus doses of chemotherapeutic agents (Migliorati et al., 2006, Lalla et al., 2008, Lilleby et al., 2006, Vokurka et al., 2011, Chaveli-López and Bagán-Sebastián, 2016). Several studies have demonstrated that placing ice chips in the patient's mouth for 5-10 minutes before, 15-35 minutes during and up to 30 minutes after the administration of chemotherapy, significantly reduces the incidence of OM

(Chaveli-López and Bagán-Sebastián, 2016, Katranci et al., 2012, Vokurka et al., 2011, Papadeas et al., 2007). Although the precise underlying mechanism is ill-defined, studies imply that local vasoconstriction decreases direct toxicity to the oral mucosa by reducing blood flow and exposure of the oral mucosa to the cytostatic agent (Scully et al., 2006, Cidon, 2017). The MASCC/ISOO guidelines recommend the use of 30 minutes of oral cryotherapy to prevent OM in patients receiving 5-FU and high-dose melphalan (Elad et al., 2020), but its use is not indicated in oxaliplatin-treated patients due to the consequential development of dysesthesia, mandibular stiffness and laryngopharyngeal spasms (Harris et al., 2008, Cidon, 2017).

Molgramostim

Molgramostim is a recombinant granulocyte-macrophage colony-stimulating factor (GM-CSF) that has been shown to shorten the duration of OM and reduce symptoms. Anecdotal reports propose that molgramostim promotes neutrophil activation and proliferation of keratinocyte and fibroblasts, ultimately enhancing wound healing (Sharma et al., 2005a). Henja and colleagues observed that topical application of molgramostism shortened the duration of OM by approximately 3 days (p=0.0008), in patients receiving 5-FU treatment, compared to the control group treated with a topical antiseptic agent (povidone-iodine) (Hejna et al., 2001). Similarly, another study highlighted rapid resolution of grade 3 OM in patients, after a twice-daily molgramostim mouthwash treatment for 3 consecutive days following 5-FU treatment, as opposed to patients receiving supportive care. Despite supporting evidence, inferences drawn from these studies are disputable on account of the small and underpowered sample size, and the selection of patients who have previously had severe OM (Sharma et al., 2005a). Due to the lack of evidence, the MASCC/ISOO guidelines recommend that CM-CSF should not be used for the prevention of OM in cancer patients undergoing hematopoietic stem-cell transplantation (Elad et al., 2020; Logan et al., 2020).

Antimicrobial and Anti-Inflammatory Agents

Antimicrobial agents can reduce the duration and severity of OM, and prevent bacterial colonization evidenced in patients with late-stage ulcerative mucositis (Lalla et al., 2014, Harris et al., 2008; Saunders et al., 2020). For example, a 30% decrease in OM was evident in patients who rinsed their mouth with povidone-iodine, compared to sterile water rinses (Potting et al., 2006). Implementation of antimicrobial rinses in the management of OM is not justified and may only be beneficial in the late stages of OM when the risk of bacterial infection is greater (Chaveli-López and Bagán-Sebastián, 2016). The systematic review of anti-inflammatory agents revealed that benzydamine was proven effective in the treatment of OM (Ariyawardana et al., 2019). Therefore, the MASCC/ISOO guidelines recommend the use of benzydamine mouthwash for the prevention of OM in head and neck cancer patients receiving a moderate dose of radiotherapy with or without a combination with chemotherapy (Elad et al., 2020). No guidelines were developed for the use of any other anti-inflammatory agents due to inadequate and/or conflicting clinical reports (Ariyawardana et al., 2019). Additional well-designed research is needed on other (class of agents) interventions and in other cancer treatment settings.

Glutamine

Glutamine is required for the maintenance of mucosal surfaces (Sharma et al., 2005a). Administered via the parental, enteral and intravenous routes and available as a mouth rinse, glutamine has been indicated in the treatment and prevention of mucositis (Pavesi et al., 2011). In a double-blind randomised trial, a decrease in mucositis and gastric ulcerations was examined in metastatic colorectal cancer patients treated with glutamine via the parenteral route versus placebo (Rubenstein, 2004). Furthermore, a randomized, double-blind, controlled phase III study executed by Peterson et al. (2007) analysed the efficacy of daily 2.5 g/5 mL doses of Saforis (oral suspension of L-glutamine). Findings observed a significant decrease in the severity of OM compared to placebo (Peterson et al., 2007). Limited mucosal injury associated with glutamine can be attributed to enhanced uptake of amino acids into epithelial cells, diminished production of pro-inflammatory cytokines and cytokine related apoptosis, and augmented fibroblast and collagen synthesis, inevitably promoting healing (Lalla et al., 2008, Coëffier et al., 2002, Evans et al., 2003). Glutamine has been reported to significantly improve gut score in patients receiving stem cell transplants, maintain nutritional status, and prevent against intestinal permeability and chemotherapy-induced gut toxicity (Gibson et al., 2013, Blijlevens et al., 2005, Sornsuvit et al., 2008, Li et al., 2006). MASCC/ISOO guidelines recommend oral glutamine for the prevention of OM in patients with head and neck cancer receiving radio and chemotherapy but not for patients undergoing hematopoietic stem-cell transplantation (Elad et al., 2020; Yarom et al., 2019).

Low-Level Laser Therapy

Multiple studies have indicated that low-level laser therapy (LLLT) also known as photobiomodulation is proficient in decreasing the incidence, pain and severity of mucositis (Worthington et al., 2011, Evans et al., 2003; Freitas et al., 2014, Kuhn et al., 2009, Chaveli-López and Bagán-Sebastián, 2016; Migliorati et al., 2013). Due to systemic complications associated with other treatments of mucositis, LLLT is a preferred alternative to other approaches, due to its trophic, anti-inflammatory, and analgesic properties (Abramoff et al., 2008). It was speculated that LLLT may reduce levels of ROS and/or pro-inflammatory cytokines that contribute to the etiopathogenesis of mucositis, thereby accelerating tissue regeneration and healing (Lalla et al., 2008, Migliorati et al., 2006, Worthington et al., 2011, Clarkson et al., 2010). For example, Abramoff et al. (2008) ascertained marked pain relief and diminished severity of OM in patients treated with LLLT (Abramoff et al., 2008). Most studies showed that LLLT (photobiomodulation) itself does not induce adverse effects, and does not increase the risk of tumor recurrences and metastasis (de Pauli Paglioni et al., 2019). In the wake of sufficiency in supportive data, the MASCC/ISOO guidelines recommend the use of LLLT (photobiomodulation) in patients subjected to hematopoietic stem cell transplantation and in adult patients with head and neck cancer receiving radiotherapy alone or in combination with chemotherapy (Elad et al., 2020). The use of LLLT (photobiomodulation) for the prevention of OM in cancer patients should follow the MASCC/ISOO recommended protocol and safety considerations unique to patients with oral cancer (Zadik et al., 2019). However, LLLT (photobiomodulation) has been used mostly for the treatment, prevention, and management of OM predominantly in head and neck cancer patients (Sonis et al., 2016; Antunes et al., 2017; Brandao et al., 2018). Therefore, no guidelines were possible for the application of LLLT (photobiomodulation) in other cancers and for other light sources. Therefore, further studies to evaluate the efficacy and determine the most appropriate doses of laser and other light therapies for treating and preventing OM in various cancers are warranted (Migliorati et al., 2013; Peralta-Mamani et al., 2019).

Anesthetics and Analgesics

Pain is a prominent symptom associated with OM and GI mucositis. No drug has been successful in eliminating mucositis; thus, pain management is a crucial component of any mucositis management strategy in order to preserve patient QoL (Lalla et al., 2008). In a clinical setting, the use of anaesthetic solutions that contain diphenhydramine, viscous xylocaine or lidocaine; potent analgesics such as morphine rinses; and the application of sublingual methadone or fentanyl patches, may afford the patient short-term relief from the oral discomfort (Harris et al., 2008, Worthington et al., 2011, Clarkson et al., 2008). The MASCC/ISOO guidelines recommend topical morphine 0.2% mouthwash for the treatment of pain associated with OM in head and neck cancer patients receiving radio and chemotherapy (Elad et al., 2020). No guidelines were made in relation to the management of mucositis-associated pain in patients with other cancers; further studies need to address this in order to develop the appropriate guidelines.

Palifermin

Although Palifermin is not directly effective in the prevention of GI mucositis, it has however demonstrated its potency in reducing the number of days with moderate diarrhoea in patients with non-Hodgkin and Hodgkin lymphoma (Herbers et al., 2014b). In a similar setting, a control-matched cohort study observed the contrary - Palifermin did not prevent clinically meaningful GI mucositis. These discrepancies in findings across studies make it difficult to draw the guidelines (Bowen et al., 2019).

Chemotherapy-Induced Constipation

Constipation is a frequent and underestimated manifestation of GI mucositis. The subjective nature of constipation as a sensation impedes the acceptance of a universal consensus definition. Broadly, constipation is clinically recognised as unsatisfactory defaecation due to difficulty passing stool owing to decreased bowel motility and increased stool consistency (Connolly and Larkin, 2012, McIlfatrick et al., 2019). Research on cancer patient-report outcomes indicates that chemotherapy-induced constipation (CIC) is the third most common debilitating adverse effect of chemotherapy (31.9%), after CINV (59.6%) and anorexia (46%) (Gibson and Keefe, 2006b, Sánchez-Lara et al., 2013, Toygar et al., 2020). Additionally, following the administration of cisplatin, thalidomide, and vinca alkaloids (vincristine, vinblastine and vinorelbine), CIC rates are said to be as high as 80-90%, with an overall prevalence of 16%; 5% classified as severe and 11% as moderate (Anthony and Chauhan, 2018, Yamagishi et al., 2009, Escalante et al., 2017, Stojanovska et al., 2015). In a clinical observation, 57% of children (up to 21 years of age) who received cisplatin/vincristine therapy combined with opiates acquired CIC, further accentuating the burden of CIC on all cancer patients (Kato et al., 1998; Pashankar et al., 2011).

Constipation is classified as either normal-transit constipation, defecatory disorder or slow-transit constipation. Normal transit-constipation is the most prevalent of the three, and presents as bloating, discomfort and abdominal pain. Afflicted patients experience normal colonic evacuation, yet endure difficulty defecating due to the presence of hard stools (Lembo and Camilleri, 2003, McQuade et al., 2017). Although exhibiting similar symptoms, slow-transit constipation is consequential of less frequent urges to defecate. Defecatory disorders are commonly due to an impaired pelvic floor and/or anal sphincter from prolonged avoidance to defecate, because of the pain associated with the passage of large and/or hard stool, resulting in anal fissures and haemorrhoids (Escalante et al., 2017, McQuade et al., 2017, Bassotti and Villanacci, 2011, Lembo and Camilleri, 2003).

Chronic post-treatment constipation has been estimated to persist for up to 10 years following cessation of cancer treatment (Denlinger and Barsevick, 2009). As a result, the long-term consequences of CIC are associated with physical and psychosocial patient costs ultimately culminating in a suboptimal QoL (Dennison et al., 2005). For example, constipated patients may experience rectal tearing, haemorrhoids and rectal fissures, and if left untreated, it may progress to obstipation, faecal impaction and bowel obstruction (Leung et al., 2011, McQuade et al., 2016a). These life-threatening complications are exacerbated as intraluminal pressure increases within the bowel, potentially inducing ischaemic necrosis of the mucosa, pain, bleeding, and perforation (McQuade et al., 2016a). The worsening of symptoms escalates confusion, predominately in the elderly population, as well as irritability and aggression. There is accumulating evidence to suggest that CIC affects the tolerability and efficacy of anti-cancer treatment by triggering rapid onset nausea with or without vomiting adversely influencing the absorption of oral drugs (Lembo and Camilleri, 2003, McQuade et al., 2016a).

Mechanisms of Chemotherapy-Induced Constipation

Despite recent major progress in understanding the mechanisms of CINV and OM, the scarcity of literature accentuates that little is known about CIC, as much of the literature available is based on clinical observation and limited scientific findings (Gibson and Keefe, 2006b). Nonetheless, it has been postulated that damage to the ENS innervating the GI tract and controlling intestinal motility and secretion has been implicated in severe constipation including CIC (Knowles et al., 2013; Stojanovska et al., 2015, Escalante et al., 2017; McQuade et al., 2016a). As mentioned earlier, the GI tract is innervated by the ENS, together with fibres from extrinsic sympathetic, parasympathetic (vagus nerve) and sensory afferent neurons (McQuade et al., 2016a, Phillips and Powley, 2007). Within the ENS, two major ganglionated plexi exist – the myenteric (Auerbach's) and submucosal (Meissner's) – which function to control GI absorption, secretion, motility and vascular tone (Costa and Brookes, 2008; Bornstein et al., 2012; Furness, 2012; Bon-Frauches and Boesmans, 2020; Fleming et al., 2020). The interplay between the enteric neurons, glial cells and interstitial cells of Cajal (ICCs), generates myogenic and neurogenic activity, which in turn coordinates internal circular and external longitudinal smooth muscles. This allows for the expression of phasic and tonic contractile activity contributing to segmenting contractions and peristalsis (Dinning et al., 2009, Huizinga and Lammers, 2009, Kuizenga et al., 2015).

Changes to the morphology, neurochemistry, and connectivity of this tightly knit network have been identified following treatment with platinum-based chemotherapeutic agents. Studies in animals treated with cisplatin revealed significant damage and loss of enteric neurons, damage to neuronal processes, changes in enteric glial cells, expression of neuropeptides, their receptors, and neuromuscular transmission in the GI tract; these changes persisted long after the treatment (Vera et al., 2011, Pini et al., 2016, Uranga et al., 2017; Nardini et al., 2020). Treatment with cisplatin caused ultrastructural damage to ICCs; and altered the expression of the c-kit/stem cell factor and the gap junction protein connexin 43 in ICCs (Li et al., 2020). Mice presenting with slow-transit constipation induced by oxaliplatin exhibited a reduced number of myenteric neurons but an increased proportion of inhibitory neuronal nitric oxide synthase (nNOS)-immunoreactive neurons in the proximal (16%) and distal colon (43%), and reduced number of enteric glial cells (Wafai et al., 2013; McQuade et al., 2016c; Robinson et al., 2016; Stojanovska et al., 2018a; McQuade et al., 2018). Higher proportions of nNOS-immunoreactive myenteric and submucosal neurons and reduced expression of calcitonin gene-related peptide (CGRP)-IR neurons have been observed in the gastric fundus and colon from cisplatin-treated rats and mice, and vincristine-treated rats (Vera et al., 2011; Pini et al., 2016; López-Gómez et al., 2018). Increased size of nNOS-immunoreactive myenteric neurons has been found in the colons of patients treated with oxaliplatin combined with leucovorin and 5-FU (FOLFOX) (Carbone et al., 2016).

Furthermore, it was revealed that these cisplatin-induced changes correlate with reduced upper GI transit time and obliteration of colonic contractile activities observed in CIC (Pini et al., 2016). Oxaliplatin-induced enteric neuropathy was associated with augmented cytochrome *c* release, increased superoxide production, and reduced muscle tone of the distal colon (McQuade et al., 2016c). These findings suggest that oxidative stress is one of the key mechanisms of enteric neuropathy associated with platinum-based chemotherapy. Other mechanisms involve mucosal injury, activation of pro-inflammatory immune cells, increased cytokine release leading to ENS remodelling observed in animals treated with cisplatin (Nardini et al., 2020), changes in microbiota observed in mice treated with oxaliplatin (Stojanovska et al., 2018b), and possibly direct toxicity due to accumulation of platinum in the ENS (Stojanovska et al., 2017). Thus, a clear rationale exists between enteric neuronal integrity and optimal GI function.

Risk Factors Associated with Chemotherapy-Induced Constipation

Recently, research has hinted that the risk of constipation can be partly attributed to the emetogenic potential of an anticancer regimen (Hanai et al., 2016). For instance, Kimura et al. (2014) in corroboration with Takei and colleagues reported that 5-FU-epidoxorubicin-cyclophosphamide (a high emetogenic regime) increased the risk of CIC by 84%, compared with low emetic risk drugs (50%) (Kimura et al., 2014, Hanai et al., 2016). Although CIC is a significant health concern among people with cancer, the incidence is frequently underreported in clinical trials, due to the lack of measures to distinguish between true CIC and the occurrence of secondary constipation (Hanai et al., 2016, Gibson and Keefe, 2006b). Secondary constipation arises from drugs administered to inhibit other chemotherapy-induced or cancer-related symptoms, including anti-emetics to combat CINV and opioids to entice analgesic effects (Escalante et al., 2017, Gibson and Keefe, 2006b, McQuade et al., 2014, ALMouaalamy, 2021).

Current Treatments for Chemotherapy-Induced Constipation

Constipation management can be divided into two broad categories: non-pharmacological and pharmacological interventions (McIlfatrick et al., 2019). Non-pharmacological management of CIC is most favourable and consists of lifestyle alterations, such as increasing exercise, and consumption of dietary fibre and liquid intake (Escalante et al., 2017, McQuade et al., 2016a). In support of this, a recent study on cisplatin-treated rats highlighted that physical exercise improves autonomic dysfunction and prevents gastric emptying delay (Silva et al., 2021). This rather general intervention facilitates bowel movement, which in turn enhances defaecation whilst eliminating any underlying medical factors synonymous with constipation (Vasanwala, 2009, Hamaguchi et al., 2008, Jim et al., 2011, Hanai et al., 2016). The pharmacological approach involves the administration of both oral and/or rectal laxatives: bulk-forming, osmotic/saline, emollient, stimulant and lubricant laxatives (Escalante et al., 2017, McQuade et al., 2016a, ALMouaalamy, 2021). Polypharmacy associated with cancer treatment undermines the pharmacological avenue of CIC management futile, as it often perpetuates symptoms of dehydration, bloating and abdominal pain (Costilla and Foxx-Orenstein, 2014, Hanai et al., 2016, Escalante et al., 2017). Thus, there is a need for attainable clinical guidelines, prevention strategies, and a comprehensive assessment of prescribed laxatives to bridge gaps in the pre-existing fragmented approaches (McIlfatrick et al., 2019). It is important to note that there is little evidence to support the use of the following treatments in patients undergoing platinum-based anti-cancer regimens, as such, this next section covers a broader spectrum of chemotherapy treatments.

Stimulant Laxatives

Stimulant laxatives include diphenylmethane derivatives (phenolphthalein, sodium picosulfate, anthranoids (senna and cascara) and ricinoleic acid (castor oil) (McQuade et al., 2016a). These laxatives are more potent in liquefying stools to allow for defecation, when compared to other types of laxatives (osmotic and bulk-forming) (Dosh, 2002, Scarlett, 2004). The proposed mechanism of action suggests that stimulant laxatives reduce net absorption of water and electrolytes, whilst concurrently irritating sensory nerve endings to stimulate peristalsis (Twycross et al., 2012, McQuade et al., 2016a). The rapid onset of drug activity (6-12 hours via oral route; 15-60 minutes via rectal administration), and minimal adverse effects (abdominal cramping and hypokalaemia) render stimulant laxatives advantageous in the management of iatrogenic constipation (Ruston et al., 2013, Avila, 2004).

American Gastroenterological Association Institute Clinical Guidelines Committee recommends stimulant laxatives as the first-line treatment for opioid-induced constipation (Crockett et al., 2019), which is common in advanced cancer patients (ALMouaalamy, 2021). Several randomised controlled trials have hinted at the prophylactic benefits of Bisacodyl (3 tablets/day) which is also used as a stimulant laxative. The European Society for Medical Oncology (ESMO) recommends the short-term use of Bisacodyl and sodium picosulfate in situations of refractory constipation (Larkin et al., 2018). Bisacodyl has been shown to raise the number of spontaneous bowel movements and improve QoL in cancer and non-cancer patients with opioid-induced constipation (Alnaeem et al., 2018, Ishihara et al., 2012, Masri et al., 2010, Müller-Lissner et al., 2017). Despite these positive effects, some patients receiving 10 mg Bisacodyl experience dose-limiting side effects such as diarrhoea and abdominal pain (Kamm et al., 2011, Corsetti et al., 2021). Similarly, the most common adverse effect of sodium picosulfate is diarrhoea occurring in >30% of constipated patients treated with sodium picosulfate (Müller-Lissner et al., 2010). Therefore, stimulant laxatives should be limited to 2-3 times per week (Corsetti et al., 2021).

Osmotic/Saline Laxatives

Lactulose, sorbitol, polyethylene glycol (PEG) compounds, and saline laxatives (e.g., magnesium hydroxide), draw fluid osmotically into the intestinal lumen to stimulate propulsion and motility (Twycross et al., 2012, Scarlett, 2004). The differences in potencies of the aforementioned compounds have been studied. Analysis of several studies has demonstrated an improved stool consistency, texture, more bowel movements per week, decreased abdominal pain and need for additional laxatives associated with PEG compared to lactulose (Ford and Suares, 2011, Dipalma et al., 2007, Belsey et al., 2010, Lee-Robichaud et al., 2010). It was evident that PEG is a superior osmotic laxative to lactulose (Brenner and Shah, 2016). Saline osmotic laxatives include agents that contain magnesium, sulphate, phosphate and citrate ions. These ions draw fluid into the gut through the semipermeable membrane of the small intestine, ultimately heightening intraluminal pressure producing a mechanical stimulus that increases intestinal motility (Costilla and Foxx-Orenstein, 2014, Avila, 2004). Their therapeutic effect is seen 24-72 hours after the drug has entered the intestinal lumen. However, adverse effects such as abdominal pain, flatulence, cramping and distension may arise shortly after ingestion but subside after several days (Costilla and Foxx-Orenstein, 2014, McQuade et al., 2016a, Ford and Suares, 2011). Osmotic laxatives are often used to prevent or treat opioid-induced constipation, which is common in cancer patients undergoing pain treatment with opioids (ALMouaalamy, 2021). ESMO and MASCC recommend PEG laxatives as the first-line treatment for constipation in patients with advanced cancer (Larkin et al., 2018, Davies et al., 2020). However, the patient survey showed that osmotic laxatives do not alleviate opioid-induced constipation and are associated with side effects, such as diarrhoea and abdominal distension (Emmanuel et al., 2017).

Bulk-Forming Laxatives

Bulk-forming laxatives are commonly used against the constipating effects of anticancer agents (Avila, 2004). Available as natural or semisynthetic hydrophilic polysaccharides, cellulose derivatives, or polyacrylic resins; methylcellulose, psyllium, and polycarbophil exert their effect by promoting GI evacuation (McQuade et al., 2016a). These agents dissolve or swell in the intestinal fluid, forming a viscous liquid that stimulates peristalsis, facilitates the transport of intestinal constituents, and reduces GI transit time. Moreover, bulk-forming agents induce a stretch reflex in the GI wall, which increases absorption of water, colonic motility, and bacterial proliferation in the colon, leading to stool softening (ALMouaalamy, 2021). Bulk-forming agents take 2-4 days to exert their effects, calling into question the feasibility of their administration in the initial management of symptomatic constipation (Avila, 2004). Although efficacious in most forms of mild constipation, the excessive bulk formation can often reverse mild or transient constipation, consequentially worsening symptoms of bloating, distension, and abdominal pain (Scarlett, 2004, Costilla and Foxx-Orenstein, 2014). However, these symptoms are foreseen and often resolve within the first few weeks or by gradually increasing dosage (Doughty, 2002). In addition, the use of bulk-forming laxatives is contraindicated in elderly patients and those with advanced cancer, as it may predispose them to faecal impaction and bowel obstruction, as a result of their inability to adequately hydrate (goal of fluid intake being 30 mL/kg per day) (Scarlett, 2004, Avila, 2004). It has been concluded that bulk-forming laxatives are not effective in cancer patients with chronic constipation, especially those taking opioid or anticholinergic drugs (Wickham, 2017, ALMouaalamy, 2021), and not recommended in patients with advanced cancer (Larkin et al., 2018).

Emollient and Lubricant Laxatives

Emollient and lubricant laxatives, such as Docusate (Colace, Surfak) and mineral oil (liquid paraffin), often referred to as stool softeners, are first-line therapies used simultaneously with stimulant laxatives or bulk-forming agents to avoid painful defaecation and straining (Avila, 2004). They are composed of anionic surfactants that increase the wetting efficacy of intestinal fluids and facilitate the intermixing of aqueous and fatty substances, effectively softening stools to enable easy evacuation. Docusate is a stool softener that increases fluid uptake, which facilitates stool softening. It is found in three forms - docusate calcium, docusate sodium, and docusate potassium, and takes 1-2 days and in some cases, 5 days to elicit a therapeutic effect (McQuade et al., 2016a, Avila, 2004). Discrepancies in data exist for the use of docusate to manage CIC. For example, in a randomized, double-blind, placebo-controlled trial, cancer patients undergoing chemotherapy and treated with docusate did not show significant differences in the volume, consistency, difficulty, or completeness of evacuation, compared to the placebo group. It was concluded that docusate should be considered on an individual basis (Tarumi et al., 2013). Lubricant laxatives prevent straining associated with evacuation via emulsion into faecal mass and disruption of colonic water absorption (Avila, 2004, McQuade et al., 2016a). Mineral oil, which is administered orally or as an enema, is the leading lubricant laxative in clinical settings for the treatment of constipation in non-cancer and cancer patients undergoing platinum-based or other anti-cancer therapy experiencing CIC and opioid-induced constipation. Its use as a long-term lubricating agent is deemed inappropriate, due to its reported association with anal leakage inducing perianal irritation, break in the anorectal mucosa, lipoid pneumonia and malabsorption of fat-soluble vitamins, which is amplified with the concurrent use of docusate (McQuade et al., 2016a, Avila, 2004, Costilla and Foxx-Orenstein, 2014), and therefore, not recommended in patients with advanced cancer (Larkin et al., 2018).

Rectal Laxatives

The use of rectal laxatives in combination with digital stimulation to treat faecal impaction and constipation induced by neurogenic bowel dysfunction is broadly endorsed (McQuade et al., 2016a). Rectal laxatives comprise bisacodyl (stimulant) for evacuation of soft stool, sodium phosphate (saline), glycerin (osmotic) for evacuation of hard stools, and mineral oil (lubricant) (Avila, 2004). They are all available as suppositories or enemas, thus their use in neutropenic and thrombocytopenic patients is contraindicated (O'Mahony et al., 2001). However, for most cancer patients this treatment is reserved for more severe episodes of constipation, and for those who cannot tolerate long-term administration of oral laxatives (Mancini and Bruera, 1998). Sodium phosphate enemas are commonly used in cancer patients in palliative care and are considered relatively safe. However, even standard doses of sodium phosphate enemas might cause acute and life-threatening hyperphosphatemia within 24-72 hours, especially in elderly patients or patients with renal insufficiency leading to significant morbidity and mortality (Xing and Soffer, 2001). Enema retention time >30 minutes has been correlated with hyperphosphatemia due to the absorption of phosphate from the colon into the blood circulation (Wickham, 2017). It has been recommended to avoid sodium phosphate enemas in patients with fecal impaction, bowel obstruction, paralytic ileus, and fluid-electrolyte disturbances (Wickham, 2017).

Lubiprostone

Lubiprostone is a bicyclic fatty acid metabolite derived from prostaglandin E_1 that activates chloride type 2 channels (McQuade et al., 2016a, Lacy and Levy, 2008). This substrate-receptor complex stimulates a paracellular pathway that causes an efflux of chloride, sodium and water into the lumen of the GI tract, achieving isotonic equilibrium (Jun, 2013, Lacy and Levy, 2008). The resulting luminal distension from increased intestinal fluid enhances GI motility and softens the faecal mass, thereby promoting intestinal and colonic transit (Camilleri et al., 2006). Currently, oral lubiprostone is approved as a treatment for CIC at doses of 24 μg twice a day in women who do not respond to laxatives (Davis and Gamier, 2015). MASCC recommends the use of lubiprostone in cancer patients with constipation who do not respond to optimal dosing of first-line conventional laxatives (Davies et al., 2020). A study conducted by Sada et al. (2020) evidenced that approximately 70% of patients treated with combination chemotherapy experienced an increase in initial bowel movements within 24 h after administration of lubiprostone. Although no serious adverse effects were reported, numerous patients were subject to diarrhoea and nausea (Sada et al., 2020). However, due to the lack of evidence, lubiprostone has not been recommended as first-line therapy for opioid-induced constipation in cancer and non-cancer patients by the American Gastroenterological Association Institute Clinical Guidelines Committee (Crockett et al., 2019; ALMouaalamy, 2021).

Peripheral Opioid Antagonists

Peripherally acting μ-opioid receptor antagonists (PAMORAs) are not laxatives, however, they effectively stimulate bowel movements due to the block of μ-opioid receptors in the ENS innervating the GI tract. They act only peripherally, without affecting the CNS, therefore, do not suppress the effects of opioids used to inhibit pain in cancer patients. PAMORAs, such as methylnaltrexone, naldemedine, and naloxegol, have been approved by

ESMO, MASCC, and the American Gastroenterological Association Institute Clinical Guidelines Committee for the treatment of opioid-induced constipation in patients with advanced cancer who failed to respond to laxatives (Larkin et al., 2018, Davies et al., 2020, ALMouaalamy, 2021). Methylnaltrexone stimulates bowel movement 4 hours after the initial dose, higher stool regularity with minimal side effects (Siemens and Becker, 2016). Naloxegol relieves constipation for up to 1 year and improves the QoL of cancer patients (Cobo Dols et al., 2021). However, naloxegol-induced side effects such as headache, nausea, vomiting, flatulence, abdominal pain, diarrhoea, and arthralgia have been reported (ALMouaalamy, 2021). Naldemedine has been shown to be effective and safe to use in cancer patients (Osaka et al., 2019). However, side effects including nausea, abdominal pain, gastroenteritis, and diarrhoea might occur; patients with liver dysfunction should avoid using naldemedine (ALMouaalamy, 2021). Moreover, patients using peripheral opioid antagonists need to be monitored for opioids withdrawal symptoms.

Chemotherapy-Induced Diarrhoea

Chemotherapy-induced diarrhoea (CID) is a frequently under-recognised yet debilitating adverse effect of chemotherapy, which occurs in 50-80% of people undergoing cancer therapy (Stein et al., 2010, Benson et al., 2004, Gibson and Stringer, 2009; Bossi et al., 2018). In severe cases, CID episodes can persist up to 10 years after the cessation of treatment (Schneider et al., 2007, Denlinger and Barsevick, 2009, Kim et al., 2012). The severity of CID is clinically categorized into grades; from grade 1 (uncomplicated) to grade 5 (complicated) (Table 4) (Richardson and Dobish, 2007). Uncomplicated diarrhoea encompasses grades 1 and 2 which are characterised by defecation of up to 4-6 stools per day over baseline, and complicated diarrhoea (> 7 stools per day above baseline) induces life-threatening ramifications that could potentially culminate in death (grade 3-5) (Table 4) (Escalante et al., 2017, McQuade et al., 2016a). If left untreated, CID can result in the depletion of fluids and electrolytes, malnutrition, dehydration, and hospitalisation, some of which can compromise cardiovascular function and lead to death (Stein et al., 2010).

A correlation between cumulative dose, drug administration and schedule has been linked to the severity of CID; with high dose regimens and the combined use of chemotherapy and radiotherapy with targeted agents or immunotherapy amplifying the risk of CID incidence (McQuade et al., 2016a, Verstappen et al., 2003, Bowen et al., 2019, Elad et al., 2020). A strong link between topoisomerase I inhibitors (eg. irinotecan), anti-metabolites (e.g., a thymidylate synthase inhibitor 5-FU and its prodrug, capecitabine, that converts enzymatically to active 5-FU once absorbed from the gastrointestinal tract) and platinum-based regimens (cisplatin ± docetaxel, oxaliplatin) to CID has been observed (Stein et al., 2010, Keefe et al., 2007). For instance, FOLFOX had higher frequencies of grade 3/4 diarrhea in comparison to 5-FU/LV (McQuade et al., 2017, De Gramont et al., 2000); while 87% of patients treated with 5-FU/leucovorin experienced diarrhea (1/3 experiencing grade 3/4 diarrhoea); 52% of patients hospitalised and consequentially prescribed dose reductions and intravenous hydration, leaving a further 5% of the cohort terminally ill (McQuade et al., 2017). Moreover, 5-FU administration by bolus injection as opposed to intravenous infusion has been found to intensify pre-existing CID (Vincenzi et al., 2008, Stein et al., 2010). Similarly, 60-80% of patients treated with irinotecan suffer immediate-onset diarrhoea in the first 24 hours following treatment and, another 80% endure delayed-onset diarrhoea approximately 24-48 hours post-treatment (Gibson and Keefe, 2006b, McQuade et al., 2017, Gibson and Stringer, 2009, Gibson et al., 2003). In further support of this notion, a retrospective study conducted by Abu-Sbeih et al. (2020), revealed that patients receiving carboplatin (47%), cisplatin (31%) and oxaliplatin (22%) developed mucosal ulceration, non-ulcerative inflammation and colonic perforation that required surgical intervention. They also noted that colonic perforation occurred more frequently in patients receiving oxaliplatin and cisplatin therapy than those undergoing carboplatin treatment. While this is the case, carboplatin and cisplatin-treated patients had a longer duration of colitis and diarrhoea symptoms, in contrast to those receiving oxaliplatin (Abu-Sbeih et al., 2020). Other studies demonstrated that patients receiving liposomal irinotecan + 5-FU/LV, and FOLFIRINOX (non-liposomal irinotecan + oxaliplatin + 5-FU/LV) endured diarrhoea as a result of anti-cancer treatment (Conroy et al., 2011, Wang-Gillam et al., 2019, Wainberg et al., 2021).

Mechanisms of Chemotherapy-Induced Diarrhoea

The pathophysiology of CID is complex due to the intertwining of several mechanisms and a variety of different types of diarrhoea with varying symptomology – secretory, osmotic, malabsorptive, exudative, inflammatory and hypermotility (McQuade et al., 2014, Stringer et al., 2007, Bowen et al., 2019). Although mechanisms underlying the pathophysiology of CID have been overlooked for many years, it is now well studied and believed to stem from GI mucositis, and alterations in intestinal microflora and mucin secretion (Stein et al., 2010, McQuade et al., 2014, Stringer et al., 2007). Study of animal models treated with platinum-based chemotherapeutic regimes have shown pronounced crypt ablation in the jejunum and colon, villus blunting, epithelial atrophy, depletion of intestinal enzymes, metaplasia of goblet cells and excessive mucous secretion, all of which contribute to the malabsorption and hypersecretion evident in CID (McQuade et al., 2016a, Logan et al., 2008, Stein et al., 2010, Stringer et al., 2009a, Stringer et al., 2007, Gibson et al., 2003, Richardson and Dobish, 2007). This biochemical imbalance alters the osmotic gradient of the gut owing to the heightened proportion of immature secretory cells resulting in hypersecretion, and a corresponding decrease in the absorptive capacity of damaged intestinal villi – whose normal function is active fluid absorption (McQuade et al., 2016a, Viele, 2003). Furthermore, luminal retention of non-absorbable compounds and reduced chloride absorption in response to damaged intestinal crypt cells triggers an osmotic shift of water into the lumen to maintain luminal potential. Increased luminal constituents overwhelm the absorptive capacity of the colon, resulting in osmotic CID (Richardson and Dobish, 2007, Stringer et al., 2009a, McQuade et al., 2014).

As outlined earlier, antineoplastic therapies induce GI mucositis, and subsequent upregulation of prostaglandins, leukotrienes and cytokines coupled with the activation of nuclear factor kappa B (NFκB). This aggravates intestinal epithelium damage and disrupts intestinal water-ion homeostasis, leading to enhanced fluid secretion thus, secretory diarrhoea (McQuade et al., 2014, Richardson and Dobish, 2007, Ferrell et al., 2015, Lawrence, 2009, Bowen and Wardill, 2022). The impact of chemotherapeutics on enteric neurons and GI toxicity has been overlooked, until recently, cisplatin and irinotecan-induced enteric neuropathy has been proposed to underly secretory and motility disturbances experienced in GI toxicity (McQuade et al., 2014, Vera et al., 2011, Pini et al., 2016). Myenteric neuronal loss, elevated numbers of choline acetyltransferase immunoreactive (ChAT-IR) neurons and vesicular acetylcholine transporter (vAChT)-IR fibres in the myenteric plexus following irinotecan treatment (30mg/kg), has been shown to amplify the contractions of the gastric fundus strips, increase gastric and intestinal emptying times, and faecal water content in mice – symptomatic of diarrhoea (McQuade et al., 2017, Thorpe et al., 2020). In support of this, a study of tumour-bearing rats by Thorpe et al. (2020) established that high doses of irinotecan (175mg/kg), destroyed S100β-IR submucosal and myenteric glia in the jejunum and colon, resulting in hypersecretion of mucous, contributing to irinotecan induced diarrhoea (Thorpe et al., 2020).

Table 4. Diarrhoea and Consitpation Toxicity Criteria (adapted from the National Cancer Council) (McQuade et al., 2014, McQuade et al., 2016a, Stein et al., 2010)

Toxicity	Grade 1	Grade 2	Grade 3	Grade 4	Grade 5
Constipation	Occasional or intermittent symptoms; occasional use of stool softeners, laxatives, dietary modification, or enema	Persistent symptoms with regular use of laxatives or enemas; limiting daily life activities	Obstipation with manual evacuation indicated, limiting self-care and daily life activities	Life-threatening consequences: urgent intervention indicated	Death
Diarrhoea	Increase of <4 stools per day over baseline; mild increase in ostomy output compared to baseline	Increase of 4–6 stools per day over baseline; moderate increase in ostomy output compared to baseline	Increase of ≥7 stools per day over baseline; incontinence; hospitalization indicated; severe increase in ostomy output compared to baseline	Life-threatening consequences. Urgent intervention indicated.	Death

Gut microbiota plays a principal role in the maintenance of the structural integrity of the gut mucosal barrier and modulation of inflammatory responses through its interaction with TLRs and stimulation of NFκB (McQuade et al., 2016a, Van Vliet et al., 2010, Jandhyala et al., 201, Wardill et al., 2016, Al-Qadami et al., 2022, Bowen and Wardill, 2022). If not regulated, changes in intestinal microflora can promote mucositis culminating in CID. Current research suggests that the composition of intestinal microflora is easily manipulated by anticancer analogues namely, oxaliplatin, 5-FU and irinotecan (Stringer et al., 2008, Stringer et al., 2009a, Stringer et al., 2009b, Stojanovska et al., 2018b, Al-Qadami et al., 2022). Irinotecan has been associated with a shift in levels of β-glucuronidase- producing bacteria, a decrease in beneficial bacteria, *Lactobacillus* spp. and *Bifidobacterium* spp. and a concurrent increase in *Staphylococcus* spp., *Clostridium* spp. and *E. coli* (Stringer et al.,

2007, Stringer et al., 2008). This is consistent with previous findings that reveal the presence of excess free intestinal luminal and faecal 7-ethyl-10-hydroxycamptothecin (SN38) – an active metabolite of irinotecan (Stringer et al., 2007, Stringer et al., 2008, Stein et al., 2010). Upon metabolism, irinotecan is converted by hepatic and peripheral carboxylesterase into SN38. Thereafter, SN38 is deactivated through glucuronidation by hepatic uridine diphosphate glucuronosyltransferase-1A1 (UDP-GT 1A1), to SN38-glucuronide (SN38G). However, SN38G can undergo deconjugation by bacterial ß-glucuronidase to reform into the active metabolite, SN38. Noteworthy, is the profusion of SN38 relative to SN38G in faeces of patients treated with irinotecan, suggesting the abundance of ß-glucuronidase in the human intestinal lumen (McQuade et al., 2016a, Stein et al., 2010, Stringer et al., 2007, Stringer et al., 2008). As such, several animal studies have drawn a direct link between excess SN38 and mucosal damage, mucous hypersecretions and water-electrolyte imbalance contributing to CID (Stein et al., 2010). Equally, Stringer and colleagues (2009), noted a decline in *Enterococcus spp., Lactobacillus spp.* and *Streptococcus spp.* in rats treated with 5-FU (Stringer et al., 2009a). Interestingly, the combination of 5-FU with irinotecan confirmed an increase in the presence of *Clostridium cluster XI* and *Enterobacteriaceae* (Stringer et al., 2009b). In a study by Stojanovska and colleagues (2018), it was observed that oxaliplatin treatment was correlated with reductions in *Parabacteroides* and *Prevotellal*, and a concomitant increase in *Prevotella2* and *Odoribacter* (Stojanovska et al., 2018b). Furthermore, the interaction between microbial constituents and TLRs is implicated in intestinal mucositis, and stems from the increased expression and morphological changes noted in TLRs following anticancer drug therapy (Ferreira et al., 2012, Stringer et al., 2009b; Wardill et al., 2016; Wardill et al., 2021, Bowen and Wardill, 2022).

Whether chemotherapy induces microbial injury or the changes in the gut microbiome are simply a form of collateral damage resulting from mucosal injury, is a topic of intense investigation (Nayak et al., 2021, Da Silva Ferreira et al., 2020). In a different light, the baseline composition of the microbiome is strongly correlated with an individual's increased risk of mucosal injury caused by chemotherapy (Shi et al., 2020, Zhang et al., 2020, Wardill and Tissing, 2017, Wardill et al., 2021, Al-Qadami et al., 2022). Consistent with this rationale, antibiotic use before cancer therapy causes disruption of the microbiome and exacerbates chemotherapy-induced mucosal injury and gastrointestinal toxicity (Wardill et al., 2020, Reyna et al., 2015, Shouval et al., 2019). This has been most elegantly demonstrated by Wardill et al. (2021) in male Wistar rats who endured severe mucosal injury, and exacerbated villous atrophy, leading to an increase in severe diarrhoea and mortality after being treated with antibiotics before methotrexate. Importantly, these detrimental effects were reversed with autologous FMT, which restored the microbiome (Wardill et al., 2021). Albeit great advancements in knowledge of the mechanisms underlying CID, further research needs to home in on microbial factors that control mucosa recovery in the context of chemotherapy treatment.

Risk Factors Associated with Chemotherapy-Induced Diarrhea

The likelihood of developing CID is highly unpredictable, but some patients may be predisposed to higher risk owing to individual and treatment factors. Vincenzi et al. (2008) proposed that weekly administration of irinotecan, poor performance status, neutropenia, high serum creatinine levels, age > 70 and genetic polymorphism, is predictive of irinotecan-related diarrhoea (Vincenzi et al., 2008, McQuade et al., 2014). As an example, polymorphisms of uridine diphosphate glucuronyltransferase 1A1 (UGT1A1 - UGT1A1*28, UGT1A1*6) have been associated with a high incidence of severe toxicity among patients prescribed with irinotecan (Teh et al., 2012). This type of genetic polymorphism is common in Asian and Caucasian populations who are said to experience more intense episodes of neutropenia and diarrhoea following irinotecan treatment (Teh et al., 2012, Liu et al., 2007, Campbell et al., 2017). It has been suggested that gender (females), race (Caucasian) and comorbid conditions including, diabetes and bowel pathologies are prognostic of 5-FU-induced diarrhoea (Stein et al., 2010, Meyerhardt et al., 2004, McCollum et al., 2002). Genetic polymorphism of the dihydropyrimidine-dehydrogenase (DPD) and thymidylate synthase is associated with an increased risk of CID induced by fluoropyrimidines and platinum-based therapies (Campbell et al., 2016). A deficient DPD gene hinders drug clearance, subjecting the gut to periods of prolonged exposure to 5-FU, ultimately intensifying the severity of CID (Stein et al., 2010). Polymorphism of several other genes and their pathways involved in the metabolism of various chemotherapeutic drugs has been described (Coller et al., 2015, Reyes-Gibby et al., 2017, Korver et al., 2019, Wardill et al., 2020). Accompanying this, certain chemotherapeutic drugs, their combinations, and administration regimes have been found to increase susceptibility, severity and prevalence of CID, including the combination of 5-FU/LV with irinotecan and oxaliplatin (McQuade et al., 2014). Knowledge of populations at risk of CID may enable informed dosing, targeted surveillance, prophylactic measures, and personalised medicine (Campbell et al., 2017).

Current Treatments for Chemotherapy-Induced Diarrhea

Patients suffering from persistent CID often develop malnutrition, dehydration, cachexia, renal insufficiency, haemorrhoids and perianal skin breakdown contributing to treatment disruptions, which may lead to life-threatening sequelae (McQuade et al., 2014, McQuade et al., 2016a, Mitchell, 2006, Shafi and Bresalier, 2010, Benson et al., 2004, Stein et al., 2010). As such, 60% of patients with CID have alterations of anti-cancer treatment; 22% receive dose reductions, 28% experience dose delays, and 15% discontinue chemotherapy (Dranitsaris et al., 2005, McQuade et al., 2014, Russo et al., 2013). Aggressive symptomatology of CID impairs patient QoL and prolongs hospitalisation by approximately 8 days, indicating that CID has a substantial economic impact on both the patient and healthcare resources (McQuade et al., 2014, Dranitsaris et al., 2005, Arbuckle et al., 2000, Viele, 2003). Extended periods of hospitalisation interfere with the daily activities of >30% CID sufferers. Lack of independence in oncological patients has been shown to give rise to psychological disorders such as depression, anxiety, low self-esteem, social isolation, and irregular sleep patterns (McQuade et al., 2014, Stein et al., 2010, Viele, 2003).

Well-structured and updated guidelines developed by ASCO, ESMO and MASCC involve the use of loperamide, octreotide, deodorized tincture of opium (DTO) and other treatment approaches to manage CID (Benson et al., 2004, Stein et al., 2010, Bossi et al., 2018; Bowen et al., 2019). Although effective, they are associated with an excessive amount of side effects that sustain pre-existing damage to the ENS (Escalante et al., 2017).

Loperamide and Deodorized Tincture of Opium

Loperamide is the standard first-line therapy for CID. It is a synthetic opioid derivative that does not cross the blood-brain barrier at therapeutic doses, but decreases intestinal motility and increases gastric transit time by antagonising μ-opioid receptors of the myenteric plexus (McQuade et al., 2014, Stein et al., 2010, Benson et al., 2004, Regnard et al., 2011). It also exhibits anti-secretory effects by inhibiting thromboxane-A2 (McQuade et al., 2014). It is recommended that cancer patients with grade 1 or 2 diarrhoea without other complications are managed conservatively with oral hydration and loperamide

(Benson et al., 2004, Bossi et al., 2018). High-dose loperamide is recommended for patients with irinotecan-induced diarrhoea – an initial dose of 4mg followed by an additional 2mg for each subsequent diarrhoeal episode, 8 hours after irinotecan administration (Gibson and Keefe, 2006a, Sharma et al., 2005a). Its use leads to a variety of side effects including severe constipation, bloating, abdominal pain, nausea, vomiting, and dizziness at high doses, paralytic ileus (Stein et al., 2010, Lenfers et al., 1999, Sharma et al., 2005a, Richardson and Dobish, 2007).

Similar to loperamide, deodorized tincture of opium (DTO) antagonises the ENS μ-opioid receptors thereby slowing intestinal peristalsis, enhancing intestinal transit time and promoting fluid reabsorption (Richardson and Dobish, 2007, McQuade et al., 2016a). Despite the paucity of data regarding the efficacy and safety of DTO in CID management, DTO is available by prescription and is considered second-line therapy for persistent and uncomplicated diarrhoea (Richardson and Dobish, 2007). DTO contains the equivalent of 10 mg/mL morphine and the guidelines recommend dose for CID is 10–15 drops in water every 3–4 hours; if not effective after 48 hours, other drugs should be considered for CID treatment (Bossi et al., 2018). DTO induces a wide range of side effects including stomach/abdominal pain, seizures, severe constipation, euphoria or dysphoria, vomiting, nausea, psychological dependence, physical dependence, miosis, and respiratory depression (Benson et al., 2004, Richardson and Dobish, 2007, McQuade et al., 2014).

Octreotide

Octreotide is a synthetically engineered somatostatin analogue that exerts its therapeutic effect by inhibiting adenylyl cyclase, thereby decreasing the secretion of pancreatic and intestinal hormones such as insulin, glucagon, serotonin, and vasoactive intestinal peptide (VIP), as well as gastric acid secretion. As a result, intestinal transit time and water absorption are increased and mesenteric blood flow and secretion of fluids and electrolytes are decreased (Jansman et al., 2001, Rubenstein et al., 2004, Gibson and Keefe, 2006a, Stein et al., 2010). It is reserved as second-line therapy for patients who are unresponsive to loperamide (after 48 hours), despite increments in dosage and patients with mild to moderate diarrhoea complicated by bleeding or dehydration, cramping, nausea and vomiting, fever, sepsis, neutropenia, and patients with severe diarrhoea (Bossi et al., 2018). Although a standard octreotide dosage is not well defined, guidelines recommend a dose of 100–150 μg subcutaneously with dose escalation up to 500 μg until diarrhoea is controlled or 25–50 μg/h intravenously three times a day if the patient is severely dehydrated (Stein et al., 2010; Gibson et al., 2013; Bossi et al., 2018; Bowen et al., 2019). Of note, the severe side effects are experienced by 10% of the patients treated with octreotide (Hovind et al., 2010). These adverse effects include vomiting, nausea, headaches, dizziness, severe abdominal pain, constipation, enlarged thyroid, tachycardia and arrhythmia (McQuade et al., 2014). Octreotide injections may worsen GI symptoms, such as diarrhoea or rectal bleeding, in patients undergoing radiotherapy (Bossi et al., 2018).

Probiotics, Antibiotics, and β-Glucuronidase Inhibitors

The implication between intestinal microbiota and mucositis highlights the potentially promising therapeutic action against CID that may arise from probiotics and antibiotics. The suggestion in favour of probiotics by MASCC/ISOO Clinical Practice Guidelines for Gastrointestinal Mucositis has been maintained. They propose that probiotics containing *Lactobacillus* spp. may be beneficial for the prevention of radiotherapy and CID (Elad et al., 2020). This rationale has been confirmed in preliminary studies which observed a 15% reduction in the severity of grade 3/4 fluorouracil/ leucovorin-induced diarrhea, following treatment with *Lactobacillus rhamnosus* and fibre (Chong et al., 1997, McQuade et al., 2016a). A mixed probiotic formulation containing 10 billion colony-forming units of bacteria (*Bifidobacterium breve, Bifidobacterium bifidum, Bifidobacterium longum, Lactobacillus rhamnosus, Lactobacillus acidophilus, Lactobacillus casei, Lactobacillus plantarum, Streptococcus thermophilus, Lactobacillus brevis, Bifidobacterium infantis*) and additives inulin, maltodextrine, magnesium stearate, and ascorbic acid to be taken thrice a day for 12 weeks, has shown strong potency against irinotecan-induced diarrhoea. As such, the MASCC/ISOO maintains suggestions in favour of probiotics based on supporting evidence of significantly reduced incidence of severe and overall chemoradiation-induced diarrhoea (Bowen et al., 2019). In addition, oral administration of bacterial β-glucuronidase inhibitors has been found to reduce the severity and frequency of grade 3/4 irinotecan-induced diarrhoea (Wallace et al., 2010, Wardill et al., 2018). However, the use of probiotics for the prevention of CID is controversial. Despite their protective effect on the intestinal barrier, which reduces diarrhoea and abdominal discomfort, probiotics might increase the risk of severe infections in immunocompromised patients (Bossi et al., 2018).

Chloride Channel Inhibitors

Secretory diarrhoea is the result of a combination of excessive secretion drive by chloride channels and reduced reabsorption in the intestinal lumen (McQuade et al., 2016a, Thiagarajah and Verkman, 2013). Thus, the calculated inhibition of calcium-activated chloride channels located on enterocytes throughout the intestines reduces secretion of chloride and, therefore, secondary movement of water and sodium into the intestinal lumen, mitigating symptoms of CID (Thiagarajah et al., 2015). An animal study conducted by Ko et al. (2014) demonstrated that inhibition of calcium-activated chloride channels via red wine extract reduced intestinal fluid secretion, alleviating symptoms of diarrhoea induced by rotavirus (Ko et al., 2014, Bible et al., 2012). Nevertheless, to date, there are no data to support the use of red wine extract in the treatment of CID.

Secondary Complications of Gastrointestinal Toxicities Induced by Platinum-Based Therapies and Their Combinations

GI toxicities are prevalent during and post-chemotherapy treatments, and as a result, they impose a significant challenge for anticancer treatment. In this chapter, the prominent GI toxicities of platinum-based chemotherapeutics have been defined as nausea and vomiting, constipation, and mucositis as a precursor of diarrhoea. However, these adverse effects of chemotherapy at large, give rise to other detrimental and life-threatening secondary complications as collateral damage; these include malnutrition (including weight loss), dehydration, and infection. The secondary complications of GI toxicities induced by platinum-based and other chemotherapeutics will be discussed below.

Malnutrition

The WHO defines malnutrition as an umbrella term that refers to deficiencies, excesses, or imbalances in a person's intake of energy and/or nutrients. The term malnutrition encompasses undernutrition, overweight, obesity, and diet-related non-communicable diseases, such as cancer. Malnutrition is a common phenomenon among cancer patients with reports ranging from 30% to 85%

(Bozzetti et al., 2012, Hébuterne et al., 2014, WHO, 2012, Muscaritoli et al., 2017). These figures may not be an exact representation of the burden of disease, as historically there was no consensus on the definition of malnutrition and surrogate markers such as weight loss, low body mass index (BMI), and serum albumin levels were employed to establish an indistinct benchmark of measurement. Therefore, reports of occurrence may be underreported or overreported in different populations (Attar et al., 2012, Baldwin et al., 2012, Marian and August, 2014, Muscaritoli et al., 2017). In a retrospective longitudinal descriptive study, patients treated with 4-6 cycles of platinum-based chemotherapy for non-small cell lung cancer (NSCLC) had their nutritional status assessed (Sirichanchuen et al., 2019). Malnutrition was classified as having a BMI under 18.5 kg/m^2 and weight greater than 5% of their body weight. Of 114 patients, 85% suffered malnutrition, with the docetaxel regimen showing the highest incidence of malnutrition. Furthermore, patients treated with a combination of carboplatin and paclitaxel expressed the highest change in BMI (-0.6 kg/m^2) (Sirichanchuen et al., 2019). In corroboration with the previous study, Morio et al. (2016) established a significant positive correlation between weight loss and the incidence of neutropenia and leukopenia in patients receiving platinum-based chemotherapy. Another study examining the tolerability and safety of carboplatin-based combination chemotherapy revealed that the malnourished lung cancer patients completed fewer chemotherapy cycles and experienced poorer outcomes than the well-nourished group (Fujio et al., 2019). Similar results were observed in patients with advanced tumours receiving platinum-containing chemotherapy (carboplatin, cisplatin and oxaliplatin) (Gao et al., 2020). It is now well established that patients undergoing chemotherapy endure changes in nutritional status which may worsen chemotherapy-induced toxicities, QoL, and overall disease prognosis. Recently, it has been proposed that a Mediterranean diet may lessen the GI toxicities discussed above. An observational study presented a significant decrease in the frequency and gravity of nausea, stomach pain, abdominal bloating, and interference with daily activities in patients with a high Mediterranean diet serving score whilst undergoing platinum-based chemotherapy (Ghisoni et al., 2019). As such, appropriate nutritional screening, evaluation, advice, and treatment should be accessible to all cancer patients to improve the patient's nutritional status and treatment outcomes.

Dehydration

Dehydration is the excessive loss of water and other fluids that impedes the body's normal functioning. Among cancer patients, dehydration is commonly caused by severe diarrhoea and vomiting – both of which are principal GI toxicities caused by many chemotherapeutic drugs, including platinum-based anti-cancer drugs and their combinations (Erickson et al., 2018). To show the gravity of the matter, a population-based cancer registry study showed that the most common adverse events leading to hospitalization in elderly patients treated with adjuvant platinum-based chemotherapy were dehydration, anaemia, and infection (Sigel et al., 2013). Additionally, other studies have also deemed dehydration as a prominent cause of admissions to hospitals among patients treated with adjuvant chemotherapy (Wisnivesky et al., 2011, Malhotra et al., 2015). Furthermore, it is estimated that 20% to 30% of elderly people may suffer from cisplatin-induced dehydration (Manz et al., 2011, Duan et al., 2020).

Studies have endorsed that CINV is a precursor of dehydration. Failure to effectively treat CINV may lengthen hospital stays due to a greater need for artificial hydration with intravenous saline solution, weaken the body, reduce appetite, contribute to electrolyte imbalances, and ultimately reduce their nutritional status increasing the risk of patient consented cessation of treatment (Hamadani et al., 2007). As such, drugs to diminish CINV in an attempt to prevent the downstream cascade of events that may occur are commonly used. Of particular interest is palonosetron, which mitigates acute and delayed CINV. Nevertheless, palonosetron has been implicated in increasing hydration rate in patients with cancer who were receiving chemotherapy and an antiemetic combination including either palonosetron or granisetron extended-release subcutaneous (GERSC) injection. The proportion of patients who received/needed unscheduled hydration was significantly higher in patients treated with palonosetron than GERSC (54 vs 33%, respectively). This finding suggests that GERSC is a superior antiemetic to palonosetron by reducing the demand for unscheduled hydration, thus, reducing health care costs and the patients' financial burden (Erickson et al., 2018). Complementary to this, mannitol is a diuretic that has underlying nephroprotective effects by presumably reducing the concentration of cisplatin in the kidneys. However, it was reported that these nephroprotective benefits are only felt by patients receiving high doses of cisplatin (e.g., 100 mg/m^2), whilst others may experience dehydration, inadequate renal perfusion, thus further deteriorating renal function (Santoso et al., 2003, Crona et al., 2017, Duan et al., 2020).

Therefore, it is of utmost importance that treatment schemes are tailored to the patient in order to inhibit the domino effect caused by the interplay between drug metabolism and polypharmacy.

Infection

Infection remains one of the most prominent complications of mucositis that accompanies cytotoxic therapy (van der Velden et al., 2010, Herbers et al., 2014a). Perturbation of the normal innate immune system at the mucosal barriers has been shown to distort host-microbe interactions, by promoting local invasion and systemic dissemination of commensal microorganisms – all of which cause local infection and systemic bacteraemia. Several studies have shown that mucositis-induced infections are due to opportunistic pathogens that inhabit the oral and GI tract (Rolston, 2004, Klastersky et al., 2007, Tomblyn et al., 2009, van der Velden et al., 2014, Bowen and Wardill, 2022). For instance, bacteraemia in up to 39% of patients receiving high-dose chemotherapy was due to oral viridans streptococci (*Streptococcus oralis* and *Streptococcus mitis*) (Sobue et al., 2018).

Integration of patient characteristics is vital to estimate the risk of infection complications. This includes inquiring about patients' characteristics (gene predisposition, age, gender) and treatment characteristics (type of chemotherapy, schedule, and intensity). For example, children with acute lymphoblastic leukaemia with polymorphisms in MBL2 (mannose-binding lectin), TLR4 and CLEC7A (dectin-1) are at increased risk of systemic bacterial and fungal infections induced by anti-cancer therapies (Miedema et al., 2011, Bochud et al., 2008, Chai et al., 2011, van der Velden et al., 2014).

Besides the physical and mental burden of infection, patients also endure a significant economic impact. It was reported that patients diagnosed with mucositis related to anti-neoplastic therapy had almost twice higher total median medical cost compared to patients without therapy-induced mucositis (Nonzee et al., 2008, Carlotto et al., 2013). The largest contributor to disparities in medical cost among cohorts was attributed to the potential sequelae of mucositis, such as infection or nutritional deficiency (Novak and Amini, 2021). It is therefore apparent that it is crucial to develop therapeutic approaches that re-establish the intricate balance between the host and the microbiota (van der Velden et al., 2014, Al-Qadami et al., 2022, Bowen and Wardill, 2022).

Conclusion

Platinum-based and other chemotherapeutic agents have shown significant anti-tumour efficacy, however, these drugs are positively correlated with an abundance of concomitant GI symptoms including CINV, mucositis, diarrhoea and constipation. Chemotherapy-induced GI dysfunction is an under-acknowledged and insufficiently researched clinical hurdle that contributes to dose delays, reductions and, in severe cases, treatment termination. Further understanding of the dynamic interplay between the gut microbiota, genetic, inflammatory, epithelial, and neuronal systems in the aetiology of chemotherapy-induced GI dysfunction, might lead to defining risk factors and potential therapeutic targets for alleviating the debilitating adverse effects of cytotoxic drugs. Understanding the mechanisms underlying chemotherapy-induced GI toxicity may perhaps provide a promising avenue for novel chemotherapeutic drug developments that will improve prognostic outcomes and patient survival with little or no adverse effects.

References

Aapro, M. 2005. 5-HT(3)-receptor antagonists in the management of nausea and vomiting in cancer and cancer treatment. *Oncology,* 69, 97-109.

Abalo, R., Uranga, J. A., Pérez-García, I., De Andrés, R., Girón, R., Vera, G., López-Pérez, A. E. & Martín-Fontelles, M. I. 2017. May cannabinoids prevent the development of chemotherapy-induced diarrhea and intestinal mucositis? Experimental study in the rat. *Neurogastroenterol Motil,* 29(3), 10.1111/nmo.12952.

Abramoff, M. M. F., Lopes, N. N. F., Lopes, L. A., Dib, L. L., Guilherme, A., Caran, E. M., Barreto, A. D., Lee, M. L. M. & Petrilli, A. S. 2008. Low-Level Laser Therapy in the Prevention and Treatment of Chemotherapy-Induced Oral Mucositis in Young Patients. *Photomedicine and Laser Surgery,* 26, 393-400.

Abu-Sbeih, H., Mallepally, N., Goldstein, R., Chen, E., Tang, T., Dike, U. K., Al-Asadi, M., Westin, S., Halperin, D. & Wang, Y. 2020. Gastrointestinal toxic effects in patients with cancer receiving platinum-based therapy. *Journal of Cancer,* 11, 3144-3150.

Adel, N. 2017. Overview of chemotherapy-induced nausea and vomiting and evidence-based therapies. *Am J Manag Care,* 23, S259-s265.

Ahn, J. H., Kang, Y. K., Kim, T. W., Bahng, H., Chang, H. M., Kang, W. C., Kim, W. K., Lee, J. S. & Park, J. S. 2002. Nephrotoxicity of heptaplatin: a randomized comparison with cisplatin in advanced gastric cancer. *Cancer Chemother Pharmacol,* 50, 104-10.

Al-Ansari, S., Zecha, J. A. E. M., Barasch, A., De Lange, J., Rozema, F. R. & Raber-Durlacher, J. E. 2015. Oral Mucositis Induced By Anticancer Therapies. *Current oral health reports,* 2, 202-211.

Al-Dasooqi, N., Gibson, R. J., Bowen, J. M., Logan, R. M., Stringer, A. M. & Keefe, D. M. 2010. Matrix metalloproteinases are possible mediators for the development of alimentary tract mucositis in the dark agouti rat. *Exp Biol Med (Maywood),* 235, 1244-56.

Alcindor, T. & Beauger, N. 2011. Oxaliplatin: a review in the era of molecularly targeted therapy. *Curr Oncol,* 18, 18-25.

Alnaeem, M., Qadire, M. & Alasad Alshraideh, J. 2018. Effects of Prophylactic Laxatives for Opioid-Induced Constipation on Constipation Severity and Quality of Life among Patients with Cancer. *Open Journal of Nursing,* 08.

ALMouaalamy N. 2021. Opioid-Induced Constipation in Advanced Cancer Patients. *Cureus, 13*(4), e14386.

Al-Qadami, G., Van Sebille, Y., Bowen, J., & Wardill, H. (2022). Oral-Gut Microbiome Axis in the Pathogenesis of Cancer Treatment-Induced Oral Mucositis. *Frontiers in oral health, 3,* 881949.

Andrea, M. S., Rachel, J. G., Joanne, M. B. & Dorothy, M. K. K. 2009. Chemotherapy-Induced Modifications to Gastrointestinal Microflora: Evidence and Implications of Change. *Current Drug Metabolism,* 10, 79-83.

Ang, K. K., Zhang, Q., Rosenthal, D. I., Nguyen-Tan, P. F., Sherman, E. J., Weber, R. S., Galvin, J. M., Bonner, J. A., Harris, J. & El-Naggar, A. K. 2014. Randomized phase III trial of concurrent accelerated radiation plus cisplatin with or without cetuximab for stage III to IV head and neck carcinoma: RTOG 0522. *Journal of Clinical Oncology,* 32, 2940.

Anthony, L. B. & Chauhan, A. 2018. Diarrhea, constipation, and obstruction in cancer management. *The MASCC Textbook of Cancer Supportive Care and Survivorship.* Springer.

Antunes, H. S., Herchenhorn, D., Small, I. A., Araújo, C., Viégas, C., de Assis Ramos, G., Dias, F. L., & Ferreira, C. G. 2017. Long-term survival of a randomized phase III trial of head and neck cancer patients receiving concurrent chemoradiation therapy with or without low-level laser therapy (LLLT) to prevent oral mucositis. *Oral Oncology, 71,* 11–15.

Arbuckle, R., Huber, S. & Zacker, C. 2000. The consequences of diarrhea occurring during chemotherapy for colorectal cancer: a retrospective study. *The Oncologist,* 5, 250-259.

Ariyawardana, A., Cheng, K., Kandwal, A., Tilly, V., Al-Azri, A. R., Galiti, D., Chiang, K., Vaddi, A., Ranna, V., Nicolatou-Galitis, O., Lalla, R. V., Bossi, P., Elad, S., & Mucositis Study Group of the Multinational Association of Supportive Care in Cancer/International Society for Oral Oncology (MASCC/ISOO). 2019. Systematic review of anti-inflammatory agents for the management of oral mucositis in cancer patients and clinical practice guidelines. *Supportive Care in Cancer: official journal of the Multinational Association of Supportive Care in Cancer, 27*(10), 3985–3995.

Atay, H., Aslan, N., Aktimur, S., Buyukkaya, P., Kelkitli, E., Turgut, M. & Haznedaroglu, I. 2015. Safety and Efficacy of Ankaferd Hemostat (ABS) in the Chemotherapy-Induced Oral Mucositis. *UHOD - Uluslararasi Hematoloji-Onkoloji Dergisi,* 25, 166-171.

Attar A, Malka D, Sabate JM, Bonnetain F, Lecomte T, Aparicio T, Locher C, Laharie D, Ezenfis J, Taieb J. 2012. Malnutrition is high and underestimated during chemotherapy in gastrointestinal cancer: an AGEO prospective cross-sectional multicenter study. *Nutr Cancer,* 64:535–542.

Avila, J. G. 2004. Pharmacologic treatment of constipation in cancer patients. *Cancer Control,* 11, 10-18.

Babic, T. & Browning, K. N. 2014. The role of vagal neurocircuits in the regulation of nausea and vomiting. *Eur J Pharmacol,* 722, 38-47.

Bajic, J. E., Johnston, I. N., Howarth, G. S. & Hutchinson, M. R. 2018. From the Bottom-Up: Chemotherapy and Gut-Brain Axis Dysregulation. *Front Behav Neurosci,* 12, 104.

Baldwin, C., Spiro, A., Ahern, R. & Emery, P. W. 2012. Oral nutritional interventions in malnourished patients with cancer: a systematic review and meta-analysis. *J Natl Cancer Inst,* 104, 371-85.

Basch, E., Prestrud, A. A., Hesketh, P. J., Kris, M. G., Feyer, P. C., Somerfield, M. R., Chesney, M., Clark-Snow, R. A., Flaherty, A. M., Freundlich, B., Morrow, G., Rao, K. V., Schwartz, R. N. & Lyman, G. H. 2011. Antiemetics: American Society of Clinical Oncology clinical practice guideline update. *J Clin Oncol,* 29, 4189-98.

Bassotti, G. & Villanacci, V. 2011. Can "functional" constipation be considered as a form of enteric neuro-gliopathy? *Glia,* 59, 345-350.

Bayo, J., Fonseca, P. J., Hernando, S., Servitja, S., Calvo, A., Falagan, S., García, E., González, I., De Miguel, M. J., Pérez, Q., Milena, A., Ruiz, A. & Barnadas, A. 2012. Chemotherapy-induced nausea and vomiting: pathophysiology and therapeutic principles. *Clinical and Translational Oncology,* 14, 413-422.

Belsey, J. D., Geraint, M. & Dixon, T. A. 2010. Systematic review and meta-analysis: polyethylene glycol in adults with non-organic constipation. *Int J Clin Pract,* 64, 944-55.

Bensinger, W., Schubert, M., Ang, K. K., Brizel, D., Brown, E., Eilers, J. G., Elting, L., Mittal, B. B., Schattner, M. A., Spielberger, R., Treister, N. S. & Trotti, A. M., 3rd 2008. NCCN Task Force Report. Prevention and management of mucositis in cancer care. *J Natl Compr Canc Netw,* 6 Suppl 1, S1-21; quiz S22-4.

Benson, A. B., 3rd, Ajani, J. A., Catalano, R. B., Engelking, C., Kornblau, S. M., Martenson, J. A., Jr., Mccallum, R., Mitchell, E. P., O'dorisio, T. M., Vokes, E. E. & Wadler, S. 2004. Recommended guidelines for the treatment of cancer treatment-induced diarrhea. *J Clin Oncol,* 22, 2918-26.

Benson, A. B., 3rd, Ajani, J. A., Catalano, R. B., Engelking, C., Kornblau, S. M., Martenson, J. A., Jr., Mccallum, R., Mitchell, E. P., O'dorisio, T. M., Vokes, E. E. & Wadler, S. 2004. Recommended guidelines for the treatment of cancer treatment-induced diarrhea. *J Clin Oncol,* 22, 2918-26.

Berger, M. J., Ettinger, D. S., Aston, J., Barbour, S., Bergsbaken, J., Bierman, P. J., Brandt, D., Dolan, D. E., Ellis, G., Kim, E. J., Kirkegaard, S., Kloth, D. D., Lagman, R., Lim, D., Loprinzi, C., Ma, C. X., Maurer, V., Michaud, L. B., Nabell, L. M., Noonan, K., Roeland, E., Rugo, H. S., Schwartzberg, L. S., Scullion, B., Timoney, J., Todaro, B., Urba, S. G., Shead, D. A. & Hughes, M. 2017. NCCN Guidelines Insights: Antiemesis, Version 2.2017. *J Natl Compr Canc Netw,* 15, 883-893.

Bible, K., Peethambaram, P., Oberg, A., Maples, W., Groteluschen, D., Boente, M., Burton, J., Dahl, L., Tibodeau, J., Isham, C., Maguire, J., Shridhar, V., Kukla, A., Voll, K.,

Mauer, M., Colevas, A., Wright, J., Doyle, L. & Erlichman, C. 2012. A Phase 2 Trial of Flavopiridol (Alvocidib) and Cisplatin in Platin-Resistant Ovarian and Primary Peritoneal Carcinoma: MC0261. *Gynecologic Oncology,* 127, 55-62.

Blijlevens, N. & Sonis, S. 2007. Palifermin (recombinant keratinocyte growth factor-1): a pleiotropic growth factor with multiple biological activities in preventing chemotherapy- and radiotherapy-induced mucositis. *Ann Oncol,* 18, 817-26.

Blijlevens, N. M., Donnelly, J. P., Naber, A. H., Schattenberg, A. V. & Depauw, B. E. 2005. A randomised, double-blinded, placebo-controlled, pilot study of parenteral glutamine for allogeneic stem cell transplant patients. *Support Care Cancer,* 13, 790-6.

Bochud, P. Y., Chien, J. W., Marr, K. A., Leisenring, W. M., Upton, A., Janer, M., Rodrigues, S. D., Li, S., Hansen, J. A., Zhao, L. P., Aderem, A. & Boeckh, M. 2008. Toll-like receptor 4 polymorphisms and aspergillosis in stem-cell transplantation. *N Engl J Med,* 359, 1766-77.

Boers-Doets, C. B., Epstein, J. B., Raber-Durlacher, J. E., Ouwerkerk, J., Logan, R. M., Brakenhoff, J. A., Lacouture, M. E. & Gelderblom, H. 2012. Oral adverse events associated with tyrosine kinase and mammalian target of rapamycin inhibitors in renal cell carcinoma: a structured literature review. *Oncologist,* 17, 135-44.

Bogunia-Kubik, K., Mazur, G., Urbanowicz, I., Wróbel, T., Kuliczkowski, K., Woźniak, M. & Lange, A. 2006. Lack of association between the TNF-alpha promoter gene polymorphism and susceptibility to B-cell chronic lymphocytic leukaemia. *Int J Immunogenet,* 33, 21-4.

Bon-Frauches, A. C., and Boesmans, W. 2020. The Enteric Nervous System: the Hub in a star Network. *Nat. Rev. Gastroenterol. Hepatol.* 17, 717–718.

Bornstein, J., Gwynne, R., and Sjövall, H. 2012. "Enteric Neural Regulation of Mucosal Secretion," in Physiology of the Gastrointestinal Tract. 5th Edition (Amsterdam, Netherlands: Elsevier).

Bossi, P., Antonuzzo, A., Cherny, N. I., Rosengarten, O., Pernot, S., Trippa, F., Schuler, U., Snegovoy, A., Jordan, K., Ripamonti, C. I., & ESMO Guidelines Committee. 2018. Diarrhoea in adult cancer patients: ESMO Clinical Practice Guidelines. *Annals of Oncology: official journal of the European Society for Medical Oncology, 29 Suppl 4*, iv126–iv142.

Bowen, J., Al-Dasooqi, N., Bossi, P., Wardill, H., Van Sebille, Y., Al-Azri, A., Bateman, E., Correa, M. E., Raber-Durlacher, J., Kandwal, A., Mayo, B., Nair, R. G., Stringer, A., Ten Bohmer, K., Thorpe, D., Lalla, R. V., Sonis, S., Cheng, K. & Elad, S. 2019. The pathogenesis of mucositis: updated perspectives and emerging targets. *Support Care Cancer,* 27, 4023-4033.

Bowen, J., Wardill, H. 2022. The science of mucositis. *Support Care Cancer* 30, 2915–2917.

Bozzetti, F., Mariani, L., Lo Vullo, S., Amerio, M. L., Biffi, R., Caccialanza, G., Capuano, G., Correja, I., Cozzaglio, L., Di Leo, A., Di Cosmo, L., Finocchiaro, C., Gavazzi, C., Giannoni, A., Magnanini, P., Mantovani, G., Pellegrini, M., Rovera, L., Sandri, G., Tinivella, M. & Vigevani, E. 2012. The nutritional risk in oncology: a study of 1,453 cancer outpatients. *Support Care Cancer,* 20, 1919-28.

Brandão, T. B., Morais-Faria, K., Ribeiro, A., Rivera, C., Salvajoli, J. V., Lopes, M. A., Epstein, J. B., Arany, P. R., de Castro, G., Jr, Migliorati, C. A., & Santos-Silva, A. R.

2018. Locally advanced oral squamous cell carcinoma patients treated with photobiomodulation for prevention of oral mucositis: retrospective outcomes and safety analyses. *Supportive Care in Cancer: official journal of the Multinational Association of Supportive Care in Cancer*, *26*(7), 2417–2423.

Brenner, D. M. & Shah, M. 2016. Chronic Constipation. *Gastroenterol Clin North Am,* 45, 205-16.

Brunner, L. S. 2010. *Brunner & Suddarth's textbook of medical-surgical nursing*, Lippincott Williams & Wilkins.

Camilleri, M., Bharucha, A. E., Ueno, R., Burton, D., Thomforde, G. M., Baxter, K., Mckinzie, S. & Zinsmeister, A. R. 2006. Effect of a selective chloride channel activator, lubiprostone, on gastrointestinal transit, gastric sensory, and motor functions in healthy volunteers. *American Journal of Physiology-Gastrointestinal and Liver Physiology,* 290, G942-G947.

Campbell, J. M., Stephenson, M. D., Bateman, E., Peters, M. D. J., Keefe, D. M. & Bowen, J. M. 2017. Irinotecan-induced toxicity pharmacogenetics: an umbrella review of systematic reviews and meta-analyses. *The Pharmacogenomics Journal,* 17, 21-28.

Campbell JM, Bateman E, Peters M, Bowen JM, Keefe DM, Stephenson MD. 2016. Fluoropyrimidine and platinum toxicity pharmacogenetics: an umbrella review of systematic reviews and meta-analyses. *Pharmacogenomics* 17(4):435–451.

Carbone, S. E., Jovanovska, V., Brookes, S. J. & Nurgali, K. 2016. Electrophysiological and morphological changes in colonic myenteric neurons from chemotherapy-treated patients: a pilot study. *Neurogastroenterol Motil,* 28, 975-84.

Carlotto, A., Hogsett, V. L., Maiorini, E. M., Razulis, J. G. & Sonis, S. T. 2013. The economic burden of toxicities associated with cancer treatment: review of the literature and analysis of nausea and vomiting, diarrhoea, oral mucositis and fatigue. *Pharmacoeconomics,* 31, 753-66.

Chai, L. Y., De Boer, M. G., Van Der Velden, W. J., Plantinga, T. S., Van Spriel, A. B., Jacobs, C., Halkes, C. J., Vonk, A. G., Blijlevens, N. M., Van Dissel, J. T., Donnelly, P. J., Kullberg, B. J., Maertens, J. & Netea, M. G. 2011. The Y238X stop codon polymorphism in the human β-glucan receptor dectin-1 and susceptibility to invasive aspergillosis. *J Infect Dis,* 203, 736-43.

Chaveli-López, B. & Bagán-Sebastián, J. V. 2016. Treatment of oral mucositis due to chemotherapy. *Journal of Clinical and Experimental Dentistry,* 8, e201-e209.

Chen, J., Rao, J. N., Zou, T., Liu, L., Marasa, B. S., Xiao, L., Zeng, X., Turner, D. J. & Wang, J. Y. 2007. Polyamines are required for expression of Toll-like receptor 2 modulating intestinal epithelial barrier integrity. *Am J Physiol Gastrointest Liver Physiol,* 293, G568-76.

Chen, L., Cao, H., Yu, C. & Feng, Y. 2018. Lobaplatin inhibits prostate cancer progression in part by impairing AR and ERG signal. *Fundam Clin Pharmacol,* 32, 548-557.

Choi, C.H., Cha, Y.J., An, C.S., Kim, K.J., Kim, K.C., Moon, S.P., Lee, Z. H. & Min, Y.D. 2004. Molecular mechanisms of heptaplatin effective against cisplatin-resistant cancer cell lines: less involvement of metallothionein. *Cancer Cell International,* 4, 6-6.

Chong, L. K., Drury, D. E., Dummer, J. F., Ghahramani, P., Schleimer, R. P. & Peachell, P. T. 1997. Protection by dexamethasone of the functional desensitization to β2-

adrenoceptor-mediated responses in human lung mast cells. *British Journal of Pharmacology,* 121, 717-722.

Cidon, E. U. 2017. Chemotherapy induced oral mucositis: prevention is possible. *Chinese Clinical Oncology,* 7, 6.

Clark, K., & Currow, D. C. 2020. Response to Davies A, Leach C, Caponero R, Dickman A, Fuchs D, Paice J, Emmanuel A. 2020. MASCC recommendations on the management of constipation in patients with advanced cancer. Support Care Cancer 28:23. *Supportive Care in Cancer: official journal of the Multinational Association of Supportive Care in Cancer*, *28*(5), 2041–2042.

Clarkson, J. E., Worthington, H. V., Furness, S., Mccabe, M., Khalid, T. & Meyer, S. 2010. Interventions for treating oral mucositis for patients with cancer receiving treatment. *Cochrane Database Syst Rev,* 2010, Cd001973.

Clarkson, J., Worthington, H. & Eden, O. 2008. Interventions for treating oral mucositis for patients with cancer receiving treatment. *Australian dental journal,* 53, 363-365.

Cobo Dols, M., Beato Zambrano, C., Cabezón-Gutiérrez, L., Chicas-Sett, R., Blancas López-Barajas, M. I., García Navalón, F. J., Fírvida Pérez, J. L., Serrano Bermúdez, G., Togores Torres, P., Delgado Mingorance, I., Giraldo Marín, A., Librán Oriol, A., Paredes Lario, A., Sánchez Mauriño, P., Higuera Gómez, O., Moreno Muñoz, D., Huerta González, I., Sanz-Yagüe, A., & Soler López, B. 2021. One-year efficacy and safety of naloxegol on symptoms and quality of life related to opioid-induced constipation in patients with cancer: KYONAL study. *BMJ supportive & palliative care*, bmjspcare-2020-002816. Advance online publication.

Coëffier, M., Marion, R., Leplingard, A., Lerebours, E., Ducrotté, P. & Déchelotte, P. 2002. Glutamine decreases interleukin-8 and interleukin-6 but not nitric oxide and prostaglandins e(2) production by human gut in-vitro. *Cytokine,* 18, 92-7.

Coller, J. K., White, I. A., Logan, R. M., Tuke, J., Richards, A. M., Mead, K. R., Karapetis, C. S., & Bowen, J. M. 2015. Predictive model for risk of severe gastrointestinal toxicity following chemotherapy using patient immune genetics and type of cancer: a pilot study. *Supportive Care in Cancer: official journal of the Multinational Association of Supportive Care in Cancer*, *23*(5), 1233–1236.

Connolly, M. & Larkin, P. 2012. Managing constipation: a focus on care and treatment in the palliative setting. *British journal of Community Nursing,* 17, 60-67.

Conroy, T., Desseigne, F., Ychou, M., Bouché, O., Guimbaud, R., Bécouarn, Y., Adenis, A., Raoul, J. L., Gourgou-Bourgade, S., De La Fouchardière, C., Bennouna, J., Bachet, J. B., Khemissa-Akouz, F., Péré-Vergé, D., Delbaldo, C., Assenat, E., Chauffert, B., Michel, P., Montoto-Grillot, C. & Ducreux, M. 2011. FOLFIRINOX versus gemcitabine for metastatic pancreatic cancer. *N Engl J Med,* 364, 1817-25.

Corsetti, M., Landes, S. & Lange, R. 2021. Bisacodyl: A review of pharmacology and clinical evidence to guide use in clinical practice in patients with constipation. *Neurogastroenterology & Motility,* 33, e14123.

Costa, A. L., Abreu, C., Pacheco, T. R., Macedo, D., Sousa, A. R., Pulido, C., Quintela, A. & Costa, L. 2015. Prevention of Nausea and Vomiting in Patients Undergoing Oral Anticancer Therapies for Solid Tumors. *BioMed Research International,* 2015, 309601.

Costa, M. & Brookes, S. H. 2008. Architecture of enteric neural circuits involved in intestinal motility. *Eur Rev Med Pharmacol Sci,* 12 Suppl 1, 3-19.

Costilla, V. C. & Foxx-Orenstein, A. E. 2014. Constipation: understanding mechanisms and management. *Clin Geriatr Med,* 30, 107-15.

Crockett, S. D., Greer, K. B., Heidelbaugh, J. J., Falck-Ytter, Y., Hanson, B. J., Sultan, S., & American Gastroenterological Association Institute Clinical Guidelines Committee. 2019. American Gastroenterological Association Institute Guideline on the Medical Management of Opioid-Induced Constipation. *Gastroenterology*, *156*(1), 218–226.

Crona, D. J., Faso, A., Nishijima, T. F., Mcgraw, K. A., Galsky, M. D. & Milowsky, M. I. 2017. A Systematic Review of Strategies to Prevent Cisplatin-Induced Nephrotoxicity. *The Oncologist,* 22, 609-619.

Da Silva Ferreira, A. R., Wardill, H. R., Tissing, W. J. E. & Harmsen, H. J. M. 2020. Pitfalls and novel experimental approaches to optimize microbial interventions for chemotherapy-induced gastrointestinal mucositis. *Curr Opin Support Palliat Care,* 14, 127-134.

Da Silva Santos, P. S., Coracin, F. L., Barros, J. C. D. A., Dulley, F. L., Nunes, F. D. & Magalhães, M. G. 2011. Impact of oral care prior to HSCT on the severity and clinical outcomes of oral mucositis. *Clinical Transplantation,* 25, 325-328.

Davies, A., Leach, C., Caponero, R., Dickman, A., Fuchs, D., Paice, J., & Emmanuel, A. 2020. MASCC recommendations on the management of constipation in patients with advanced cancer. *Supportive Care in Cancer: official journal of the Multinational Association of Supportive Care in Cancer*, *28*(1), 23–33.

Davis, M. & Gamier, P. 2015. New options in constipation management. *Current oncology reports,* 17, 1-11.

De Gramont, A., Figer, A., Seymour, M., Homerin, M., Hmissi, A., Cassidy, J., Boni, C., Cortes-Funes, H., Cervantes, A., Freyer, G., Papamichael, D., Le Bail, N., Louvet, C., Hendler, D., De Braud, F., Wilson, C., Morvan, F. & Bonetti, A. 2000. Leucovorin and fluorouracil with or without oxaliplatin as first-line treatment in advanced colorectal cancer. *J Clin Oncol,* 18, 2938-47.

Denlinger, C. S. & Barsevick, A. M. 2009. The challenges of colorectal cancer survivorship. *J Natl Compr Canc Netw,* 7, 883-93; quiz 894.

Dennison, C., Prasad, M., Lloyd, A., Bhattacharyya, S. K., Dhawan, R. & Coyne, K. 2005. The health-related quality of life and economic burden of constipation. *Pharmacoeconomics,* 23, 461-76.

de Pauli Paglioni, M., Araújo, A., Arboleda, L., Palmier, N. R., Fonsêca, J. M., Gomes-Silva, W., Madrid-Troconis, C. C., Silveira, F. M., Martins, M. D., Faria, K. M., Ribeiro, A., Brandão, T. B., Lopes, M. A., Leme, A., Migliorati, C. A., & Santos-Silva, A. R. 2019. Tumor safety and side effects of photobiomodulation therapy used for prevention and management of cancer treatment toxicities. A systematic review. *Oral Oncology*, *93*, 21–28.

Depré, M., Van Hecken, A., Oeyen, M., De Lepeleire, I., Laethem, T., Rothenberg, P., Petty, K. J., Majumdar, A., Crumley, T., Panebianco, D., Bergman, A. & De Hoon, J. N. 2005. Effect of aprepitant on the pharmacokinetics and pharmacodynamics of warfarin. *Eur J Clin Pharmacol,* 61, 341-6.

Dinning, P. G., Smith, T. K. & Scott, S. M. 2009. Pathophysiology of colonic causes of chronic constipation. *Neurogastroenterol Motil,* 21 Suppl 2, 20-30.

Dipalma, J. A., Cleveland, M. V., Mcgowan, J. & Herrera, J. L. 2007. A randomized, multicenter, placebo-controlled trial of polyethylene glycol laxative for chronic treatment of chronic constipation. *Am J Gastroenterol,* 102, 1436-41.

Dosh, S. A. 2002. Evaluation and treatment of constipation.(Clinical Update). *Journal of Family Practice,* 51, 555-560.

Doughty, D. B. 2002. When fiber is not enough: current thinking on constipation management. *Ostomy/wound Management,* 48, 30-41.

Dranitsaris, G., Maroun, J. & Shah, A. 2005. Estimating the cost of illness in colorectal cancer patients who were hospitalized for severe chemotherapy-induced diarrhea. *Can J Gastroenterol,* 19, 83-7.

Duan, Z., Cai, G., Li, J. & Chen, X. 2020. Cisplatin-induced renal toxicity in elderly people. *Ther Adv Med Oncol,* 12, 1758835920923430.

Dupuis, L. L., Robinson, P. D., Boodhan, S., Holdsworth, M., Portwine, C., Gibson, P., Phillips, R., Maan, C., Stefin, N. & Sung, L. 2014. Guideline for the prevention and treatment of anticipatory nausea and vomiting due to chemotherapy in pediatric cancer patients. *Pediatric Blood & Cancer,* 61, 1506-1512.

Eisenberg, P., Figueroa-Vadillo, J., Zamora, R., Charu, V., Hajdenberg, J., Cartmell, A., Macciocchi, A. & Grunberg, S. 2003. Improved prevention of moderately emetogenic chemotherapy-induced nausea and vomiting with palonosetron, a pharmacologically novel 5-HT3 receptor antagonist: results of a phase III, single-dose trial versus dolasetron. *Cancer,* 98, 2473-82.

El-Akawi, Z., Abu-Hadid, M., Perez, R., Glavy, J., Zdanowicz, J., Creaven, P. J. & Pendyala, L. 1996. Altered glutathione metabolism in oxaliplatin resistant ovarian carcinoma cells. *Cancer Lett,* 105, 5-14.

Elad, S., Cheng, K. K. F., Lalla, R. V., Yarom, N., Hong, C., Logan, R. M., Bowen, J., Gibson, R., Saunders, D. P., Zadik, Y., Ariyawardana, A., Correa, M. E., Ranna, V. & Bossi, P. 2020. MASCC/ISOO clinical practice guidelines for the management of mucositis secondary to cancer therapy. *Cancer,* 126, 4423-4431.

Elad S, Zadik Y. 2016. Chronic oral mucositis after radiotherapy to the head and neck: a new insight. *Support Care Cancer.* 24(11):4825-30.

Elting, L. S., Cooksley, C., Chambers, M., Cantor, S. B., Manzullo, E. & Rubenstein, E. B. 2003. The burdens of cancer therapy. Clinical and economic outcomes of chemotherapy-induced mucositis. *Cancer,* 98, 1531-9.

Emmanuel, A., Johnson, M., McSkimming, P., & Dickerson, S. 2017. Laxatives Do Not Improve Symptoms of Opioid-Induced Constipation: Results of a Patient Survey. *Pain medicine (Malden, Mass.)*, *18*(10), 1932–1940.

Epstein, J. B., Thariat, J., Bensadoun, R. J., Barasch, A., Murphy, B. A., Kolnick, L., Popplewell, L. & Maghami, E. 2012. Oral complications of cancer and cancer therapy: from cancer treatment to survivorship. *CA Cancer J Clin,* 62, 400-22.

Erickson, R., Nebughr, N., Mosier, M. C. & Nibley, W. 2018. Hydration requirements in Patients Receiving Highly Emetogenic Chemotherapy. *Future Oncology,* 15, 753-761.

Escalante, J., Mcquade, R. M., Stojanovska, V. & Nurgali, K. 2017. Impact of chemotherapy on gastrointestinal functions and the enteric nervous system. *Maturitas,* 105, 23-29.

Evans, M. E., Jones, D. P. & Ziegler, T. R. 2003. Glutamine prevents cytokine-induced apoptosis in human colonic epithelial cells. *The Journal of nutrition,* 133, 3065-3071.

Feeney, K., Cain, M. & Nowak, A. K. 2007. Chemotherapy induced nausea and vomiting--prevention and treatment. *Aust Fam Physician,* 36, 702-6.

Ferreira, T. M., Leonel, A. J., Melo, M. A., Santos, R. R., Cara, D. C., Cardoso, V. N., Correia, M. I. & Alvarez-Leite, J. I. 2012. Oral supplementation of butyrate reduces mucositis and intestinal permeability associated with 5-Fluorouracil administration. *Lipids,* 47, 669-78.

Ferrell, B. R., Coyle, N. & Paice, J. 2015. *Oxford Textbook of Palliative Nursing*, Oxford University Press.

Fleming, M. A., Ehsan, L., Moore, S. R., and Levin, D. E. 2020. The Enteric Nervous System and its Emerging Role as a Therapeutic Target. *Gastroenterol. Res. Pract.* 2020, 8024171.

Ford, A. C. & Suares, N. C. 2011. Effect of laxatives and pharmacological therapies in chronic idiopathic constipation: systematic review and meta-analysis. *Gut,* 60, 209-18.

Fram, R. J. 1992. Cisplatin and platinum analogues: recent advances. *Curr Opin Oncol,* 4, 1073-9.

Freitas, A. C. C., Campos, L., Brandao, T. B., Cristófaro, M., Eduardo, F. D. P., Luiz, A. C., Marques, M. M., Eduardo, C. D. P. & Simoes, A. 2014. Chemotherapy-induced oral mucositis: effect of LED and laser phototherapy treatment protocols. *Photomedicine and Laser surgery,* 32, 81-87.

Fujio, T., Nakashima, K., Naito, T., Kobayashi, H., Omori, S., Wakuda, K., Ono, A., Kenmotsu, H., Murakami, H. & Takahashi, T. 2019. Platinum Combination Chemotherapy Is Poorly Tolerated in Malnourished Advanced Lung Cancer Patients with Poor Performance Status. *Nutrition and Cancer,* 71, 767-771.

Furness, J. B. 2012. The enteric nervous system and neurogastroenterology. *Nat Rev Gastroenterol Hepatol,* 9, 286-94.

Furness, J. B., Callaghan, B. P., Rivera, L. R. & Cho, H. J. 2014. The enteric nervous system and gastrointestinal innervation: integrated local and central control. *Adv Exp Med Biol,* 817, 39-71.

Gao, H., Liu, D., Tong, J., Han, J., Liu, B., Zhu, S., Huang, L., Yao, Y., Yu, S. & Fu, Q. 2020. Weight Loss and Gastrointestinal Symptoms in Advanced Cancer Patients Treated with Platinum-based Chemotherapy. *Journal of Nutritional Oncology,* 5, 97-104.

Garcia-Recio, S. & Gascón, P. 2015. Biological and Pharmacological Aspects of the NK1-Receptor. *Biomed Res Int,* 2015, 495704.

Gelevert, T., Messerschmidt, J., Meinardi, M. T., Alt, F., Gietema, J. A., Franke, J. P., Sleijfer, D. T. & Uges, D. R. 2001. Adsorptive voltametry to determine platinum levels in plasma from testicular cancer patients treated with cisplatin. *Ther Drug Monit,* 23, 169-73.

Ghisoni, E., Casalone, V., Giannone, G., Mittica, G., Tuninetti, V. & Valabrega, G. 2019. Role of Mediterranean diet in preventing platinum based gastrointestinal toxicity in gynecolocological malignancies: A single Institution experience. *World Journal of Clinical Oncology,* 10, 391-401.

Gibson, R. J. & Keefe, D. M. 2006a. Cancer chemotherapy-induced diarrhoea and constipation: mechanisms of damage and prevention strategies. *Support Care Cancer,* 14, 890-900.

Gibson, R. J. & Keefe, D. M. K. 2006b. Cancer chemotherapy-induced diarrhoea and constipation: mechanisms of damage and prevention strategies. *Supportive Care in Cancer,* 14, 890.

Gibson, R. J. & Stringer, A. M. 2009. Chemotherapy-induced diarrhoea. *Curr Opin Support Palliat Care,* 3, 31-5.

Gibson, R. J., Bowen, J. M., Inglis, M. R., Cummins, A. G. & Keefe, D. M. 2003. Irinotecan causes severe small intestinal damage, as well as colonic damage, in the rat with implanted breast cancer. *Journal of Gastroenterology and Hepatology,* 18, 1095-1100.

Gibson, R. J., Keefe, D. M. K., Lalla, R. V., Bateman, E., Blijlevens, N., Fijlstra, M., King, E. E., Stringer, A. M., Van Der Velden, W. J. F. M., Yazbeck, R., Elad, S., Bowen, J. M. & For The Mucositis Study Group Of The Multinational Association Of Supportive Care In Cancer/International Society Of Oral Oncology (MASCC/ISOO). 2013. Systematic review of agents for the management of gastrointestinal mucositis in cancer patients. *Supportive Care in Cancer,* 21, 313-326.

Goh, I., Lai, O., & Chew, L. 2018. Prevalence and Risk of Polypharmacy Among Elderly Cancer Patients Receiving Chemotherapy in Ambulatory Oncology Setting. *Current oncology reports*, 20(5), 38.

Goldstein, A. M., Hofstra, R. M. W. & Burns, A. J. 2013. Building a brain in the gut: development of the enteric nervous system. *Clinical genetics,* 83, 307-316.

Gralla, R., Lichinitser, M., Van Der Vegt, S., Sleeboom, H., Mezger, J., Peschel, C., Tonini, G., Labianca, R., Macciocchi, A. & Aapro, M. 2003. Palonosetron improves prevention of chemotherapy-induced nausea and vomiting following moderately emetogenic chemotherapy: results of a double-blind randomized phase III trial comparing single doses of palonosetron with ondansetron. *Ann Oncol,* 14, 1570-7.

Grimison, P., Mersiades, A., Kirby, A., Lintzeris, N., Morton, R., Haber, P., Olver, I., Walsh, A., Mcgregor, I., Cheung, Y., Tognela, A., Hahn, C., Briscoe, K., Aghmesheh, M., Fox, P., Abdi, E., Clarke, S., Della-Fiorentina, S., Shannon, J., Gedye, C., Begbie, S., Simes, J. & Stockler, M. 2020. Oral THC:CBD cannabis extract for refractory chemotherapy-induced nausea and vomiting: a randomised, placebo-controlled, phase II crossover trial. *Ann Oncol,* 31, 1553-1560.

Grunberg, S. M., Slusher, B. & Rugo, H. S. 2013. Emerging Treatments in Chemotherapy-Induced Nausea and Vomiting. *Clinical Advances in Hematology & Oncology* 11, 1–18.

Grunberg, S., Chua, D., Maru, A., Dinis, J., Devandry, S., Boice, J. A., Hardwick, J. S., Beckford, E., Taylor, A., Carides, A., Roila, F. & Herrstedt, J. 2011. Single-dose fosaprepitant for the prevention of chemotherapy-induced nausea and vomiting associated with cisplatin therapy: randomized, double-blind study protocol--EASE. *J Clin Oncol,* 29, 1495-501.

Grundy, D. & Brookes, S. 2011. Neural control of gastrointestinal function. Colloquium Series on Integrated Systems Physiology: From Molecule to Function, Morgan & Claypool Life Sciences, 1-134.

Hamadani, M., Chaudhary, L., Awan, F., Khan, J., Kojouri, K., Ozer, H. & Tfayli, A. 2007. Management of platinum-based chemotherapy-induced acute nausea and vomiting: Is there a superior serotonin receptor antagonist? *Journal of Oncology Pharmacy Practice: official publication of the International Society of Oncology Pharmacy Practitioners,* 13, 69-75.

Hamaguchi, T., Fukudo, S., Kanazawa, M., Tomiie, T., Shimizu, K., Oyama, M. & Sakurai, K. 2008. Changes in salivary physiological stress markers induced by muscle stretching in patients with irritable bowel syndrome. *BioPsychoSocial Medicine,* 2, 1-8.

Hanai, A., Ishiguro, H., Sozu, T., Tsuda, M., Arai, H., Mitani, A. & Tsuboyama, T. 2016. Effects of a self-management program on antiemetic-induced constipation during chemotherapy among breast cancer patients: a randomized controlled clinical trial. *Breast Cancer Research and Treatment,* 155, 99-107.

Hanigan, M. H., Frierson, H. F., Jr., Brown, J. E., Lovell, M. A. & Taylor, P. T. 1994. Human ovarian tumors express gamma-glutamyl transpeptidase. *Cancer Res,* 54, 286-90.

Harris, D. J., Eilers, J., Harriman, A., Cashavelly, B. J. & Maxwell, C. 2008. Putting evidence into practice®: evidence-based interventions for the management of oral mucositis. *Clinical Journal of Oncology Nursing,* 12, 141-152.

Hashimoto, H., Abe, M., Tokuyama, O., Mizutani, H., Uchitomi, Y., Yamaguchi, T., Hoshina, Y., Sakata, Y., Takahashi, T. Y., Nakashima, K., Nakao, M., Takei, D., Zenda, S., Mizukami, K., Iwasa, S., Sakurai, M., Yamamoto, N. & Ohe, Y. 2020. Olanzapine 5 mg plus standard antiemetic therapy for the prevention of chemotherapy-induced nausea and vomiting (J-FORCE): a multicentre, randomised, double-blind, placebo-controlled, phase 3 trial. *Lancet Oncol,* 21, 242-249.

Hawkins, R. & Grunberg, S. 2009. Chemotherapy-induced nausea and vomiting: challenges and opportunities for improved patient outcomes. *Clin J Oncol Nurs,* 13, 54-64.

He, M., Xu, R., Liu, M., Zhang, Y., Yi, F., Wei, Y., Liu, Q. & Zhang, W. 2021. Use of dexamethasone and a 5-HT3 receptor antagonist with or without aprepitant to prevent chemotherapy-induced nausea and vomiting among patients with lung cancer who are treated with platinum-based chemotherapy: a systematic review and meta-analysis of randomized controlled trials. *Annals of Palliative Medicine,* 10, 4308-4319.

Hébuterne, X., Lemarié, E., Michallet, M., De Montreuil, C. B., Schneider, S. M. & Goldwasser, F. 2014. Prevalence of Malnutrition and Current Use of Nutrition Support in Patients With Cancer. *Journal of Parenteral and Enteral Nutrition,* 38, 196-204.

Hegerova, L. T., Leal, A. D., Grendahl, D. C., Seisler, D. K., Sorgatz, K. M., Anderson, K. J., Hilger, C. R. & Loprinzi, C. L. 2015. An analysis of fosaprepitant-induced venous toxicity in patients receiving highly emetogenic chemotherapy. *Supportive Care in Cancer: official journal of the Multinational Association of Supportive Care in Cancer,* 23, 55-59.

Hejna, M., Köstler, W., Raderer, M., Steger, G., Brodowicz, T., Scheithauer, W., Wiltschke, C. & Zielinski, C. 2001. Decrease of duration and symptoms in chemotherapy-induced oral mucositis by topical GM-CSF: results of a prospective randomised trial. *European Journal of Cancer,* 37, 1994-2002.

Herbers, A. H. E., Van Der Velden, W. J. F. M., De Haan, A. F. J., Donnelly, J. P. & Blijlevens, N. M. A. 2014b. Impact of palifermin on intestinal mucositis of HSCT recipients after BEAM. *Bone Marrow Transplantation,* 49, 8-10.

Herbers, A. H., De Haan, A. F., Van Der Velden, W. J., Donnelly, J. P. & Blijlevens, N. M. 2014a. Mucositis not neutropenia determines bacteremia among hematopoietic stem cell transplant recipients. *Transpl Infect Dis,* 16, 279-85.

Herrstedt, J. & Dombernowsky, P. 2007. Anti-emetic therapy in cancer chemotherapy: current status. *Basic Clin Pharmacol Toxicol,* 101, 143-50.

Herrstedt, J. 2008. Antiemetics: an update and the MASCC guidelines applied in clinical practice. *Nat Clin Pract Oncol,* 5, 32-43.

Herrstedt, J., Lindberg, S. & Petersen, P. C. 2022. Prevention of Chemotherapy-Induced Nausea and Vomiting in the Older Patient: Optimizing Outcomes. *Drugs & Aging. 39*(1), 1–21.

Hesketh, P. J. 2008. Chemotherapy-induced nausea and vomiting. *N Engl J Med,* 358, 2482-94.

Hesketh, P. J., Aapro, M., Street, J. C. & Carides, A. D. 2010. Evaluation of risk factors predictive of nausea and vomiting with current standard-of-care antiemetic treatment: analysis of two phase III trials of aprepitant in patients receiving cisplatin-based chemotherapy. *Support Care Cancer,* 18, 1171-7.

Hesketh, P. J., Kris, M. G., Basch, E., Bohlke, K., Barbour, S. Y., Clark-Snow, R. A., Danso, M. A., Dennis, K., Dupuis, L. L., Dusetzina, S. B., Eng, C., Feyer, P. C., Jordan, K., Noonan, K., Sparacio, D. & Lyman, G. H. 2020. Antiemetics: ASCO Guideline Update. *J Clin Oncol,* 38, 2782-2797.

Hesketh, P. J., Palmas, M. & Nicolas, P. 2018. Preventing chemotherapy-induced nausea and vomiting in patients with lung cancer: efficacy of NEPA (netupitant-palonosetron), the first combination antiemetic. *Supportive Care in Cancer: official journal of the Multinational Association of Supportive Care in Cancer,* 26, 1151-1159.

Hesketh, P. J., Van Belle, S., Aapro, M., Tattersall, F. D., Naylor, R. J., Hargreaves, R., Carides, A. D., Evans, J. K. & Horgan, K. J. 2003. Differential involvement of neurotransmitters through the time course of cisplatin-induced emesis as revealed by therapy with specific receptor antagonists. *Eur J Cancer,* 39, 1074-80.

Ho, C. M., Ho, S. T., Wang, J. J., Tsai, S. K. & Chai, C. Y. 2004. Dexamethasone has a central antiemetic mechanism in decerebrated cats. *Anesth Analg,* 99, 734-9, table of contents.

Hocking, C. M. & Kichenadasse, G. 2014. Olanzapine for chemotherapy-induced nausea and vomiting: a systematic review. *Support Care Cancer,* 22, 1143-51.

Hong, C., Gueiros, L. A., Fulton, J. S., Cheng, K., Kandwal, A., Galiti, D., Fall-Dickson, J. M., Johansen, J., Ameringer, S., Kataoka, T., Weikel, D., Eilers, J., Ranna, V., Vaddi, A., Lalla, R. V., Bossi, P., Elad, S., & Mucositis Study Group of the Multinational Association of Supportive Care in Cancer/International Society for Oral Oncology (MASCC/ISOO). 2019. Systematic review of basic oral care for the management of oral mucositis in cancer patients and clinical practice guidelines. *Supportive Care in Cancer: official journal of the Multinational Association of Supportive Care in Cancer, 27*(10), 3949–3967.

Hornby, P. J. 2001. Central neurocircuitry associated with emesis. *Am J Med,* 111 Suppl 8A, 106s-112s.

Hovind, P., Simonsen, L. & Bülow, J. 2010. Decreased leg glucose uptake during exercise contributes to the hyperglycaemic effect of octreotide. *Clinical Physiology and Functional Imaging,* 30, 141-145.

Howard, P., Twycross, R., Shuster, J., Mihalyo, M. & Wilcock, A. 2014. Benzodiazepines. *Journal of Pain and Symptom Management,* 47, 955-964.

Huizinga, J. D. & Lammers, W. J. 2009. Gut peristalsis is governed by a multitude of cooperating mechanisms. *Am J Physiol Gastrointest Liver Physiol,* 296, G1-8.

Ishihara, M., Ikesue, H., Matsunaga, H., Suemaru, K., Kitaichi, K., Suetsugu, K., Oishi, R., Sendo, T., Araki, H. & Itoh, Y. 2012. A multi-institutional study analyzing effect of prophylactic medication for prevention of opioid-induced gastrointestinal dysfunction. *Clin J Pain,* 28, 373-81.

Ito, Y., Karayama, M., Inui, N., Kuroishi, S., Nakano, H., Nakamura, Y., Yokomura, K., Toyoshima, M., Shirai, T., Masuda, M., Yamada, T., Yasuda, K., Hayakawa, H., Suda, T. & Chida, K. 2014. Aprepitant in patients with advanced non-small-cell lung cancer receiving carboplatin-based chemotherapy. *Lung Cancer,* 84, 259-264.

Jandhyala, S. M., Talukdar, R., Subramanyam, C., Vuyyuru, H., Sasikala, M. & Nageshwar Reddy, D. 2015. Role of the normal gut microbiota. *World Journal of Gastroenterology,* 21, 8787-8803.

Janelsins, M. C., Tejani, M. A., Kamen, C., Peoples, A. R., Mustian, K. M. & Morrow, G. R. 2013. Current pharmacotherapy for chemotherapy-induced nausea and vomiting in cancer patients. *Expert Opin Pharmacother,* 14, 757-66.

Janowitz, T., Kleeman, S. & Vonderheide, R. H. 2021. Reconsidering Dexamethasone for Antiemesis when Combining Chemotherapy and Immunotherapy. *The Oncologist,* 26, 269-273.

Jansman, F. G., Sleijfer, D. T., De Graaf, J. C., Coenen, J. L. & Brouwers, J. R. 2001. Management of chemotherapy-induced adverse effects in the treatment of colorectal cancer. *Drug Safety,* 24, 353-367.

Jemal, A., Bray, F., Center, M. M., Ferlay, J., Ward, E. & Forman, D. 2011. Global cancer statistics. *CA Cancer J Clin,* 61, 69-90.

Jim, H. S., Small, B., Faul, L. A., Franzen, J., Apte, S. & Jacobsen, P. B. 2011. Fatigue, depression, sleep, and activity during chemotherapy: daily and intraday variation and relationships among symptom changes. *Annals of Behavioral Medicine,* 42, 321-333.

Jordan, K., Schmoll, H. J. & Aapro, M. S. 2007a. Comparative activity of antiemetic drugs. *Critical Reviews in Oncology/Hematology,* 61, 162-175.

Jordan, K., Sippel, C. & Schmoll, H. J. 2007b. Guidelines for antiemetic treatment of chemotherapy-induced nausea and vomiting: past, present, and future recommendations. *Oncologist,* 12, 1143-50.

Jun, J. Y. 2013. Role of lubiprostone on gastrointestinal motility. *J Neurogastroenterol Motil,* 19, 277-278.

Kamm, M. A., Mueller-Lissner, S., Wald, A., Richter, E., Swallow, R. & Gessner, U. 2011. Oral bisacodyl is effective and well-tolerated in patients with chronic constipation. *Clin Gastroenterol Hepatol,* 9, 577-83.

Kashiwazaki, H., Matsushita, T., Sugita, J., Shigematsu, A., Kasashi, K., Yamazaki, Y., Kanehira, T., Yamamoto, S., Kondo, T. & Endo, T. 2012. Professional oral health care reduces oral mucositis and febrile neutropenia in patients treated with allogeneic bone marrow transplantation. *Supportive Care in Cancer,* 20, 367-373.

Kato, T., Sawamura, Y., Tada, M., Ikeda, J., Ishii, N. & Abe, H. 1998. Cisplatin/vincristine chemotherapy for hypothalamic/visual pathway astrocytomas in young children. *J Neurooncol,* 37, 263-70.

Katranci, N., Ovayolu, N., Ovayolu, O. & Sevinc, A. 2012. Evaluation of the effect of cryotherapy in preventing oral mucositis associated with chemotherapy–a randomized controlled trial. *European Journal of Oncology Nursing,* 16, 339-344.

Keefe, D. M., Schubert, M. M., Elting, L. S., Sonis, S. T., Epstein, J. B., Raber-Durlacher, J. E., Migliorati, C. A., Mcguire, D. B., Hutchins, R. D. & Peterson, D. E. 2007. Updated clinical practice guidelines for the prevention and treatment of mucositis. *Cancer,* 109, 820-831.

Kenward, H., Elliott, J., Lee, T. & Pelligand, L. 2017. Anti-nausea effects and pharmacokinetics of ondansetron, maropitant and metoclopramide in a low-dose cisplatin model of nausea and vomiting in the dog: a blinded crossover study. *BMC Veterinary Research,* 13, 244.

Kim, A. R., Cho, J., Hsu, Y.-J., Choi, M. G., Noh, J. H., Sohn, T. S., Bae, J. M., Yun, Y. H. & Kim, S. 2012. Changes of quality of life in gastric cancer patients after curative resection: a longitudinal cohort study in Korea. *Annals of Surgery,* 256, 1008-1013.

Kim, D. K., Kim, G., Gam, J., Cho, Y. B., Kim, H. T., Tai, J. H., Kim, K. H., Hong, W. S. & Park, J. G. 1994. Synthesis and antitumor activity of a series of [2-substituted-4,5-bis(aminomethyl)-1,3-dioxolane]platinum(II) complexes. *J Med Chem,* 37, 1471-85.

Kim, Y., Kim, S. H., Whang, K. Y., Kim, Y. J. & Oh, S. 2008. Inhibition of Escherichia coli O157:H7 attachment by interactions between lactic acid bacteria and intestinal epithelial cells. *J Microbiol Biotechnol,* 18, 1278-85.

Kimura, M., Usami, E., Kanematsu, T., Iwai, M., Yoshimura, T., Mori, H., Sugiyama, T. & Teramachi, H. 2014. Safety and continuity of second- and third-line therapy with paclitaxel or irinotecan for advanced and recurrent gastric cancer. *Mol Clin Oncol,* 2, 466-472.

Klastersky, J., Ameye, L., Maertens, J., Georgala, A., Muanza, F., Aoun, M., Ferrant, A., Rapoport, B., Rolston, K. & Paesmans, M. 2007. Bacteraemia in febrile neutropenic cancer patients. *Int J Antimicrob Agents,* 30 Suppl 1, S51-9.

Knowles, C. H., Lindberg, G., Panza, E. & De Giorgio, R. 2013. New perspectives in the diagnosis and management of enteric neuropathies. *Nature Reviews Gastroenterology & Hepatology,* 10, 206.

Ko, E.A., Jin, B.J., Namkung, W., Ma, T., Thiagarajah, J. R. & Verkman, A. 2014. Chloride channel inhibition by a red wine extract and a synthetic small molecule prevents rotaviral secretory diarrhoea in neonatal mice. *Gut,* 63, 1120-1129.

Korver, S. K., Gibson, R. J., Bowen, J. M., & Coller, J. K. 2019. Toll-like receptor/ interleukin-1 domain innate immune signalling pathway genetic variants are candidate predictors for severe gastrointestinal toxicity risk following 5-fluorouracil-based chemotherapy. *Cancer Chemotherapy and Pharmacology*, *83*(2), 217–236.

Krishna, S. G., Zhao, W., Grazziutti, M. L., Sanathkumar, N., Barlogie, B. & Anaissie, E. J. 2011. Incidence and risk factors for lower alimentary tract mucositis after 1529 courses of chemotherapy in a homogenous population of oncology patients. *Cancer,* 117, 648-655.

Kuebler, J. P., Colangelo, L., O'connell, M. J., Smith, R. E., Yothers, G., Begovic, M., Robinson, B., Seay, T. E. & Wolmark, N. 2007. Severe enteropathy among patients with stage II/III colon cancer treated on a randomized trial of bolus 5-fluorouracil/leucovorin plus or minus oxaliplatin: a prospective analysis. *Cancer,* 110, 1945-1950.

Kuhn, A., Porto, F. A., Miraglia, P. & Brunetto, A. L. 2009. Low-level infrared laser therapy in chemotherapy-induced oral mucositis: a randomized placebo-controlled trial in children. *Journal of Pediatric Hematology/Oncology,* 31, 33-37.

Kuiken, N. S. S., Rings, E. H. H. M. & Tissing, W. J. E. 2015. Risk analysis, diagnosis and management of gastrointestinal mucositis in pediatric cancer patients. *Critical Reviews in Oncology/Hematology,* 94, 87-97.

Kuizenga, M. H., Sia, T. C., Dodds, K. N., Wiklendt, L., Arkwright, J. W., Thomas, A., Brookes, S. J., Spencer, N. J., Wattchow, D. A. & Dinning, P. G. 2015. Neurally mediated propagating discrete clustered contractions superimposed on myogenic ripples in ex vivo segments of human ileum. *American Journal of Physiology-Gastrointestinal and Liver Physiology,* 308, G1-G11.

Lacy, B. E. & Levy, L. C. 2008. Lubiprostone: a novel treatment for chronic constipation. *Clin Interv Aging,* 3, 357-64.

Lalla, R. V. & Peterson, D. E. 2005. Oral mucositis. *Dent Clin North Am,* 49, 167-84, ix.

Lalla, R. V., Bowen, J., Barasch, A., Elting, L., Epstein, J., Keefe, D. M., Mcguire, D. B., Migliorati, C., Nicolatou-Galitis, O. & Peterson, D. E. 2014. MASCC/ISOO clinical practice guidelines for the management of mucositis secondary to cancer therapy. *Cancer,* 120, 1453-1461.

Lalla, R. V., Sonis, S. T. & Peterson, D. E. 2008. Management of oral mucositis in patients who have cancer. *Dental Clinics of North America,* 52, 61-viii.

Larkin, P. J., Cherny, N. I., La Carpia, D., Guglielmo, M., Ostgathe, C., Scotté, F., Ripamonti, C. I., & ESMO Guidelines Committee (2018). Diagnosis, assessment and management of constipation in advanced cancer: ESMO Clinical Practice Guidelines. *Annals of Oncology: official journal of the European Society for Medical Oncology*, *29*(Suppl 4), iv111–iv125.

Lawrence, T. 2009. The nuclear factor NF-kappaB pathway in inflammation. *Cold Spring Harb Perspect Biol,* 1, a001651.

Lee-Robichaud, H., Thomas, K., Morgan, J. & Nelson, R. L. 2010. Lactulose versus Polyethylene Glycol for Chronic Constipation. *Cochrane Database Syst Rev,* Cd007570.

Lembo, A. & Camilleri, M. 2003. Chronic constipation. *New England Journal of Medicine,* 349, 1360-1368.

Lenfers, B., Loeffler, T., Droege, C. & Hausamen, T. 1999. Substantial activity of budesonide in patients with irinotecan (CPT-11) and 5-fluorouracil induced diarrhea and failure of loperamide treatment. *Annals of Oncology,* 10, 1251-1253.

Leung, L., Riutta, T., Kotecha, J. & Rosser, W. 2011. Chronic constipation: an evidence-based review. *J Am Board Fam Med,* 24, 436-51.

Li, Y., Yu, Z., Liu, F., Tan, L., Wu, B. & Li, J. 2006. Oral glutamine ameliorates chemotherapy-induced changes of intestinal permeability and does not interfere with the antitumor effect of chemotherapy in patients with breast cancer: a prospective randomized trial. *Tumori,* 92, 396-401.

Li, H., Xu, W., Liu, X., Ye, J., Li, P., Shang, F., & Yu, X. 2020. Curcumin Alleviates the Side Effects of Cisplatin on Gastric Emptying of Mice by Inhibiting the Signal Changes of Acetylcholine and Interstitial Cells of Cajal. *Journal of Medicinal Food, 23*(9), 920–927.

Lilleby, K., Garcia, P., Gooley, T., Mcdonnnell, P., Taber, R., Holmberg, L., Maloney, D., Press, O. & Bensinger, W. 2006. A prospective, randomized study of cryotherapy during administration of high-dose melphalan to decrease the severity and duration of oral mucositis in patients with multiple myeloma undergoing autologous peripheral blood stem cell transplantation. *Bone Marrow Transplantation,* 37, 1031-1035.

Lin, X. B., Dieleman, L. A., Ketabi, A., Bibova, I., Sawyer, M. B., Xue, H., Field, C. J., Baracos, V. E. & Gänzle, M. G. 2012. Irinotecan (CPT-11) Chemotherapy Alters Intestinal Microbiota in Tumour Bearing Rats. *PLOS ONE,* 7, e39764.

Liu, J. Y., Qu, K., Sferruzza, A. D. & Bender, R. A. 2007. Distribution of the UGT1A1*28 polymorphism in Caucasian and Asian populations in the US: a genomic analysis of 138 healthy individuals. *Anticancer Drugs,* 18, 693-6.

Logan, R. M., Gibson, R. J., Bowen, J. M., Stringer, A. M., Sonis, S. T. & Keefe, D. M. 2008. Characterisation of mucosal changes in the alimentary tract following administration of irinotecan: implications for the pathobiology of mucositis. *Cancer Chemother Pharmacol,* 62, 33-41.

Logan, R. M., Gibson, R. J., Sonis, S. T. & Keefe, D. M. 2007. Nuclear factor-kappaB (NF-kappaB) and cyclooxygenase-2 (COX-2) expression in the oral mucosa following cancer chemotherapy. *Oral Oncol,* 43, 395-401.

Logan, R. M., Al-Azri, A. R., Bossi, P., Stringer, A. M., Joy, J. K., Soga, Y., Ranna, V., Vaddi, A., Raber-Durlacher, J. E., Lalla, R. V., Cheng, K., Elad, S., & Mucositis Study Group of the Multinational Association of Supportive Care in Cancer/International Society of Oral Oncology (MASCC/ISOO). 2020. Systematic review of growth factors and cytokines for the management of oral mucositis in cancer patients and clinical practice guidelines. *Supportive Care in Cancer: official journal of the Multinational Association of Supportive Care in Cancer, 28*(5), 2485–2498.

López-Gómez, L., Díaz-Ruano, S., Girón, R., López-Pérez, A. E., Vera, G., Herradón Pliego, E., López-Miranda, V., Nurgali, K., Martín-Fontelles, M. I., Uranga, J. A. & Abalo, R. 2018. Preclinical evaluation of the effects on the gastrointestinal tract of the antineoplastic drug vincristine repeatedly administered to rats. *Neurogastroenterol Motil,* 30, e13399.

Malhotra, J., Mhango, G., Gomez, J. E., Smith, C., Galsky, M. D., Strauss, G. M. & Wisnivesky, J. P. 2015. Adjuvant chemotherapy for elderly patients with stage I non-small-cell lung cancer ≥4 cm in size: an SEER–Medicare analysis. *Annals of Oncology,* 26, 768-773.

Mancini, I. & Bruera, E. 1998. Constipation in advanced cancer patients. *Supportive Care in Cancer,* 6, 356-364.

Manz, F., Johner, S., Wentz, A., Boeing, H. & Remer, T. 2011. Water balance throughout the adult life span in a German population. *The British Journal of Nutrition,* 107, 1673-81.

Marian, M. & August, D. A. 2014. Prevalence of malnutrition and current use of nutrition support in cancer patient study. *JPEN J Parenter Enteral Nutr,* 38, 163-5.

Martin, B. R. & Wiley, J. L. 2004. Mechanism of action of cannabinoids: how it may lead to treatment of cachexia, emesis, and pain. *J Support Oncol,* 2, 305-14; discussion 314-6.

Martins, F., De Oliveira, M. A., Wang, Q., Sonis, S., Gallottini, M., George, S. & Treister, N. 2013. A review of oral toxicity associated with mTOR inhibitor therapy in cancer patients. *Oral Oncol,* 49, 293-8.

Masri, Y., Abubaker, J. & Ahmed, R. 2010. Prophylactic use of laxative for constipation in critically ill patients. *Ann Thorac Med,* 5, 228-31.

Matsumoto, M. & Benno, Y. 2007. The relationship between microbiota and polyamine concentration in the human intestine: a pilot study. *Microbiol Immunol,* 51, 25-35.

Mccollum, A. D., Catalano, P. J., Haller, D. G., Mayer, R. J., Macdonald, J. S., Benson, A. B., 3rd & Fuchs, C. S. 2002. Outcomes and toxicity in african-american and caucasian patients in a randomized adjuvant chemotherapy trial for colon cancer. *J Natl Cancer Inst,* 94, 1160-7.

Mcilfatrick, S., Muldrew, D. H. L., Beck, E., Carduff, E., Clarke, M., Finucane, A., Graham-Wisener, L., Larkin, P., Mccorry, N. K., Slater, P. & Hasson, F. 2019. Examining constipation assessment and management of patients with advanced cancer receiving specialist palliative care: a multi-site retrospective case note review of clinical practice. *BMC Palliat Care,* 18, 57.

Mcquade, R. M., Stojanovska, V., Abalo, R., Bornstein, J. C. & Nurgali, K. 2016a. Chemotherapy-Induced Constipation and Diarrhea: Pathophysiology, Current and Emerging Treatments. *Front Pharmacol,* 7, 414.

Mcquade, R. M., Stojanovska, V., Bornstein, J. C. & Nurgali, K. 2017. Colorectal Cancer Chemotherapy: The Evolution of Treatment and New Approaches. *Curr Med Chem,* 24, 1537-1557.

Mcquade, R. M., Stojanovska, V., Donald, E., Abalo, R., Bornstein, J. C. & Nurgali, K. 2016b. Gastrointestinal dysfunction and enteric neurotoxicity following treatment with anticancer chemotherapeutic agent 5-fluorouracil. *Neurogastroenterol Motil,* 28, 1861-1875.

McQuade, R. M., Carbone, S. E., Stojanovska, V., Rahman, A., Gwynne, R. M., Robinson, A. M., Goodman, C. A., Bornstein, J. C., & Nurgali, K. 2016c. Role of oxidative stress in oxaliplatin-induced enteric neuropathy and colonic dysmotility in mice. *British Journal of Pharmacology*, *173*(24), 3502–3521.

McQuade. R., Bornstein. J. & Nurgali. K. 2014. Anti-Colorectal Cancer Chemotherapy-Induced Diarrhoea: Current Treatments and Side Effects. *International Journal of Clinical Medicine*, 5, 393-406.

McQuade, R. M., Stojanovska V., Donald, E. L., Rahman, A. A., Campelj, D. G., Abalo, R., Rybalka, E., Bornstein, J. C., & Nurgali, K. 2017. Irinotecan-Induced Gastrointestinal Dysfunction Is Associated with Enteric Neuropathy, but Increased Numbers of Cholinergic Myenteric Neurons. *Frontiers in Physiology*, 8, 391.

McQuade, R. M., Stojanovska, V., Stavely, R., Timpani, C., Petersen, A. C., Abalo, R., Bornstein, J. C., Rybalka, E., & Nurgali K. 2018. Oxaliplatin-induced enteric neuronal loss and intestinal dysfunction is prevented by co-treatment with BGP-15. *British Journal of Pharmacology*, 175(4), 656-677.

Meiri, E., Jhangiani, H., Vredenburgh, J. J., Barbato, L. M., Carter, F. J., Yang, H. M. & Baranowski, V. 2007. Efficacy of dronabinol alone and in combination with ondansetron versus ondansetron alone for delayed chemotherapy-induced nausea and vomiting. *Curr Med Res Opin,* 23, 533-43.

Meyerhardt, J. A., Tepper, J. E., Niedzwiecki, D., Hollis, D. R., Mccollum, A. D., Brady, D., O'connell, M. J., Mayer, R. J., Cummings, B., Willett, C., Macdonald, J. S., Benson, A. B., 3rd & Fuchs, C. S. 2004. Impact of body mass index on outcomes and treatment-related toxicity in patients with stage II and III rectal cancer: findings from Intergroup Trial 0114. *J Clin Oncol,* 22, 648-57.

Miedema, K. G., Te Poele, E. M., Tissing, W. J., Postma, D. S., Koppelman, G. H., De Pagter, A. P., Kamps, W. A., Alizadeh, B. Z., Boezen, H. M. & De Bont, E. S. 2011. Association of polymorphisms in the TLR4 gene with the risk of developing neutropenia in children with leukemia. *Leukemia,* 25, 995-1000.

Migliorati, C. A., Oberle-Edwards, L. & Schubert, M. 2006. The role of alternative and natural agents, cryotherapy, and/or laser for management of alimentary mucositis. *Supportive Care in Cancer,* 14, 533-540.

Migliorati, C., Hewson, I., Lalla, R. V., Antunes, H. S., Estilo, C. L., Hodgson, B., Lopes, N. N., Schubert, M. M., Bowen, J., Elad, S., & Mucositis Study Group of the Multinational Association of Supportive Care in Cancer/International Society of Oral Oncology (MASCC/ISOO). 2013. Systematic review of laser and other light therapy for the management of oral mucositis in cancer patients. *Supportive Care in Cancer: official journal of the Multinational Association of Supportive Care in Cancer*, *21*(1), 333–341.

Miranzadeh, S., Adib-Hajbaghery, M., Soleymanpoor, L. & Ehsani, M. 2014. A New mouthwash for Chemotherapy Induced Stomatitis. *Nursing and Midwifery Studies,* 3, e20249-e20249.

Mitchell, E. P. 2006. Gastrointestinal Toxicity of Chemotherapeutic Agents. *Seminars in Oncology,* 33, 106-120.

Mlcouskova, J., Stepankova, J. & Brabec, V. 2012. Antitumor carboplatin is more toxic in tumor cells when photoactivated: enhanced DNA binding. *Journal of Biological Inorganic Chemistry: JBIC: a publication of the Society of Biological Inorganic Chemistry,* 17, 891-898.

Molassiotis, A., Aapro, M., Dicato, M., Gascon, P., Novoa, S. A., Isambert, N., Burke, T. A., Gu, A. & Roila, F. 2014. Evaluation of risk factors predicting chemotherapy-related nausea and vomiting: results from a European prospective observational study. *J Pain Symptom Manage,* 47, 839-848.e4.

Morio, K., Minami, T., Sozu, T., Niki, K., Kijima, T., Uejima, E. & Morio, K. 2016. Weight Loss Associated with Platinum-Based Chemotherapy in Patients with Advanced Lung Cancer. *Chemotherapy,* 61, 256-261.

Mortimer, T. L., Mabin, T. & Engelbrecht, A. M. 2019. Cannabinoids: the lows and the highs of chemotherapy-induced nausea and vomiting. *Future Oncol,* 15, 1035-1049.

Motoori, M., Yano, M., Miyata, H., Sugimura, K., Saito, T., Omori, T., Fujiwara, Y., Miyoshi, N., Akita, H., Gotoh, K., Takahashi, H., Kobayashi, S., Noura, S., Ohue, M., Asahara, T., Nomoto, K., Ishikawa, O. & Sakon, M. 2017. Randomized study of the effect of synbiotics during neoadjuvant chemotherapy on adverse events in esophageal cancer patients. *Clinical Nutrition,* 36, 93-99.

Mueller-Lissner, S., Kamm, M. A., Wald, A., Hinkel, U., Koehler, U., Richter, E. & Bubeck, J. 2010. Multicenter, 4-week, double-blind, randomized, placebo-controlled trial of sodium picosulfate in patients with chronic constipation. *Am J Gastroenterol,* 105, 897-903.

Mukhopadhyay, S., Kwatra, G., Alice K, P. & Badyal, D. 2017. Role of olanzapine in chemotherapy-induced nausea and vomiting on platinum-based chemotherapy patients: a randomized controlled study. *Supportive Care in Cancer,* 25, 145-154.

Müller-Lissner, S., Bassotti, G., Coffin, B., Drewes, A. M., Breivik, H., Eisenberg, E., Emmanuel, A., Laroche, F., Meissner, W. & Morlion, B. 2017. Opioid-Induced Constipation and Bowel Dysfunction: A Clinical Guideline. *Pain Medicine (Malden, Mass.),* 18, 1837-1863.

Muscaritoli, M., Lucia, S., Farcomeni, A., Lorusso, V., Saracino, V., Barone, C., Plastino, F., Gori, S., Magarotto, R., Carteni, G., Chiurazzi, B., Pavese, I., Marchetti, L., Zagonel, V., Bergo, E., Tonini, G., Imperatori, M., Iacono, C., Maiorana, L., Pinto, C., ... PreMiO Study Group. 2017. Prevalence of malnutrition in patients at first medical oncology visit: the PreMiO study. *Oncotarget*, *8*(45), 79884–79896.

Naidu, M. U. R., Ramana, G. V., Rani, P. U., Mohan, I. K., Suman, A. & Roy, P. 2004. Chemotherapy-induced and/or radiation therapy-induced oral mucositis--complicating the treatment of cancer. *Neoplasia (New York, N.Y.),* 6, 423-431.

Nardini, P., Pini, A., Bessard, A., Duchalais, E., Niccolai, E., Neunlist, M., & Vannucchi, M. G. 2020. GLP-2 Prevents Neuronal and Glial Changes in the Distal Colon of Mice Chronically Treated with Cisplatin. *International Journal of Molecular Sciences*, *21*(22), 8875.Navari, R. M. & Aapro, M. 2016. Antiemetic Prophylaxis for Chemotherapy-Induced Nausea and Vomiting. *N Engl J Med,* 374, 1356-67.

Navari, R. M. 2014. Olanzapine for the prevention and treatment of chronic nausea and chemotherapy-induced nausea and vomiting. *Eur J Pharmacol,* 722, 180-6.

Navari, R. M., Qin, R., Ruddy, K. J., Liu, H., Powell, S. F., Bajaj, M., Dietrich, L., Biggs, D., Lafky, J. M. & Loprinzi, C. L. 2016. Olanzapine for the Prevention of Chemotherapy-Induced Nausea and Vomiting. *New England Journal of Medicine,* 375, 134-142.

Navari, R. M. & Aapro, M. 2016. Antiemetic Prophylaxis for Chemotheraphy-Induced Nausea and Vomiting. *The New England Journal of Medicine*, 374(14), 1356-1367.

Nayak, R. R., Alexander, M., Deshpande, I., Stapleton-Gray, K., Rimal, B., Patterson, A. D., Ubeda, C., Scher, J. U. & Turnbaugh, P. J. 2021. Methotrexate impacts conserved pathways in diverse human gut bacteria leading to decreased host immune activation. *Cell Host Microbe,* 29, 362-377.e11.

Niioka, T., Uno, T., Yasui-Furukori, N., Takahata, T., Shimizu, M., Sugawara, K. & Tateishi, T. 2007. Pharmacokinetics of low-dose nedaplatin and validation of AUC prediction in patients with non-small-cell lung carcinoma. *Cancer Chemother Pharmacol,* 59, 575-80.

Nishii, M., Soutome, S., Kawakita, A., Yutori, H., Iwata, E., Akashi, M., Hasegawa, T., Kojima, Y., Funahara, M., Umeda, M., & Komori, T. 2020. Factors associated with severe oral mucositis and candidiasis in patients undergoing radiotherapy for oral and oropharyngeal carcinomas: a retrospective multicenter study of 326 patients. *Supportive care in cancer: official journal of the Multinational Association of Supportive Care in Cancer*, *28*(3), 1069–1075.

Nonzee, N. J., Dandade, N. A., Patel, U., Markossian, T., Agulnik, M., Argiris, A., Patel, J. D., Kern, R. C., Munshi, H. G., Calhoun, E. A. & Bennett, C. L. 2008. Evaluating the supportive care costs of severe radiochemotherapy-induced mucositis and pharyngitis: results from a Northwestern University Costs of Cancer Program pilot study with head and neck and nonsmall cell lung cancer patients who received care at a county hospital, a Veterans Administration hospital, or a comprehensive cancer care center. *Cancer,* 113, 1446-52.

Novak, J. A. & Amini, A. 2021. Mucositis. *In:* TODD, K. H., THOMAS, J. C. R. & ALAGAPPAN, K. (eds.) *Oncologic Emergency Medicine: Principles and Practice.* Cham: Springer International Publishing.

O'mahony, S., Coyle, N. & Payne, R. 2001. Current management of opioid-related side effects. *Oncology (Williston Park, NY),* 15, 61-73.

Okabe, K., Beppu, T., Haraoka, K., Oh-Uchida, Y., Yamamura, S., Tomiyasu, S., Yamanaka, T., Sano, O., Masuda, T., Chikamoto, A., Fujiyama, S. & Baba, H. 2011. Safety and Short-term Therapeutic Effects of Miriplatin–Lipiodol Suspension in Transarterial Chemoembolization (TACE) for Hepatocellular Carcinoma. *Anticancer Research,* 31, 2983.

Osaka, I., Ishiki, H., Yokota, T., Tada, Y., Sato, H., Okamoto, M., & Satomi, E. 2019. Safety and efficacy of naldemedine in cancer patients with opioid-induced constipation: a pooled, subgroup analysis of two randomised controlled studies. *ESMO open*, *4*(4), e000527.

Oun, R., Moussa, Y. E. & Wheate, N. J. 2018. The side effects of platinum-based chemotherapy drugs: a review for chemists. *Dalton Transactions,* 47, 6645-6653.

Papadeas, E., Naxakis, S., Riga, M. & Kalofonos, C. 2007. Prevention of 5-fluorouracil-related stomatitis by oral cryotherapy: a randomized controlled study. *European Journal of Oncology Nursing,* 11, 60-65.

Parkhill, A. L. 2013. Oral Mucositis and Stomatitis Associated with Conventional and Targeted Anticancer Therapy. *Journal of Pharmacovigilance,* 1:4.

Pashankar, F. D., Season, J. H., Mcnamara, J. & Pashankar, D. S. 2011. Acute Constipation in Children Receiving Chemotherapy for Cancer. *Journal of Pediatric Hematology/Oncology,* 33.

Passik, S. D., Navari, R. M., Jung, S. H., Nagy, C., Vinson, J., Kirsh, K. L. & Loehrer, P. 2004. A phase I trial of olanzapine (Zyprexa) for the prevention of delayed emesis in cancer patients: a Hoosier Oncology Group study. *Cancer Invest,* 22, 383-8.

Patel, P., Robinson, P. D., Thackray, J., Flank, J., Holdsworth, M. T., Gibson, P., Orsey, A., Portwine, C., Freedman, J., Madden, J. R., Phillips, R., Sung, L. & Dupuis, L. L. 2017. Guideline for the prevention of acute chemotherapy-induced nausea and vomiting in pediatric cancer patients: A focused update. *Pediatr Blood Cancer,* 64.

Pavesi, V. C., Lopez, T. C., Martins, M. A., Sant'ana Filho, M., Bussadori, S. K., Fernandes, K. P., Mesquita-Ferrari, R. A. & Martins, M. D. 2011. Healing action of topical chamomile on 5-fluoracil induced oral mucositis in hamster. *Support Care Cancer,* 19, 639-46.

Peery, A. F., Dellon, E. S., Lund, J., Crockett, S. D., Mcgowan, C. E., Bulsiewicz, W. J., Gangarosa, L. M., Thiny, M. T., Stizenberg, K., Morgan, D. R., Ringel, Y., Kim, H. P., Dibonaventura, M. D., Carroll, C. F., Allen, J. K., Cook, S. F., Sandler, R. S., Kappelman, M. D. & Shaheen, N. J. 2012. Burden of gastrointestinal disease in the United States: 2012 update. *Gastroenterology,* 143, 1179-1187.e3.

Peralta-Mamani, M., da Silva, B. M., da Silva Pinto, A. C., Rubira-Bullen, I., Honório, H. M., Rubira, C., & da Silva Santos, P. S. 2019. Low-level laser therapy dosimetry most used for oral mucositis due to radiotherapy for head and neck cancer: a systematic review and meta-analysis. *Critical reviews in Oncology/Hematology*, *138*, 14–23.

Perwitasari, D. A., Wessels, J. A. M., Van Der Straaten, R. J. H. M., Baak-Pablo, R. F., Mustofa, M., Hakimi, M., Nortier, J. W. R., Gelderblom, H. & Guchelaar, H.-J. 2011. Association of ABCB1, 5-HT3B Receptor and CYP2D6 Genetic Polymorphisms with Ondansetron and Metoclopramide Antiemetic Response in Indonesian Cancer Patients Treated with Highly Emetogenic Chemotherapy. *Japanese Journal of Clinical Oncology,* 41, 1168-1176.

Peterson, D. E., Jones, J. B. & Petit, R. G. 2007. Randomized, placebo-controlled trial of Saforis for prevention and treatment of oral mucositis in breast cancer patients receiving anthracycline-based chemotherapy. *Cancer,* 109, 322-331.

Peterson, D. E., O'shaughnessy, J. A., Rugo, H. S., Elad, S., Schubert, M. M., Viet, C. T., Campbell-Baird, C., Hronek, J., Seery, V., Divers, J., Glaspy, J., Schmidt, B. L. & Meiller, T. F. 2016. Oral mucosal injury caused by mammalian target of rapamycin inhibitors: emerging perspectives on pathobiology and impact on clinical practice. *Cancer Medicine,* 5, 1897-1907.

Phillips, R. J. & Powley, T. L. 2007. Innervation of the gastrointestinal tract: patterns of aging. *Auton Neurosci,* 136, 1-19.

Phillips, R. S., Friend, A. J., Gibson, F., Houghton, E., Gopaul, S., Craig, J. V. & Pizer, B. 2016. Antiemetic medication for prevention and treatment of chemotherapy-induced nausea and vomiting in childhood. *Cochrane Database Syst Rev,* 2, Cd007786.

Pini, A., Garella, R., Idrizaj, E., Calosi, L., Baccari, M. C. & Vannucchi, M. G. 2016. Glucagon-like peptide 2 counteracts the mucosal damage and the neuropathy induced by chronic treatment with cisplatin in the mouse gastric fundus. *Neurogastroenterology & Motility,* 28, 206-216.

Potting, C., Uitterhoeve, R., Op Reimer, W. S. & Van Achterberg, T. 2006. The effectiveness of commonly used mouthwashes for the prevention of chemotherapy-induced oral mucositis: a systematic review. *European Journal of Cancer Care,* 15, 431-439.

Raber-Durlacher, J. E., Elad, S. & Barasch, A. 2010. Oral mucositis. *Oral Oncol,* 46, 452-6.

Ranganath, P., Einhorn, L. & Albany, C. 2015. Management of Chemotherapy Induced Nausea and Vomiting in Patients on Multiday Cisplatin Based Combination Chemotherapy. *BioMed Research International,* 2015, 943618-943618.

Ranna, V., Cheng, K. K. F., Castillo, D. A., Porcello, L., Vaddi, A., Lalla, R. V., Bossi, P. & Elad, S. 2019. Development of the MASCC/ISOO clinical practice guidelines for mucositis: an overview of the methods. *Support Care Cancer,* 27, 3933-3948.

Rao, K. V. & Faso, A. 2012. Chemotherapy-induced nausea and vomiting: optimizing prevention and management. *American Health & Drug Benefits,* 5, 232-240.

Rapoport, B. L. 2014. Efficacy of a triple antiemetic regimen with aprepitant for the prevention of chemotherapy-induced nausea and vomiting: effects of gender, age, and region. *Curr Med Res Opin,* 30, 1875-81.

Rapoport, B. L. 2017. Delayed Chemotherapy-Induced Nausea and Vomiting: Pathogenesis, Incidence, and Current Management. *Frontiers in Pharmacology,* 8, 19-19.

Raymond, E., Faivre, S., Woynarowski, J. M. & Chaney, S. G. 1998. Oxaliplatin: mechanism of action and antineoplastic activity. *Semin Oncol,* 25, 4-12.

Regnard, C., Twycross, R., Mihalyo, M., & Wilcock, A. 2011. Loperamide. *Journal of Pain and Symptom Management, 42*(2), 319–323.

Reyes-Gibby CC, Melkonian SC, Wang J, Yu RK, Shelburne SA, Lu C, Gunn GB, Chambers MS, Hanna EY, Yeung S-CJ, Shete S. 2017. Identifying novel genes and biological processes relevant to the development of cancer therapy-induced mucositis: an informative gene network analysis. *PLoS One.* 12(7):e0180396.

Reyna, J., Luna-Aguilar, F., Cardoso-Yah, G., Rivera-Salgado, M., Limon-Rojas, A. & Galindo-Delgado, P. 2015. Gastric wall perforation secondary to presumed aspergillosis in a pediatric patient with aplastic anemia: A case report. *Journal of Infection in Developing Countries,* 9, 431-4.

Richardson, G. & Dobish, R. 2007. Chemotherapy induced diarrhea. *J Oncol Pharm Pract,* 13, 181-98.

Rivera, L. R., Poole, D. P., Thacker, M. & Furness, J. B. 2011. The involvement of nitric oxide synthase neurons in enteric neuropathies. *Neurogastroenterology & Motility,* 23, 980-988.

Robinson, A. M., Stojanovska, V., Rahman, A. A., Mcquade, R. M., Senior, P. V. & Nurgali, K. 2016. Effects of Oxaliplatin Treatment on the Enteric Glial Cells and Neurons in the Mouse Ileum. *J Histochem Cytochem,* 64, 530-45.

Rojas, C., Stathis, M., Thomas, A. G., Massuda, E. B., Alt, J., Zhang, J., Rubenstein, E., Sebastiani, S., Cantoreggi, S., Snyder, S. H. & Slusher, B. 2008. Palonosetron exhibits unique molecular interactions with the 5-HT3 receptor. *Anesth Analg,* 107, 469-78.

Rojas, C., Thomas, A. G., Alt, J., Stathis, M., Zhang, J., Rubenstein, E. B., Sebastiani, S., Cantoreggi, S. & Slusher, B. S. 2010. Palonosetron triggers 5-HT(3) receptor internalization and causes prolonged inhibition of receptor function. *Eur J Pharmacol,* 626, 193-9.

Rolston, K. V. 2004. The Infectious Diseases Society of America 2002 guidelines for the use of antimicrobial agents in patients with cancer and neutropenia: salient features and comments. *Clin Infect Dis,* 39 Suppl 1, S44-8.

Rubenstein, E. B. 2004. Mucositis Study Section of the Multinational Association for Supportive Care in Cancer; International Society for Oral Oncology. Clinical practice guidelines for the prevention and treatment of cancer therapy-induced oral and gastrointestinal mucositis. *Cancer,* 100, 2026-2046.

Rubenstein, E. B., Peterson, D. E., Schubert, M., Keefe, D., Mcguire, D., Epstein, J., Elting, L. S., Fox, P. C., Cooksley, C. & Sonis, S. T. 2004. Clinical practice guidelines for the prevention and treatment of cancer therapy–induced oral and gastrointestinal mucositis. *Cancer: Interdisciplinary International Journal of the American Cancer Society,* 100, 2026-2046.

Russo, F., Linsalata, M., Clemente, C., D'attoma, B., Orlando, A., Campanella, G., Giotta, F. & Riezzo, G. 2013. The effects of fluorouracil, epirubicin, and cyclophosphamide (FEC60) on the intestinal barrier function and gut peptides in breast cancer patients: an observational study. *BMC Cancer,* 13, 56.

Ruston, T., Hunter, K., Cummings, G. & Lazarescu, A. 2013. Efficacy and side-effect profiles of lactulose, docusate sodium, and sennosides compared to PEG in opioid-induced constipation: a systematic review. *Canadian Oncology Nursing Journal/Revue canadienne de soins infirmiers en oncologie,* 23, 236-240.

Ryan, J. L. 2010. Treatment of Chemotherapy-Induced Nausea in Cancer Patients. *Eur Oncol,* 6, 14-16.

Sada, H., Kajizono, M., Ushio, S., Esumi, S., Kitamura, Y. & Sendo, T. 2020. The Efficacy and Safety of Lubiprostone for Constipation in Cancer Patients Compared with Non-cancer Patients: A Retrospective Cohort Study. *Biological and Pharmaceutical Bulletin,* 43, 1699-1706.

Saito, H., Yoshizawa, H., Yoshimori, K., Katakami, N., Katsumata, N., Kawahara, M. & Eguchi, K. 2013. Efficacy and safety of single-dose fosaprepitant in the prevention of chemotherapy-induced nausea and vomiting in patients receiving high-dose cisplatin: a multicentre, randomised, double-blind, placebo-controlled phase 3 trial. *Ann Oncol,* 24, 1067-73.

Saito, M., Aogi, K., Sekine, I., Yoshizawa, H., Yanagita, Y., Sakai, H., Inoue, K., Kitagawa, C., Ogura, T. & Mitsuhashi, S. 2009. Palonosetron plus dexamethasone versus granisetron plus dexamethasone for prevention of nausea and vomiting during chemotherapy: a double-blind, double-dummy, randomised, comparative phase III trial. *Lancet Oncol,* 10, 115-24.

Sak, K. 2012. Chemotherapy and dietary phytochemical agents. *Chemotherapy Research and Practice,* 2012.

Sánchez-Lara, K., Ugalde-Morales, E., Motola-Kuba, D. & Green, D. 2013. Gastrointestinal symptoms and weight loss in cancer patients receiving chemotherapy. *British Journal of Nutrition,* 109, 894-897.

Sanchez, R. I., Wang, R. W., Newton, D. J., Bakhtiar, R., Lu, P., Chiu, S. H., Evans, D. C. & Huskey, S. E. 2004. Cytochrome P450 3A4 is the major enzyme involved in the metabolism of the substance P receptor antagonist aprepitant. *Drug Metab Dispos,* 32, 1287-92.

Sanger, G. J. 2004. Neurokinin NK1 and NK3 receptors as targets for drugs to treat gastrointestinal motility disorders and pain. *Br J Pharmacol,* 141, 1303-12.

Santoso, J. T., Lucci, J. A., 3rd, Coleman, R. L., Schafer, I. & Hannigan, E. V. 2003. Saline, mannitol, and furosemide hydration in acute cisplatin nephrotoxicity: a randomized trial. *Cancer Chemother Pharmacol,* 52, 13-8.

Saunders, D. P., Rouleau, T., Cheng, K., Yarom, N., Kandwal, A., Joy, J., Bektas Kayhan, K., van de Wetering, M., Brito-Dellan, N., Kataoka, T., Chiang, K., Ranna, V., Vaddi, A., Epstein, J., Lalla, R. V., Bossi, P., Elad, S., & Mucositis Study Group of the Multinational Association of Supportive Care in Cancer/International Society of Oral Oncology (MASCC/ISOO). 2020. Systematic review of antimicrobials, mucosal coating agents, anesthetics, and analgesics for the management of oral mucositis in cancer patients and clinical practice guidelines. *Supportive care in cancer: official journal of the Multinational Association of Supportive Care in Cancer*, *28*(5), 2473–2484.

Scarlett, Y. 2004. Medical management of fecal incontinence. *Gastroenterology,* 126, S55-S63.

Schmoll, H. J., Aapro, M. S., Poli-Bigelli, S., Kim, H. K., Park, K., Jordan, K., Von Pawel, J., Giezek, H., Ahmed, T. & Chan, C. Y. 2006. Comparison of an aprepitant regimen with a multiple-day ondansetron regimen, both with dexamethasone, for antiemetic efficacy in high-dose cisplatin treatment. *Ann Oncol,* 17, 1000-6.

Schneider, E. C., Malin, J. L., Kahn, K. L., Ko, C. Y., Adams, J. & Epstein, A. M. 2007. Surviving colorectal cancer. *Cancer,* 110, 2075-2082.

Schwab, M., Zanger, U. M., Marx, C., Schaeffeler, E., Klein, K., Dippon, J., Kerb, R., Blievernicht, J., Fischer, J., Hofmann, U., Bokemeyer, C. & Eichelbaum, M. 2008. Role of genetic and nongenetic factors for fluorouracil treatment-related severe toxicity: a prospective clinical trial by the German 5-FU Toxicity Study Group. *J Clin Oncol,* 26, 2131-8.

Scully, C., Sonis, S. & Diz, P. D. 2006. Oral mucositis. *Oral Dis,* 12, 229-41.

Shafi, M. A. & Bresalier, R. S. 2010. The gastrointestinal complications of oncologic therapy. *Gastroenterol Clin North Am,* 39, 629-47.

Shan, L., Bai, B., Lv, Y., Xie, B., Huang, X. & Zhu, H. 2018. Lobaplatin suppresses proliferation and peritoneal metastasis of colorectal cancer in a preclinical model. *Biomed Pharmacother,* 108, 486-491.

Sharma, R., Tobin, P. & Clarke, S. J. 2005a. Management of chemotherapy-induced nausea, vomiting, oral mucositis, and diarrhoea. *Lancet Oncol,* 6, 93-102.

Sharma, R., Tobin, P. & Clarke, S. J. 2005b. Management of chemotherapy-induced nausea, vomiting, oral mucositis, and diarrhoea. *The Lancet Oncology,* 6, 93-102.

Shelke, A., Mustian, K. & Morrow, G. 2004. The pathophysiology of treatment-related nausea and vomiting in cancer patients: Current models. *Indian Journal of Physiology and Pharmacology,* 48, 256-68.

Shi, W., Shen, L., Zou, W., Wang, J., Yang, J., Wang, Y., Liu, B., Xie, L., Zhu, J. & Zhang, Z. 2020. The Gut Microbiome Is Associated With Therapeutic Responses and Toxicities of Neoadjuvant Chemoradiotherapy in Rectal Cancer Patients—A Pilot Study. *Frontiers in Cellular and Infection Microbiology,* 10, 562463.

Shimada, M., Itamochi, H. & Kigawa, J. 2013. Nedaplatin: a cisplatin derivative in cancer chemotherapy. *Cancer Management and Research,* 5, 67-76.

Shouval, R., Kouniavski, E., Fein, J., Danylesko, I., Shem-Tov, N., Geva, M., Yerushalmi, R., Shimoni, A. & Nagler, A. 2019. Risk factors and implications of oral mucositis in recipients of allogeneic hematopoietic stem cell transplantation. *Eur J Haematol,* 103, 402-409.

Siemens, W., & Becker, G. 2016. Methylnaltrexone for opioid-induced constipation: review and meta-analyses for objective plus subjective efficacy and safety outcomes. *Therapeutics and Clinical Risk Management*, *12*, 401–412.

Sigel, K., Mhango, G., Cohen, J., Halm, E. A., Mandeli, J., Strauss, G. & Wisnivesky, J. 2013. Outcomes After Adjuvant Platinum-based Chemotherapy in Elderly NSCLC Patients with T4 Disease. *Annals of Surgical Oncology,* 20, 1013-1019.

Silva, M. S., De Andrade Gomes, Y., De Sousa Cavalcante, M. L., Telles, P. V. N., Da Silva, A. C. A., Severo, J. S., De Oliveira Santos, R., Dos Santos, B. L. B., Cavalcante, G. L., Rocha, C. H. L., Palheta-Junior, R. C., De Cássia Meneses Oliveira, R., Dos Santos, R. F., Sabino, J. P. J., Dos Santos, A. A. & Tolentino, M. 2021. Exercise and pyridostigmine prevents gastric emptying delay and increase blood pressure and cisplatin-induced baroreflex sensitivity in rats. *Life Sci,* 267, 118972.

Sirichanchuen, B., Thanomsakcharoen, J., Kaewpan, Y. & Sornsuvit, C. 2019. Chemotherapy Regimen and Incidence of Malnutrition after Chemotherapy in Non-small Cell Lung Cancer. *Journal of Pharmacy and Nutrition Sciences,* 9, 60-65.

Sobue, T., Bertolini, M., Thompson, A., Peterson, D. E., Diaz, P. I. & Dongari-Bagtzoglou, A. 2018. Chemotherapy-induced oral mucositis and associated infections in a novel organotypic model. *Molecular Oral Microbiology,* 33, 212-223.

Soga, Y., Yamasuji, Y., Kudo, C., Matsuura-Yoshimoto, K., Yamabe, K., Sugiura, Y., Maeda, Y., Ishimaru, F., Tanimoto, M., Nishimura, F. & Takashiba, S. 2009. Febrile neutropenia and periodontitis: lessons from a case periodontal treatment in the intervals between chemotherapy cycles for leukemia reduced febrile neutropenia. *Support Care Cancer,* 17, 581-7.

Sommariva, S., Pongiglione, B. & Tarricone, R. 2016. Impact of chemotherapy-induced nausea and vomiting on health-related quality of life and resource utilization: A systematic review. *Crit Rev Oncol Hematol,* 99, 13-36.

Sonis, S. T. 2004. The pathobiology of mucositis. *Nat Rev Cancer,* 4, 277-84.

Sonis, S. T. 2007. Pathobiology of oral mucositis: novel insights and opportunities. *J Support Oncol,* 5, 3-11.

Sonis, S. T. 2009. Mucositis: The impact, biology and therapeutic opportunities of oral mucositis. *Oral Oncol,* 45, 1015-20.

Sonis, S., Treister, N., Chawla, S., Demetri, G. & Haluska, F. 2010. Preliminary characterization of oral lesions associated with inhibitors of mammalian target of rapamycin in cancer patients. *Cancer,* 116, 210-5.

Sonis, S. T., Hashemi, S., Epstein, J. B., Nair, R. G., & Raber-Durlacher, J. E. 2016. Could the biological robustness of low level laser therapy (Photobiomodulation) impact its use in the management of mucositis in head and neck cancer patients. *Oral Oncology*, *54*, 7–14.

Sornsuvit, C., Komindr, S., Chuncharunee, S., Wanikiat, P., Archararit, N. & Santanirand, P. 2008. Pilot Study: effects of parenteral glutamine dipeptide supplementation on neutrophil functions and prevention of chemotherapy-induced side-effects in acute myeloid leukaemia patients. *J Int Med Res,* 36, 1383-91.

Sougiannis, A. T., Vanderveen, B. N., Davis, J. M., Fan, D. & Murphy, E. A. 2021. Understanding chemotherapy-induced intestinal mucositis and strategies to improve gut resilience. *American Journal of Physiology-Gastrointestinal and Liver Physiology,* 320, G712-G719.

Sougiannis, A. T., Vanderveen, B. N., Enos, R. T., Velazquez, K. T., Bader, J. E., Carson, M., Chatzistamou, I., Walla, M., Pena, M. M., Kubinak, J. L., Nagarkatti, M., Carson, J. A. & Murphy, E. A. 2019. Impact of 5 fluorouracil chemotherapy on gut inflammation, functional parameters, and gut microbiota. *Brain Behav Immun,* 80, 44-55.

Stein, A., Voigt, W. & Jordan, K. 2010. Chemotherapy-induced diarrhea: pathophysiology, frequency and guideline-based management. *Therapeutic advances in medical oncology,* 2, 51-63.

Stojanovska, V., Sakkal, S. & Nurgali, K. 2015. Platinum-based chemotherapy: gastrointestinal immunomodulation and enteric nervous system toxicity. *Am J Physiol Gastrointest Liver Physiol,* 308, G223-32.

Stojanovska, V., McQuade, R. M., Miller, S., and Nurgali, K. 2018a. Effects of Oxaliplatin Treatment on the Myenteric Plexus Innervation and Glia in the Murine Distal colon. *J. Histochem. Cytochem.* 66, 723–736.

Stojanovska, V., Mcquade, R. M., Fraser, S., Prakash, M., Gondalia, S., Stavely, R., Palombo, E., Apostolopoulos, V., Sakkal, S. & Nurgali, K. 2018b. Oxaliplatin-induced changes in microbiota, TLR4+ cells and enhanced HMGB1 expression in the murine colon. *PLoS One,* 13, e0198359.

Stojanovska, V., McQuade, R., Rybalka, E., and Nurgali, K. 2017. Neurotoxicity Associated with Platinum-Based Anti-cancer Agents: what Are the Implications of Copper Transporters? *Curr. Med. Chem*. 24, 1520–1536.

Stringer, A. M., Gibson, R. J., Bowen, J. M. & Keefe, D. M. 2009a. Chemotherapy-induced modifications to gastrointestinal microflora: evidence and implications of change. *Curr Drug Metab,* 10, 79-83.

Stringer, A. M., Gibson, R. J., Bowen, J. M., Logan, R. M., Yeoh, A. S. & Keefe, D. M. 2007. Chemotherapy-induced mucositis: the role of gastrointestinal microflora and mucins in the luminal environment. *J Support Oncol,* 5, 259-67.

Stringer, A. M., Gibson, R. J., Logan, R. M., Bowen, J. M., Yeoh, A. S. & Keefe, D. M. 2008. Faecal microflora and beta-glucuronidase expression are altered in an irinotecan-induced diarrhea model in rats. *Cancer Biol Ther,* 7, 1919-25.

Stringer, A. M., Gibson, R. J., Logan, R. M., Bowen, J. M., Yeoh, A. S. J., Laurence, J. & Keefe, D. M. K. 2009b. Irinotecan-induced mucositis is associated with changes in intestinal mucins. *Cancer Chemotherapy and Pharmacology,* 64, 123-132.

Tageja, N. & Groninger, H. 2014. Chemotherapy-induced nausea and vomiting #285. *Journal of palliative medicine,* 17, 1400-1402.

Takemoto, H., Nishimura, J., Komori, T., Kim, H. M., Ota, H., Suzuki, R., Ikenaga, M., Ikeda, M., Yamamoto, H., Satoh, T., Hata, T., Takemasa, I., Mizushima, T., Doki, Y.,

Mori, M. & Multicenter Clinical Study Group Of Osaka, C. C. T. G. 2017. Combination antiemetic therapy with aprepitant/fosaprepitant in patients with colorectal cancer receiving oxaliplatin-based chemotherapy in the SENRI trial: analysis of risk factors for vomiting and nausea. *International Journal of Clinical Oncology,* 22, 88-95.

Tan, L., Liu, J., Liu, X., Chen, J., Yan, Z., Yang, H. & Zhang, D. 2009. Clinical research of Olanzapine for prevention of chemotherapy-induced nausea and vomiting. *J Exp Clin Cancer Res,* 28, 131.

Tanihata, S., Oda, S., Nakai, S. & Uchiyama, T. 2004. Antiemetic effect of dexamethasone on cisplatin-induced early and delayed emesis in the pigeon. *Eur J Pharmacol,* 484, 311-21.

Tarumi, Y., Wilson, M. P., Szafran, O. & Spooner, G. R. 2013. Randomized, Double-Blind, Placebo-Controlled Trial of Oral Docusate in the Management of Constipation in Hospice Patients. *Journal of Pain and Symptom Management,* 45, 2-13.

Teh, L. K., Hashim, H., Zakaria, Z. A. & Salleh, M. Z. 2012. Polymorphisms of UGT1A1*6, UGT1A1*27 & UGT1A1*28 in three major ethnic groups from Malaysia. *Indian J Med Res,* 136, 249-59.

Temple, M. D., Recabarren, P., Mcfadyen, W. D., Holmes, R. J., Denny, W. A. & Murray, V. 2002. The interaction of DNA-targeted 9-aminoacridine-4-carboxamide platinum complexes with DNA in intact human cells. *Biochimica et Biophysica Acta (BBA) - Gene Structure and Expression,* 1574, 223-230.

Thiagarajah, J. R. & Verkman, A. 2013. Chloride channel-targeted therapy for secretory diarrheas. *Current Opinion in Pharmacology,* 13, 888-894.

Thiagarajah, J. R., Donowitz, M. & Verkman, A. S. 2015. Secretory diarrhoea: mechanisms and emerging therapies. *Nature reviews Gastroenterology & hepatology,* 12, 446.

Thomas, A. G., Stathis, M., Rojas, C. & Slusher, B. S. 2014. Netupitant and palonosetron trigger NK1 receptor internalization in NG108-15 cells. *Experimental Brain Research,* 232, 2637-2644.

Thorpe, D., Butler, R., Sultani, M., Vanhoecke, B. & Stringer, A. 2020. Irinotecan-Induced Mucositis Is Associated with Goblet Cell Dysregulation and Neural Cell Damage in a Tumour Bearing DA Rat Model. *Pathol Oncol Res,* 26, 955-965.

Tomblyn, M., Chiller, T., Einsele, H., Gress, R., Sepkowitz, K., Storek, J., Wingard, J. R., Young, J. A. & Boeckh, M. J. 2009. Guidelines for preventing infectious complications among hematopoietic cell transplantation recipients: a global perspective. *Biol Blood Marrow Transplant,* 15, 1143-238.

Toygar, İ., Yeşilbalkan, Ö. U., Kürkütlü, M. & Aslan, A. 2020. Complementary and alternative medicines used by cancer patients to cope with chemotherapy-induced constipation. *Complementary Therapies in Clinical Practice,* 39, 101108.

Treister, N. & Sonis, S. 2007. Mucositis: biology and management. *Curr Opin Otolaryngol Head Neck Surg,* 15, 123-9.

Trotti, A., Bellm, L. A., Epstein, J. B., Frame, D., Fuchs, H. J., Gwede, C. K., Komaroff, E., Nalysnyk, L. & Zilberberg, M. D. 2003. Mucositis incidence, severity and associated outcomes in patients with head and neck cancer receiving radiotherapy with or without chemotherapy: a systematic literature review. *Radiother Oncol,* 66, 253-62.

Tsuji, D., Suzuki, K., Kawasaki, Y., Goto, K., Matsui, R., Seki, N., Hashimoto, H., Hama, T., Yamanaka, T., Yamamoto, N. & Itoh, K. 2019. Risk factors associated with chemotherapy-induced nausea and vomiting in the triplet antiemetic regimen including palonosetron or granisetron for cisplatin-based chemotherapy: analysis of a randomized, double-blind controlled trial. *Support Care Cancer,* 27, 1139-1147.

Twycross, R., Sykes, N., Mihalyo, M. & Wilcock, A. 2012. Stimulant laxatives and opioid-induced constipation. *Journal of Pain and Symptom Management,* 43, 306-313.

Ullah, I., Subhan, F., Alam, J., Shahid, M. & Ayaz, M. 2018. Suppression of Cisplatin-Induced Vomiting by Cannabis sativa in Pigeons: Neurochemical Evidences. *Frontiers in Pharmacology,* 9, 231.

Uranga, J. A., García-Martínez, J. M., García-Jiménez, C., Vera, G., Martín-Fontelles, M. I., and Abalo, R. 2017. Alterations in the Small Intestinal wall and Motor Function after Repeated Cisplatin in Rat. *Neurogastroenterol Motil.* 29 (7), 10.1111/ nmo.13047.

Van den Broek, G. B., Balm, A. J., van den Brekel, M. W., Hauptmann, M., Schornagel, J. H., & Rasch, C. R. 2006. Relationship between clinical factors and the incidence of toxicity after intra-arterial chemoradiation for head and neck cancer. *Radiotherapy and Oncology: Journal of the European Society for Therapeutic Radiology and Oncology*, *81*(2), 143–150.

Van Der Velden, W. J. F. M., Herbers, A. H. E., Feuth, T., Schaap, N. P. M., Donnelly, J. P. & Blijlevens, N. M. A. 2010. Intestinal Damage Determines the Inflammatory Response and Early Complications in Patients Receiving Conditioning for a Stem Cell Transplantation. *PLOS ONE,* 5, e15156.

Van Der Velden, W. J. F. M., Herbers, A. H. E., Netea, M. G. & Blijlevens, N. M. A. 2014. Mucosal barrier injury, fever and infection in neutropenic patients with cancer: introducing the paradigm febrile mucositis. *British Journal of Haematology,* 167, 441-452.

Van Vliet, M. J., Harmsen, H. J., De Bont, E. S. & Tissing, W. J. 2010. The role of intestinal microbiota in the development and severity of chemotherapy-induced mucositis. *PLoS Pathog,* 6, e1000879.

Vardy, J., Chiew, K. S., Galica, J., Pond, G. R. & Tannock, I. F. 2006. Side effects associated with the use of dexamethasone for prophylaxis of delayed emesis after moderately emetogenic chemotherapy. *Br J Cancer,* 94, 1011-5.

Vasanwala, F. F. 2009. Management of chronic constipation in the elderly. *SFP,* 35, 84-92.

Vera-Llonch, M., Oster, G., Ford, C. M., Lu, J. & Sonis, S. 2007. Oral mucositis and outcomes of allogeneic hematopoietic stem-cell transplantation in patients with hematologic malignancies. *Support Care Cancer,* 15, 491-6.

Vera, G., Castillo, M., Cabezos, P. A., Chiarlone, A., Martín, M. I., Gori, A., Pasquinelli, G., Barbara, G., Stanghellini, V., Corinaldesi, R., De Giorgio, R. & Abalo, R. 2011. Enteric neuropathy evoked by repeated cisplatin in the rat. *Neurogastroenterol Motil,* 23, 370-8, e162-3.

Verstappen, C. C., Heimans, J. J., Hoekman, K. & Postma, T. J. 2003. Neurotoxic complications of chemotherapy in patients with cancer: clinical signs and optimal management. *Drugs,* 63, 1549-63.

Viele, C. S. 2003. Overview of chemotherapy-induced diarrhea. *Seminars in Oncology Nursing,* 19, 2-5.

Villa, A., Vollemans, M., De Moraes, A. & Sonis, S. 2021. Concordance of the WHO, RTOG, and CTCAE v4.0 grading scales for the evaluation of oral mucositis associated with chemoradiation therapy for the treatment of oral and oropharyngeal cancers. *Support Care Cancer,* 29, 6061-6068.

Vincenzi, B., Schiavon, G., Pantano, F., Santini, D. & Tonini, G. 2008. Predictive factors for chemotherapy-related toxic effects in patients with colorectal cancer. *Nat Clin Pract Oncol,* 5, 455-65.

Vokurka, S., Bystricka, E., Scudlova, J., Mazur, E., Visokaiova, M., Vasilieva, E., Brandejsova, R., Chvojkova, I., Vrabcova, M. & Vitkova, J. 2011. The risk factors for oral mucositis and the effect of cryotherapy in patients after the BEAM and HD-l-PAM 200 mg/m2 autologous hematopoietic stem cell transplantation. *European Journal of Oncology Nursing,* 15, 508-512.

Wafai, L., Taher, M., Jovanovska, V., Bornstein, J. C., Dass, C. R. & Nurgali, K. 2013. Effects of oxaliplatin on mouse myenteric neurons and colonic motility. *Frontiers in neuroscience,* 7, 30-30.

Wainberg, Z. A., Bekaii-Saab, T., Boland, P. M., Dayyani, F., Macarulla, T., Mody, K., Belanger, B., Maxwell, F., Moore, Y., Thiagalingam, A., Wang, T., Zhang, B. & Dean, A. 2021. First-line liposomal irinotecan with oxaliplatin, 5-fluorouracil and leucovorin (NALIRIFOX) in pancreatic ductal adenocarcinoma: A phase I/II study. *European Journal of Cancer,* 151, 14-24.

Wallace, B. D., Wang, H., Lane, K. T., Scott, J. E., Orans, J., Koo, J. S., Venkatesh, M., Jobin, C., Yeh, L. A., Mani, S. & Redinbo, M. R. 2010. Alleviating cancer drug toxicity by inhibiting a bacterial enzyme. *Science,* 330, 831-5.

Wang-Gillam, A., Hubner, R. A., Siveke, J. T., Von Hoff, D. D., Belanger, B., De Jong, F. A., Mirakhur, B. & Chen, L. T. 2019. NAPOLI-1 phase 3 study of liposomal irinotecan in metastatic pancreatic cancer: Final overall survival analysis and characteristics of long-term survivors. *Eur J Cancer,* 108, 78-87.

Wardill, H. R., Bowen, J. M., Van Sebille, Y. Z., Secombe, K. R., Coller, J. K., Ball, I. A., Logan, R. M., & Gibson, R. J. 2016. TLR4-Dependent Claudin-1 Internalization and Secretagogue-Mediated Chloride Secretion Regulate Irinotecan-Induced Diarrhea. *Molecular Cancer Therapeutics, 15*(11), 2767–2779.

Wardill, H. R. & Tissing, W. J. E. 2017. Determining risk of severe gastrointestinal toxicity based on pretreatment gut microbial community in patients receiving cancer treatment: a new predictive strategy in the quest for personalized cancer medicine. *Curr Opin Support Palliat Care,* 11, 125-132.

Wardill, H. R., Sonis, S. T., Blijlevens, N. M. A., Van Sebille, Y. Z. A., Ciorba, M. A., Loeffen, E. A. H., Cheng, K. K. F., Bossi, P., Porcello, L., Castillo, D. A., Elad, S. & Bowen, J. M. 2020. Prediction of mucositis risk secondary to cancer therapy: a systematic review of current evidence and call to action. *Support Care Cancer,* 28, 5059-5073.

Wardill, H. R., Sonis, S. T., Blijlevens, N. M. A., Van Sebille, Y. Z. A., Ciorba, M. A., Loeffen, E. A. H., Cheng, K. K. F., Bossi, P., Porcello, L., Castillo, D. A., Elad, S. & Bowen, J. M. 2020. Prediction of mucositis risk secondary to cancer therapy: a systematic review of current evidence and call to action. *Support Care Cancer,* 28, 5059-5073.

Wardill, H. R., Van Der Aa, S. A. R., Da Silva Ferreira, A. R., Havinga, R., Tissing, W. J. E. & Harmsen, H. J. M. 2021. Antibiotic-induced disruption of the microbiome exacerbates chemotherapy-induced diarrhoea and can be mitigated with autologous faecal microbiota transplantation. *European Journal of Cancer,* 153, 27-39.

Wardill, H. R., Van Sebille, Y. Z. A., Ciorba, M. A. & Bowen, J. M. 2018. Prophylactic probiotics for cancer therapy-induced diarrhoea: a meta-analysis. *Current Opinion in Supportive and Palliative Care,* 12.

Warr, D. G., Hesketh, P. J., Gralla, R. J., Muss, H. B., Herrstedt, J., Eisenberg, P. D., Raftopoulos, H., Grunberg, S. M., Gabriel, M., Rodgers, A., Bohidar, N., Klinger, G., Hustad, C. M., Horgan, K. J. & Skobieranda, F. 2005. Efficacy and tolerability of aprepitant for the prevention of chemotherapy-induced nausea and vomiting in patients with breast cancer after moderately emetogenic chemotherapy. *J Clin Oncol,* 23, 2822-30.

Watters, A. L., Epstein, J. B. & Agulnik, M. 2011. Oral complications of targeted cancer therapies: a narrative literature review. *Oral Oncol,* 47, 441-8.

Wei, L., Wen, X. S. & Xian, C. J. 2021. Chemotherapy-Induced Intestinal Microbiota Dysbiosis Impairs Mucosal Homeostasis by Modulating Toll-like Receptor Signaling Pathways. *Int J Mol Sci,* 22(17), 9474.

White, M. C., Hommers, C., Parry, S. & Stoddart, P. A. 2011. Pain management in 100 episodes of severe mucositis in children. *Paediatr Anaesth,* 21, 411-6.

WHO, W. H. O. 2012. WHO Guidelines Approved by the Guidelines Review Committee. *WHO Guidelines on the Pharmacological Treatment of Persisting Pain in Children with Medical Illnesses.* Geneva: World Health Organization.

Wickham R. J. (2017). Managing Constipation in Adults With Cancer. *Journal of the advanced practitioner in oncology*, *8*(2), 149–161.

Wiseman, L. R., Adkins, J. C., Plosker, G. L. & Goa, K. L. 1999. Oxaliplatin: a review of its use in the management of metastatic colorectal cancer. *Drugs Aging,* 14, 459-75.

Wisnivesky, J. P., Smith, C. B., Packer, S., Strauss, G. M., Lurslurchachai, L., Federman, A. & Halm, E. A. 2011. Survival and risk of adverse events in older patients receiving postoperative adjuvant chemotherapy for resected stages II-IIIA lung cancer: observational cohort study. *BMJ,* 343, d4013.

Worthington, H. V., Clarkson, J. E., Bryan, G., Furness, S., Glenny, A. M., Littlewood, A., Mccabe, M. G., Meyer, S. & Khalid, T. 2011. Interventions for preventing oral mucositis for patients with cancer receiving treatment. *Cochrane Database Syst Rev,* 2011, Cd000978.

Wuketich, S., Hienz, S. A. & Marosi, C. 2012. Prevalence of clinically relevant oral mucositis in outpatients receiving myelosuppressive chemotherapy for solid tumors. *Support Care Cancer,* 20, 175-83.

Xia, T., Zhang, J., Han, L., Jin, Z., Wang, J., Li, X., Man, S., Liu, C. & Gao, W. 2019. Protective effect of magnolol on oxaliplatin-induced intestinal injury in mice. *Phytotherapy Research,* 33, 1161-1172.

Xie, C. Y., Xu, Y. P., Jin, W. & Lou, L. G. 2012. Antitumor activity of lobaplatin alone or in combination with antitubulin agents in non-small-cell lung cancer. *Anticancer Drugs,* 23, 698-705.

Xing, J. H., & Soffer, E. E. 2001. Adverse effects of laxatives. *Diseases of the colon and rectum*, *44*(8), 1201–1209.

Yamagishi, A., Morita, T., Miyashita, M. & Kimura, F. 2009. Symptom prevalence and longitudinal follow-up in cancer outpatients receiving chemotherapy. *Journal of pain and symptom management,* 37, 823-830.

Yarom, N., Hovan, A., Bossi, P., Ariyawardana, A., Jensen, S. B., Gobbo, M., Saca-Hazboun, H., Kandwal, A., Majorana, A., Ottaviani, G., Pentenero, M., Nasr, N. M., Rouleau, T., Lucas, A. S., Treister, N. S., Zur, E., Ranna, V., Vaddi, A., Cheng, K., Barasch, A., ... Mucositis Study Group of the Multinational Association of Supportive Care in Cancer/International Society of Oral Oncology (MASCC/ISOO). 2019. Systematic review of natural and miscellaneous agents for the management of oral mucositis in cancer patients and clinical practice guidelines-part 1: vitamins, minerals, and nutritional supplements. *Supportive Care in Cancer: official journal of the Multinational Association of Supportive Care in Cancer*, *27*(10), 3997–4010.

Yeoh, A. S., Bowen, J. M., Gibson, R. J. & Keefe, D. M. 2005. Nuclear factor kappaB (NFkappaB) and cyclooxygenase-2 (Cox-2) expression in the irradiated colorectum is associated with subsequent histopathological changes. *Int J Radiat Oncol Biol Phys,* 63, 1295-303.

Yin, C. Y., Lin, X. L., Tian, L., Ye, M., Yang, X. Y. & Xiao, X. Y. 2014. Lobaplatin inhibits growth of gastric cancer cells by inducing apoptosis. *World J Gastroenterol,* 20, 17426-33.

Yoo, B. B. & Mazmanian, S. K. 2017. The Enteric Network: Interactions between the Immune and Nervous Systems of the Gut. *Immunity,* 46, 910-926.

Zadik, Y., Arany, P. R., Fregnani, E. R., Bossi, P., Antunes, H. S., Bensadoun, R. J., Gueiros, L. A., Majorana, A., Nair, R. G., Ranna, V., Tissing, W., Vaddi, A., Lubart, R., Migliorati, C. A., Lalla, R. V., Cheng, K., Elad, S., & Mucositis Study Group of the Multinational Association of Supportive Care in Cancer/International Society of Oral Oncology (MASCC/ISOO). 2019. Systematic review of photobiomodulation for the management of oral mucositis in cancer patients and clinical practice guidelines. *Supportive Care in Cancer: official journal of the Multinational Association of Supportive Care in Cancer*, *27*(10), 3969–3983.

Zhang, M., Zhou, H., Xu, S., Liu, D., Cheng, Y., Gao, B., Li, X. & Chen, J. 2020. The gut microbiome can be used to predict the gastrointestinal response and efficacy of lung cancer patients undergoing chemotherapy. *Annals of Palliative Medicine,* 9, 4211-4227.

Zhou, Z., Jiang, H., Xia, J. & Zhang, J. 2020. Comparison of the therapeutic effects of lobaplatin and carboplatin on retinoblastoma in vitro and in vivo. *Int J Oncol,* 57, 697-706.

About the Editors

Kulmira Nurgali

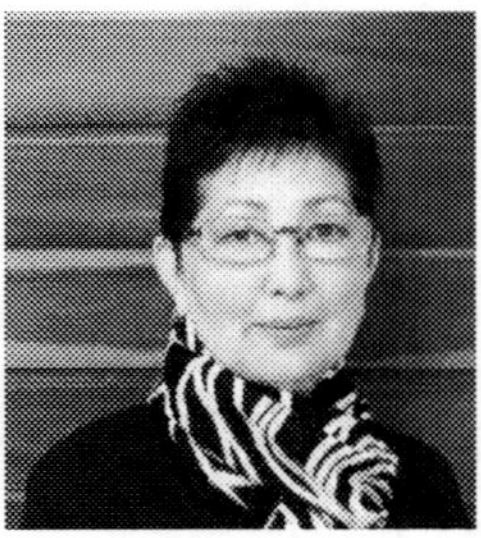

Professor Kulmira Nurgali (PhD 2004, Melbourne University) is a researcher and teaching academic at the College of Health and Biomedicine, Institute for Health and Sport, Victoria University, Australia and an Honorary Associate Professor at the Department of Medicine, University of Melbourne, Australia. She is the Head of Enteric Neuropathy Laboratory at the Centre for Health, Research and Education, Sunshine Hospital, Melbourne, Australia and Director of the Stem Cells and Regenerative Medicine Program at the Australian Institute for Musculoskeletal Science. She has an internationally-recognized prominence in the fields of Enteric Neuroscience and Neurogastroenterology. Prof Nurgali's research is focused on enteric neuropathy associated with Inflammatory Bowel Disease, colorectal cancer, and the side effects of chemotherapy. Being a medical graduate, she focuses on the development of novel treatments and pre-clinical studies that have translational value.

Further information regarding Professor Nurgali's publications and research activity can be found via ORCID ID: 0000-0002-2597-6929.

Contact e-mails: kulmira.nurgali@vu.edu.au;
kulmira.nurgali@unimelb.edu.au

Raquel Abalo

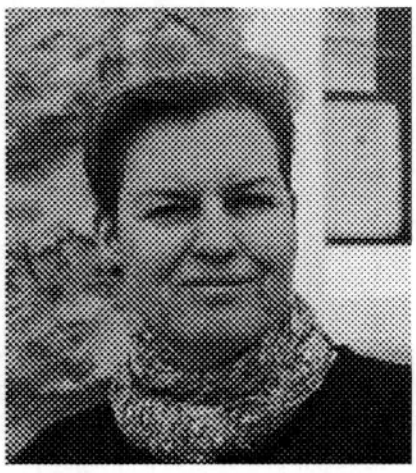

WoS Researcher ID: H-3764-2015
SCOPUS Author ID:13806228800
Open Researcher and Contributor ID (ORCID): 0000-0002-6726-8795

https://gestion2.urjc.es/pdi/ver/raquel.abalo
raquel.abalo@urjc.es

- *PhD in Biological Sciences at Universidad Complutense de Madrid (Spain, 2000)*
- *Full Professor of Pharmacology at Universidad Rey Juan Carlos (URC, Spain) from 2017*
- *Head of the High-Performance Research Group in Physiopathology and Pharmacology of the Digestive System (NeuGut-URJC) from 2019*
- *Head of the Area of Pharmacology at the Dept. of Basic Health Sciences (URJC) from 2018*
- *Coordinator of the PhD Program in Health Sciences at the URJC International Doctorate School from 2021*
- *Keywords: brain-gut axis, adverse effects of cancer chemotherapy, nutraceuticals, cannabinoids, sex-dependent differences*

List of Contributors

Mauricio A. Retamal
Ignacio A. Cortés-Fuentes
Juan G. Gormaz
Paola R. Campodónico
Aleksandra Olszewska
Monika Granica
Aleksandra Klemba
Claudine Kieda
Halina Was
Mauricio Burotto
Jaime Gonzalez-Montero
Hannah R. Wardill
Ysabella Z. A. Van Sebille
Nadeen T. Ali
Lisa B. Grech
Kristen Renee McSweeney
Laura Kate Gadanec
Anthony Zulli
Petra Semenye
Rachel McQuade
Raquel Abalo
Kulmira Nurgali

Index

A

D

E

J

K

L

M

N

O

N

O

S

T

W

X

Y

Z